Ultrasound in Reproductive Healthcare Practice

GW00775923

Ultrasound in Reproductive Healthcare Practice

Edited by

Mary Pillai
Gloucestershire Care Services NHS Trust and
Gloucestershire Hospitals NHS Foundation Trust

Paula Briggs
Southport and Ormskirk Hospital NHS Trust

Julie-Michelle Bridson
University of Liverpool

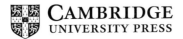
CAMBRIDGE
UNIVERSITY PRESS

CAMBRIDGE
UNIVERSITY PRESS

University Printing House, Cambridge CB2 8BS, United Kingdom

One Liberty Plaza, 20th Floor, New York, NY 10006, USA

477 Williamstown Road, Port Melbourne, VIC 3207, Australia

314-321, 3rd Floor, Plot 3, Splendor Forum, Jasola District Centre, New Delhi – 110025, India

79 Anson Road, #06-04/06, Singapore 079906

Cambridge University Press is part of the University of Cambridge.

It furthers the University's mission by disseminating knowledge in the pursuit of
education, learning, and research at the highest international levels of excellence.

www.cambridge.org
Information on this title: www.cambridge.org/9781316609736
DOI: 10.1017/9781316659410

© Cambridge University Press 2018

This publication is in copyright. Subject to statutory exception
and to the provisions of relevant collective licensing agreements,
no reproduction of any part may take place without the written
permission of Cambridge University Press.

First published 2018

Printed in the United Kingdom by Clays, St Ives plc

A catalogue record for this publication is available from the British Library.

Library of Congress Cataloging-in-Publication Data
Names: Pillai, Mary, editor. | Briggs, Paula, 1964– editor. | Bridson, Julie-Michelle, editor.
Title: Ultrasound in Reproductive Healthcare Practice /
edited by Mary Pillai, Paula Briggs, Julie-Michelle Bridson.
Description: Cambridge, United Kingdom; New York, NY: Cambridge University Press, 2018. |
Includes bibliographical references and index.
Identifiers: LCCN 2017035383 | ISBN 9781316609736 (pbk.)
Subjects: | MESH: Genital Diseases, Female – diagnostic imaging |
Ultrasonography – methods | Pregnancy Complications – diagnostic imaging
Classification: LCC RG107 | NLM WP 141 | DDC 618.1/075–dc23
LC record available at https://lccn.loc.gov/2017035383

ISBN 978-1-316-60973-6 Paperback

Cambridge University Press has no responsibility for the persistence or accuracy of URLs
for external or third-party internet websites referred to in this publication and does not
guarantee that any content on such websites is, or will remain, accurate or appropriate.

. . . .

Every effort has been made in preparing this book to provide accurate and up-to-date
information that is in accord with accepted standards and practice at the time of publication.
Although case histories are drawn from actual cases, every effort has been made to disguise
the identities of the individuals involved. Nevertheless, the authors, editors, and publishers
can make no warranties that the information contained herein is totally free from error, not
least because clinical standards are constantly changing through research and regulation.
The authors, editors, and publishers therefore disclaim all liability for direct or consequential
damages resulting from the use of material contained in this book. Readers are strongly
advised to pay careful attention to information provided by the manufacturer of any drugs or
equipment that they plan to use.

Contents

List of Contributors   *page* vii
Foreword by Diana Mansour   ix
Acknowledgments   xi

1   **A Short History of Ultrasound in Gynaecology**   1
Pat Lewis

2   **Use of the Ultrasound System**   8
Julie-Michelle Bridson

3   **Communication Skills in Ultrasound Assessment**   45
Karen Easton

4   **Ultrasound of Pelvic Anatomy Scanning Techniques and 'Normal' Findings**   49
Mary Pillai and Julie-Michelle Bridson

5   **Contrast Sonohysterography**   73
Mary Pillai

6   **Ultrasound of Abnormal Pelvic Anatomy: Benign Pathology**   87
Mary Pillai

7   **Pregnancy Ultrasound for SRH Work**   115
Mary Pillai

8   **Ultrasound Assessment of a Potential Ectopic Pregnancy**   135
Karen Easton

9   **Ultrasound Imaging of Progestogen-Only Subdermal Contraceptive Implants**   151
Paul O' Brien

10   **Ultrasound Imaging in Relation to Intrauterine Contraception**   163
Zara Haider

11   **The Role of Ultrasound Scanning in the Investigation and Management of Subfertility**   182
Paula Briggs and Gab Kovacs

12   **Polycystic Ovaries, Polycystic Ovary Syndrome and the Role of Ultrasound in Relation to This Condition**   195
Paula Briggs and Gab Kovacs

13   **Ultrasound Imaging of Women with Abnormal Uterine Bleeding (AUB)**   201
Jane Dickson

14   **The Use of Ultrasound in the Perimenopausal Patient**   218
Steven R. Goldstein

15   **Recognition of Possible Gynaecological Cancer**   225
Kathryn Hillaby

16   **Quality in SRH Ultrasound Service Provision**   234
Julie-Michelle Bridson

17   **Annotation, Archiving, Reporting and Audit**   241
Julie-Michelle Bridson

Glossary of Abbreviations and Terms   249
Index   251

v

Contributors

Julie-Michelle Bridson
Senior Lecturer, University of Liverpool
Academic Lead, Postgraduate Medical Education &
Training
Head of School, Physician Associate Studies
Former President, British Medical Ultrasound
Society

Paula Briggs
Consultant in Sexual and Reproductive Healthcare
Southport and Ormskirk Hospital NHS Trust

Jane Dickson
Consultant in Sexual and Reproductive Healthcare
Oxleas NHS Foundation Trust

Karen Easton
Nurse Consultant in Gynaecology
Gloucestershire Hospitals NHS Foundation Trust

Steven R. Goldstein
Professor of Obstetrics and Gynecology
New York University School of Medicine

Zara Haider
Consultant in Sexual Reproductive Healthcare
The Wolverton Centre, Kingston Hospital NHS Trust

Kathryn Hillaby
Consultant Gynaecological Oncologist
Gloucestershire Hospitals NHS Foundation Trust

Gab Kovacs
Professor of Obstetrics and Gynaecology
Monash University

Pat Lewis
Retired Consultant in Obstetrics and Gynaecology

Diana Mansour
Consultant in Community Gynaecology and
Reproductive Healthcare, Newcastle upon Tyne
Vice President, Clinical Quality
Faculty of Sexual and Reproductive Healthcare

Paul O'Brien
Associate Specialist
Raymede Clinic, Central North West London NHS
Foundation Trust

Mary Pillai
Consultant in Fetal Medicine and Community
Gynaecology
Gloucestershire Hospitals NHS Foundation Trust and
Gloucestershire Care Services NHS Trust

Foreword

In the twenty-first century, ultrasound scanning has become part of the gynaecological examination. Many consulting rooms have a scanner, readily available to the clinician. This has led to the evolution of a one-stop shop service and immediate management of the presenting complaint rather than repeated visits and a delay in treatment. Traditionally, theoretical and practical training in diagnostic ultrasound has focused on other areas of gynaecology and obstetrics with minimal information covering the visualisation of intra-uterine contraceptives and no inclusion of deep-sited and non-palpable contraceptive implants. There has been a significant focus on early pregnancy units with little consideration of the different context and needs where women with early pregnancy complications present to a pregnancy advisory service.

This book has been written in conjunction with the Faculty of Sexual and Reproductive Healthcare's (FSRH) accredited ultrasound theoretical course developed in collaboration with the School of Medicine, University of Liverpool. However, it will complement the wide range of medical ultrasound training courses currently available, and be particularly useful to doctors, nurses and sonographers who go on to undertake practical ultrasound training such as the FSRH Special Skills Module in Ultrasound or the RCOG ultrasound modules in early pregnancy and gynaecology. It will also be a valuable resource for those providing ultrasound within pregnancy advisory services.

This book is essential reading for all gynaecologists, obstetrics and gynaecology trainees, and consultants/specialty doctors and trainees in sexual reproductive healthcare. They will find up-to-date information about ultrasound for community/office gynaecology in a concise format. There are helpful hints and guidance on the use of ultrasound machines, scanning techniques, and lots of images of normal ultrasound scans, anatomical variants and specific pathologies. The chapters are written by subject experts and provide an evidence-based review of complex issues. The editors have a keen interest in this field and the contributors are knowledgeable and well respected.

Dr Diana Mansour

Consultant in Community Gynaecology and Reproductive Healthcare, Newcastle upon Tyne

Vice President, Clinical Quality Faculty of Sexual and Reproductive Healthcare

Acknowledgments

The artwork included in the drawn figures was by Mark Pountney, Content Developer for the Centre for Educational Development and Support, Faculty of Health and Life Sciences, University of Liverpool.

A majority of the ultrasound images used in the book were sourced during routine work by the first editor in the Sexual Health Service of Gloucestershire Care Services NHS Trust. Where ultrasound is available in a clinic setting more than 98% of referred coil problems and 99% of implant problems can be managed in a one-stop 30-minute outpatient appointment.

Chapter

1

A Short History of Ultrasound in Gynaecology

Pat Lewis

1.1 Evolution of Ultrasound in Medicine 1
1.2 Development of Ultrasound in Obstetrics and Gynaecology 3
1.3 Development of Ultrasound in Gynaecology and Its Impact 4
1.4 Training and Skills 7
1.5 Summary 7

1.1 Evolution of Ultrasound in Medicine

The history of ultrasound in medicine starts with the initial research and development of ultrasound for medical use.[1] As with many developments in medicine, it can be difficult to pinpoint exactly when they began, and ultrasound is no exception. However, there are some key events that occurred which provided the foundation for the evolution of ultrasound in medical applications.

The first real breakthrough was in 1880, when Pierre Curie discovered the piezo-electric effect in certain crystals. Paul Langevin applied this in the early twentieth century as the basis for a transducer containing a piezoelectric crystal, capable of both generating an ultrasonic beam and receiving the returning echoes from interfaces between surfaces of substances of two differing acoustic impedances. This is still fundamental to the ultrasound transducers in use today.

Ultrasound had its origins in the early twentieth century via SONAR, which was developed to detect submarines, and RADAR, which used electromagnetic waves being subsequently adapted to produce two-dimensional scan images and pulse echo metal flaw detectors.

Research was continued from the principles described in these earlier works, by many people, independently, in different countries and often in parallel. Karl Theo Dussik (University of Vienna, Austria) is regarded as the first physician to use ultrasound for medical diagnosis in the 1930s. Dussik's work in the 1940s resulted in the use of ultrasound to produce echo images of the human head. In the 1950s, an English surgeon John Wild immigrated to America and worked with an engineer (Donald Neal) to produce an A-mode device to assess the gut (Figure 1.1). An electrical engineer, John Reid, was commissioned through grant income to construct Wild's ultrasound apparatus. In 1952, Wild and Reid published their landmark paper 'Application of Echo-Ranging Techniques to the Determination of Structure of Biological Tissues'. This was followed by the first production of ultrasound images of the breast in 1953 and their invention and application of transvaginal and transrectal transducers in 1955, the precursor of the equipment used daily in SRH services across the world.

However, it was not until 1958 with the publication of Ian Donald, John McVicar and Tom Brown's seminal paper in the *Lancet*, 'The Investigation of Abdominal Masses with Pulsed Ultrasound' (Figures 1.2a, b), that ultrasound as a clinical mode of investigation really started.[2] Their paper was the first to describe contact compound 2D scanning using olive oil as a coupling medium. Their machine produced the first direct contact images, which were bi-stable (black and white) (Figure 1.3). As a result of this paper, commercial 2D scanning machines were produced and effectively signaled the real start of the use of ultrasound in medicine. From this seminal paper, further advances incorporated computer technology to improve the resolution of the image. The development of the scan

1

converter in the late 1960s allowed the display of scattered reflections to produce the grey scale image, with which we are all familiar. The initial images were analog, but they were enhanced by digitalisation, which significantly improved the grey scale quality and image resolution enabling more accurate interpretation of the images.

On the basis of the principles of industrial metal flaw technology, A-scan was initially developed and

found to be successful in locating a returning echo from gallstones insonated from outside the body and was also used to measure the bi-parietal diameter of the fetal head.

Early ultrasound systems produced static images. The images were produced by moving a transducer on a scanning arm over a part of the body using a coupling medium. The use of this equipment was very time consuming and required great skill to build up an 'impression' of a structure from multiple separate slices. An early system was the Diasonograph (Figure 1.4).

The development of real-time technology in the 1970s overcame many of these problems and allowed scanning of moving objects, for example, fetus. Real-time machines were initially mechanical sector scanners with heavy transducers and cables. Very quickly, linear and phased array scanners with smaller, more manoeuvrable and more user-friendly transducers were developed. Real-time scanning machines had other numerous advantages compared to static scanners; they were smaller in size, less expensive, were relatively easier to use and thus required less training time. While initially the real-time images were of inferior quality, with further development they produced images comparable to those of static scanners. For the operator, real-time imaging in obstetrics enabled obtaining fetal measurements much quicker and

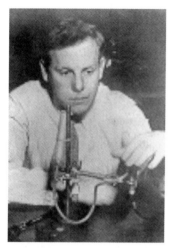

Figure 1.1 John Wild with Echoscope, circa 1953 (courtesy of Tom Brown).

(a) (b)

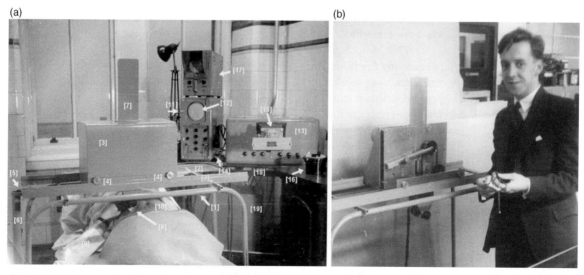

Figure 1.2 (a) Photograph of the prototype scanner used by Donald, McVicar and Brown 1958 (courtesy of Tom Brown). (b) Tom Brown (aged twenty-three), circa 1956, with the original bed table scanner which was developed in the Kelvin and Hughes research and development laboratories (courtesy of Tom Brown).

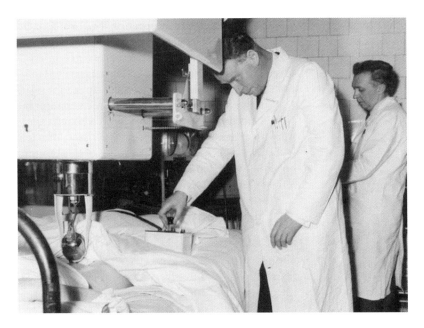

Figure 1.3 The automated scanner being operated by Professor Ian Donald, with Professor John McVicar in the background (1959) (courtesy of Tom Brown).

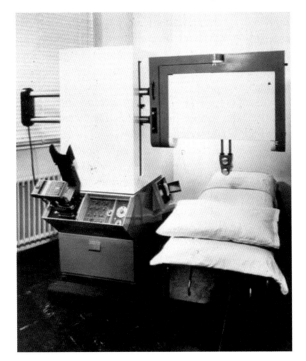

Figure 1.4 The early Kelvin and Hughes Diasonograph (circa 1965) (courtesy of Tom Brown).

easier. It was very reassuring for the mother to see her baby moving and the heart beating.

During the 1980s, Colour Doppler became available and was used in assessing vascularity in gynaecological malignancy and blood flow in fetal vessels.

This technology uses the Doppler effect described by Christian Doppler in 1842.

The 1990s saw the production of 3D ultrasound systems, which have enabled refinement of diagnosis in some fetal and uterine abnormalities. Real-time 3D ultrasound today (4D ultrasound) also has a role in maternal–fetal bonding.

Many people benefit from the use of ultrasound in medicine every day, and the remarkable advances described would not have been possible without the work of and collaboration among many talented physicists, engineers, clinicians and computer technologists.

1.2 Development of Ultrasound in Obstetrics and Gynaecology

There is no doubt that the development of ultrasound has had a major impact on obstetrics and gynaecology over the past fifty years. Notably, the aforementioned seminal paper by Ian Donald and his team in 1958 describing the first clinical use of ultrasound in obstetrics and gynaecology represented the start of this modality, and it quickly became widespread in clinical practice. The title of their paper 'The Investigation of Abdominal Masses with Pulsed Ultrasound' did not reflect that most of their work appertained to obstetrics and gynaecology and included the first images of a fetal head and of gynaecological cancer.[2] They had developed the first 2D compound contact scanner,

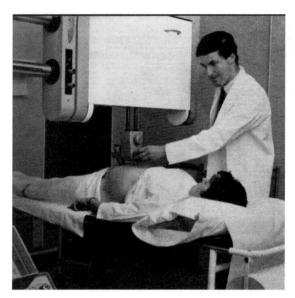

Figure 1.5 An early photograph of Professor Stuart Campbell at Queen Charlotte's Hospital, measuring a bi-parietal diameter with a Diasonograph (1968) (courtesy of Tom Brown).

upon which the first of the commercial 2D static scanning machines, the Diasonograph, was based. It was heavy and cumbersome, standing about eight feet tall, and produced static bistable, black and white images. I remember vividly using one of these machines and swinging the heavy gantry around to obtain both transverse and longitudinal single sweeps to produce an image of the fetus and placenta on the oscilloscope. Using the Diasonograph, it was possible to determine the position of the fetus, the liquor volume and the location of the placenta and to diagnose multiple pregnancies (Figure 1.5).

Following this, further advances were made in placental localisation and fetal cephalometry.[3,4] The latter was initially performed by obtaining a B-scan image and then using A-scan for measurement, but with the advent of on-screen calipers, A-scan was no longer required. Ian Donald and his team also described the 'full bladder' technique, which enabled visualisation of the pelvic organs and the uterus during the first trimester. This was a very exciting time as heretofore there was very limited knowledge of the developing pregnancy in the first trimester. So for the first time, tools existed which provided information about early pregnancy; yet no one could predict how rapidly ultrasound would advance to assist in our diagnosis and management of early pregnancy problems

(Figures 1.6 a,b,c). In his paper of 1962, Ian Donald described the early diagnosis of hydatidiform mole and ectopic pregnancy.[5] Other advantages of early pregnancy scanning were the earlier diagnosis of multiple pregnancy (Figures 1.7a,b) and 'missed miscarriage' where it became apparent that the gestation sac was either empty or not growing, even though there were no external signs of bleeding, perhaps for a few weeks. It is no surprise that as a result of this groundbreaking work, Ian Donald is known as the father of ultrasound in obstetrics and gynaecology.

1.3 Development of Ultrasound in Gynaecology and Its Impact

The impact of ultrasound on gynaecology clinical practice was equally impressive. Initially, as has been noted, the pelvic organs could be visualised by the 'full bladder' technique with uterine and ovarian masses and ascites being some of the first images to be obtained. These images, as with obstetric images, were greatly improved by the development of the scan converter and further advances in computer technology. This facilitated even better resolution of the grey scale image, thereby enhancing the ability to make differential diagnoses, particularly in gynaecological tumours. The advent of real-time scanning machines in the 1970s enhanced the service provision, as they were smaller, more mobile and were technically easier to use.

But for me, as a gynaecologist, the development of the transvaginal probe in the 1980s coupled with imaging in real-time were the most exciting advances. The transvaginal probe seemed like a natural extension of the manual gynaecological vaginal examination, but with the ability to provide much more information. Although the first commercially available endovaginal transducers were large and cumbersome (and therefore not suitable for use in all women), the images obtained were superior in resolution to those obtained via the abdominal probe. This was due to the proximity of the probe to the pelvic organs, which allowed the use of higher frequency, thus enhancing the resolution of the image. It was clear that use of the transvaginal probe would further revolutionise diagnosis and ultimately lead to ultrasound becoming the most important investigative modality in gynaecology. It would not, however, totally replace the abdominal pelvic approach, as the two remain complementary in some instances.

Transvaginal probes had been developed and used by Alfred Kratochwil in the 1960s, but their full

(a)

(b)

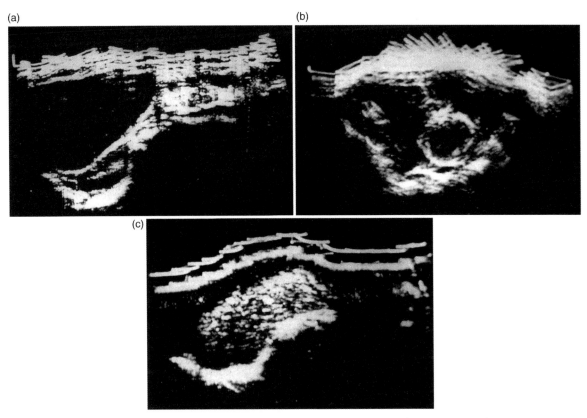

(c)

Figure 1.6 (a) Static ultrasound image of a non-pregnant uterus. (b) Static ultrasound image of an eighteen-week fetus. (c) Static ultrasound image of a hydatidiform mole.

(a)

(b)

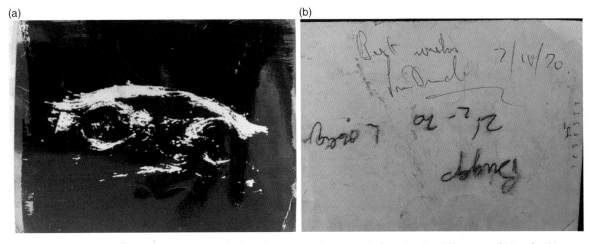

Figure 1.7 (a) Early scan of twin pregnancy (1970). (b) Signed on reverse of image by Professor Ian Donald (courtesy of Briggs family).

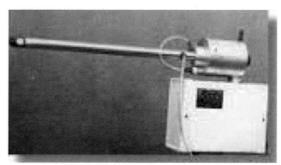

Vaginal A-scan from kretzTechnik circa 1968

Figure 1.8 Early transvaginal ultrasound probe by Kretz.

potential was not realised until real-time imaging became available. Transducer technology became progressively better, enabling a gradual reduction in the diameter of the probe. Today there are few women who are unable to tolerate vaginal ultrasound examination using a modern transvaginal probe, and it also has the advantage of avoiding the discomfort caused by a full bladder.

The transvaginal probe gave us much more detailed information about early pregnancy and its abnormalities, and enabled us to change our management of several conditions (Figure 1.8). Now we had a much-improved ability to visualise an early intrauterine gestation sac at five weeks in cases of suspected ectopic pregnancy, thus avoiding the need for invasive diagnostic laparoscopies. Subsequently, transvaginal sonography became the most accurate method of making a positive diagnosis of ectopic pregnancy, giving options of medical or surgical management. Further, in the investigation of threatened miscarriage, the ability to reliably detect the fetal heart at seven weeks gave maternal reassurance, and the earlier diagnosis of missed miscarriage gave the mother options of expectant, surgical or medical management. Confident diagnosis of hydatidiform mole at an earlier gestation has also made treatment possible with less risk.

Infertility and its management have been transformed by the development of the transvaginal probe. Monitoring follicular growth became easier and more accurate than with the abdominal probe, and the ability to assess endometrial thickness more precisely is also an advantage in the treatment of infertility. Ultrasound-guided vaginal oocyte retrieval was possible and, being more successful, quicker, less painful and completed as an outpatient, has now superseded

transabdominal oocyte collection and the previous more invasive laparoscopic retrieval. Salpingography with a positive contrast agent (HyCoSy) as a method of assessing tubal patency, which is now widely used, has also been facilitated by the endovaginal probe.

The various developments in ultrasound already described have also had a remarkable impact on the differential diagnosis of pelvic masses. It has given us greater ability to differentiate between uterine and ovarian masses, between solid and cystic ovarian lesions and also to monitor fibroids and pelvic abscesses. Also, with the transvaginal probe, ultrasound could detect pelvic tumours, which would be missed by pelvic examination alone. The use of Colour Doppler has further refined our ability to discriminate between benign and malignant lesions by the detection of angiogenesis in malignancy. Pelvic scanning, however, is still frequently a challenging area of diagnosis and remains dependent on the expertise and experience of the operator.

The ability to measure endometrial thickness more accurately with a transvaginal probe allowed a change in the management of post-menopausal bleeding, a condition that had previously necessitated invasive investigation by dilatation and curettage or hysteroscopy. It was now possible to confidently diagnose atrophic endometrium and therefore avoid the need for further investigation to exclude endometrial cancer in many cases. Endovaginal sonography has also enabled enhanced visualisation of the uterine cavity by using hydrosonography whereby a narrow catheter is inserted through the cervix and small amount of fluid (2–5 ml) is injected into the cavity to highlight any irregularity, for example, sub-mucosal fibroids or endometrial polyps.

The more recent development in the 1990s of 3D ultrasound has further contributed to our ability to detect uterine abnormalities, especially mild degrees of uterine septa. A paper by Jurkovic in 1995 indicated that 3D ultrasound was superior to 2D in demonstrating congenital uterine anomalies.[6]

In sexual and reproductive health today, as in other areas of gynaecology, ultrasound makes a significant contribution to the management of patients: assessing gestational age prior to termination and locating intrauterine devices where threads are not visible. High frequency transducers are also employed for the location of impalpable contraceptive implants. The presence of an ultrasound machine, together with the expertise to use it, is today an important adjunct to a community clinic and indeed reduces the need for hospital referral.

1.4 Training and Skills

As ultrasound developed, it became apparent that systematic training to use ultrasound machines would be necessary, given that diagnosis by ultrasound was and remains highly dependent on the skill of the operator. Initially, because the use of ultrasound machines tended to be de-centralised, standards varied widely and misdiagnosis was not uncommon. It therefore became imperative that professionals who wished to use this modality were trained and accredited. The American Institute of Ultrasound in Medicine and the British Medical Ultrasound Society were formed first, followed by the International Society of Ultrasound in Obstetrics and Gynaecology. They were, and remain, actively involved in education and training.

Training of professionals remains a fundamental aspect of ultrasound, despite the fact that current machines are easier to use and produce far superior images, and today there are many institutions that conduct their own training courses. More recently, particularly for training in transvaginal ultrasound, training simulators have become available for basic familiarisation with the technique and with ultrasound recognition of pelvic anatomy.

1.5 Summary

Ultrasound has come a long way since the first images obtained by Ian Donald and his team, and I have been privileged to be a witness to all the major advances since the days of the 2D compound scanner to our position today where ultrasound is an indispensable tool in gynaecology. I have no doubt that there will be further exciting advances in the future.

References

1. Woo J History of ultrasound. www.Ob-ultrasound.net

2. Donald I, MacVicar J, Brown TG. Investigation of abdominal masses by pulsed ultrasound. *Lancet.* 1958;1:1188–95.

3. Donald I, Abdulla S. Placentography by sonar. *J. Obstet. Gynaecol. Br. Commonw.* 1968;75:993–1006.

4. Campbell S. Prediction of fetal maturity by ultrasonic measurement of the biparietal diameter. *J. Obstet. Gynaecol. Br. Commonw.* 1969;76:603–9.

5. Donald I. Clinical applications of ultrasonic techniques in obstetrical and gynaecological diagnosis. *J. Obstet. Gynaecol. Br. Commonw.*1962;69:1036.

6. Jurkovic D,Geipel A, Gruboeck K. Jauniaux E, Natucci M, Campbell S. Three-dimensional ultrasound for the assessment of uterine anatomy and detection of congenital anomalies: a comparison with hysterosalpingography and two-dimensional sonography. *Ultrasound. Obstet. Gynecol.* 1995;5:233–7.

Chapter 2

Use of the Ultrasound System

Julie-Michelle Bridson

Part 1   The Basics   8
2.1   Introduction   8
Part 2   Clinical Cases   27
Case 2.1   Doppler in the Diagnosis of a Fibroid   28
Case 2.2   Doppler in the Diagnosis of a
             Corpus Luteum   28
Case 2.3   Doppler in the Diagnosis of
             Retained Products   28

Case 2.4   Doppler in the Diagnosis of Uterine
             Clot, in Contrast to RPCs   29
Case 2.5   Doppler in the Diagnosis of Malignant
             Pelvic Disease   29
Part 3   System Optimisation/Enhancing
             the Image   30
2.2   Ultrasound Image Formation   30
2.3   Summary   43

PART 1: THE BASICS

2.1 Introduction

Ultrasound has been used since the 1970s to produce diagnostic images. Its introduction changed the field of obstetrics and gynaecology more than any other new technology, and more widely it has found multiple applications in medicine. Understanding the physical properties of ultrasound is essential knowledge for individuals providing this service within their clinical practice.

This chapter is divided into three parts:

1 Covers the basic principles of diagnostic ultrasound imaging, the equipment, image formation, safety considerations, use of the ultrasound system and transducer care. This section is intended to provide the basics to get 'novice users started'.
2 Provides clinical cases that illustrate the use of ultrasound, including Doppler, in SRH practice.
3 Covers the physical principles and system use in greater depth focusing on optimising image quality.

2.1.1 Basic Principles of Ultrasound Imaging

A wide range of equipment for ultrasound imaging is in clinical use and can be broadly categorised as console based, laptop systems and hand-held devices (Figures 2.1a, b, c). Equipment used for gynaecological ultrasound are typically console or laptop systems and should have both transabdominal and transvaginal transducers. The latter is most commonly used in SRH applications.

Ultrasound waves are mechanical longitudinal waves produced by the ultrasound transducer. Individual waves interact by a process known as interference to produce the useful ultrasound beam, which leaves the front face of the transducer and is directed by the movement of the transducer by the operator. Think of this like shining the light beam from a torch in different directions. The image shown on the screen for conventional two-dimensional imaging represents a thin anatomical section through the patient, which is governed by the transducer position and orientation (Figures 2.2 and 2.3a).

The frequency of sound is defined as the number of complete wave cycles that pass a point in one second. The unit for frequency is Hertz. The human ear can hear sound in the range of 20–20,000 Hertz. Sound above this frequency cannot be heard and is called 'ultrasound'. Diagnostic ultrasound typically uses sound in the frequency range 2–20 MHz (million or mega Hertz), inaudible to the human ear. Frequency is important in diagnostic ultrasound since it has an impact on image quality (Section 2.1.8.4).[1]

The conventional two-dimensional ultrasound image comprises a series of grey shades, which vary

(a)   (b)   (c)

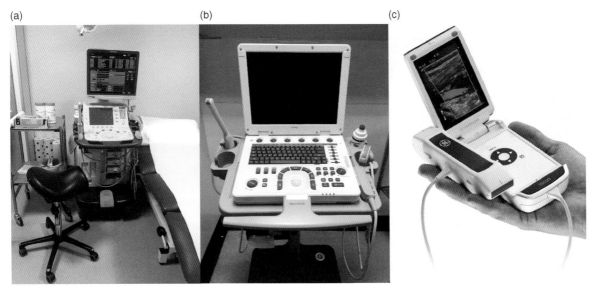

Figure 2.1 (a) Console based ultrasound system. (b) Laptop based ultrasound system. (c) Hand-held ultrasound device.

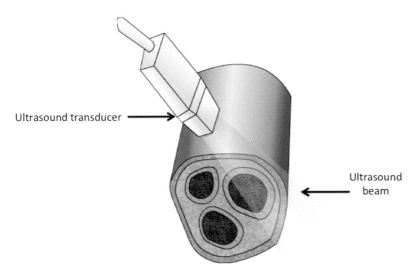

Ultrasound transducer

Ultrasound beam

Figure 2.2 Ultrasound beam transmitted from the front face of the transducer. Positioning the transducer determines the anatomical section shown on the screen.

between bright white and dark black. The grey shade corresponds to the nature of the tissues scanned (Figure 2.3b).[1]

2.1.2 Ultrasound Image Formation

Ultrasound waves are generated by a number of tiny Piezo-Electric (PE) crystals located behind the front face of the transducer (Figures 2.4 a, b).[1] The PE crystals generate ultrasound waves that interact to form the beam that is transmitted from the front face of the transducer into the body in order to produce an image. However, if the transducer is applied directly to the

skin surface, 99 per cent of the sound will be reflected straight back into the transducer at the transducer-skin interface. Thus, no ultrasound will penetrate into the body and no image will be produced. To overcome this, ultrasound gel is placed on the skin surface or applied to the front face of the transducer so that this air gap is eliminated and ultrasound propagates into the body.[1]

Ultrasound interacts with tissue in many ways and this chapter will consider only the very basics related to image formation (Figure 2.5).

Some structures such as bone and gas strongly reflect ultrasound and return strong echoes to the transducer, which will appear white on the image (Figure 2.6a).

9

(a)

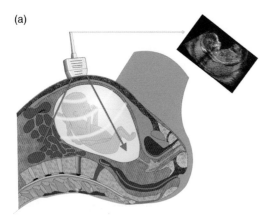

Figure 2.3a Schematic diagram showing how the transducer position and the ultrasound beam are related to a section through a patient and are then displayed on the monitor screen.

(b)

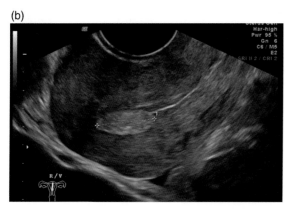

Figure 2.3b Ultrasound image showing grey scale (left) from black to white, with intermediate grey shades. This TVUS image of a retroverted uterus has good soft tissue resolution and the cavity echo, endometrium and myometrium are clearly shown. A soft tissue lesion is shown between the calipers due to good grey scale differentiation, which is key for pelvic imaging.

Weak echoes from the uterus appear as varying shades of grey (Figure 2.6b) and fluid, which is a good transmitter of ultrasound, appears black (Figure 2.6c).[1]

2.1.3 Safety Issues

Ultrasound has been used in medicine for many decades and to date, there is no evidence that diagnostic ultrasound scanning has caused any harm to patients. Current systems have a much higher power output than those used in the early days, and any consequential harm is yet to be proven. However, all ultrasound users must be aware of the key issues relating to the safe and prudent use of ultrasound.[2]

2.1.3.1 Safety Indices

There are two safety indices commonly displayed on the screen during scanning –TI and MI (Figure 2.7).[2]

2.1.3.2 TI

As ultrasound waves are absorbed, their energy is converted into heat. The TI is an on-screen guide to the user of the potential for tissue heating. The TI is an estimate of the tissue temperature rise in °C that might be possible under 'reasonable worst-case conditions'.[2] The TI is the actual acoustic power at the depth of interest divided by the estimated power required to raise the tissue temperature by 1°C.

A temperature rise of <1.5°C is not considered to be harmful to human tissue, including embryos/fetus, even when maintained indefinitely. However, temperature rises >1.5°C may cause harm and are dependent on the length of time of the temperature rise. A temperature rise of 4.0°C for five minutes may be harmful to an embryo or fetus.

(a)   (b)

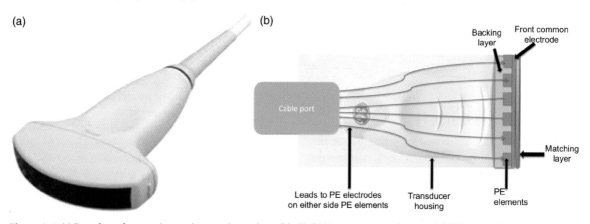

Figure 2.4 (a) Front face of a curved array ultrasound transducer (black). (b) Linear array transducer with BASIC internal structure superimposed. Simplified, there are many more crystals and components.[1]

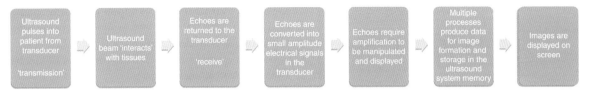

Figure 2.5 Flowchart showing the basic stages in the formation of a diagnostic ultrasound image.

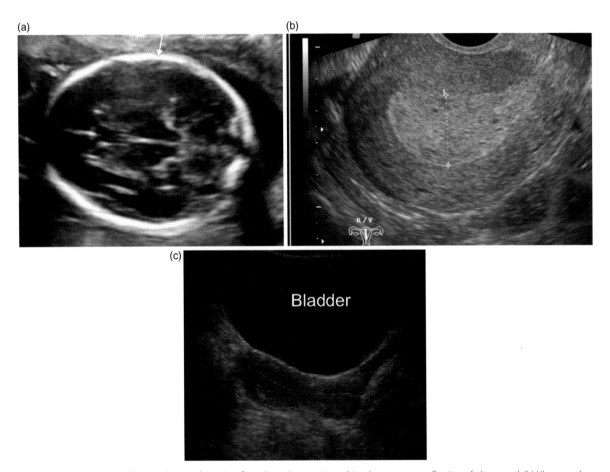

Figure 2.6 (a) Ultrasound image showing bone in a fetus (arrow) appearing white due to strong reflection of ultrasound. (b) Ultrasound image showing relatively weak echoes as varying shades of grey from the uterus. Image shows thickened endometrium between calipers. (c) Ultrasound image of fluid in the urinary bladder; fluid is a good transmitter of ultrasound and appears black. Here it is used as an acoustic window to visualise deeper pelvic structures (for example, uterus) in a transabdominal scan.

2.1.3.3 Non-thermal Effects and MI

The MI is an on-screen guide to the likelihood and magnitude of non-thermal effects. Examples of non-thermal effects include cavitation (excitation of gas bubbles).

Non-thermal damage can occur when tissues containing gas pockets are exposed to ultrasound, for example, in bowel and lung. However, the likelihood of this occurring is minimal when the MI is kept <0.3.[2]

2.1.3.4 The Exposure of the Patient to Ultrasound

While ultrasound has been used for many years without any significant proven harm to patients, the operator should be familiar with the British Medical Ultrasound Society Safety Publications.[2,3] The ALARA principle should be adopted as best practice, that is, the ultrasound 'dose' to the patient must be kept *As Low As Reasonably Achievable*.[3]

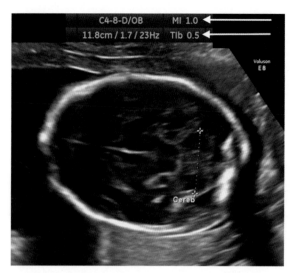

C4-8-D/OB   MI 1.0
11.8cm / 1.7 / 23Hz   TIb 0.5

Voluson
E8

Cereb

Figure 2.7 Ultrasound image of fetal cerebellum (cereb) showing the on-screen safety indices: MI and TI (arrows).

2.1.4 Infection Control and Essential Transducer Care

All transducers must be cleaned after every use. The acoustic coupling gel should be wiped off the transducer. A moistened soft cloth or wipe with approved cleansing anti-microbial substance should then be used to wipe the transducer (see Section 16.2.6). Between uses, transducers should always be stowed in the appropriate holder, which is usually an integral part of the machine (Figure 2.8a). Dropping or knocking the transducer may damage the delicate crystals, resulting in a dark line on the image due to the crystal(s) not firing (crystal drop-out) (Figure 2.8b). The transducers are plugged into ports. The connector has a series of 'pins' (Figure 2.8c) and they should not be forced into the port; otherwise damage will occur.

2.1.5 Ergonomics

Optimum assessment of the ergonomics of the scanning environment is crucial to ensure that you are comfortable and relaxed when scanning. Adverse scanning environments have resulted in work-related musculoskeletal disorders, particularly of the neck, shoulder, elbow and wrist which typically manifest as pain, dull ache, altered sensations, weakness, swelling, blurred vision and so on. Causes include: repetitive motions, awkward movement, excessive application of pressure, and poor posture and ergonomics. However, in SRH services, the ultrasound examination is usually one component of the entire

consultation and the clinician is unlikely to be scanning constantly during a clinical session and therefore may be less at risk than a sonographer. Nonetheless, all practitioners undertaking ultrasound examinations should be aware of the working standards.[4]

A few basics include:

Before you start

- Organise your workspace for efficiency and comfort.
- If you scan while seated, ensure that the height of your scanning chair is most appropriate, and where possible, the use of purpose-designed ergonomic scan chairs that encourage good posture is recommended.
- Ensure the monitor height and tilt are adjusted to suit your line of sight.

During scanning

- Position the patient close to you and where appropriate, ask the patient to roll onto his or her side, to minimise you stretching to reach the area for scanning, for example – left flank.
- Keep your scanning arm as close to your body as possible to reduce arm abduction.
- Where appropriate, rest your 'scanning arm', on the patient, always ensuring that the reason is explained and that the patient is accepting.
- Adopt a power grip (not a pinch grip) around the transducer (Figure 2.9a, b). Do not tightly grip the transducer; try to relax your hand.
- Avoid twisting your neck and trunk (for example, position the monitor directly in front of you).
- Be mindful of scanning technique when examining high BMI patients. Avoid pressing for long periods when scanning transabdominally and vary patient position to displace fat from scan area.
- Adjust heights of couch, monitor and seat to ensure that they suit you.
- Take regular breaks and vary the type of examinations performed if possible.

The Operator

Ultrasound scanning is a very operator-dependent technique and requires significant education, training and skills. The Chief Medical Officer (1994) stated that the greatest risk to the patient is not from exposure to the ultrasound beam, but from the operator. It is the practitioners' responsibility to ensure that they are operating within the boundaries of their knowledge

(a)

(b)

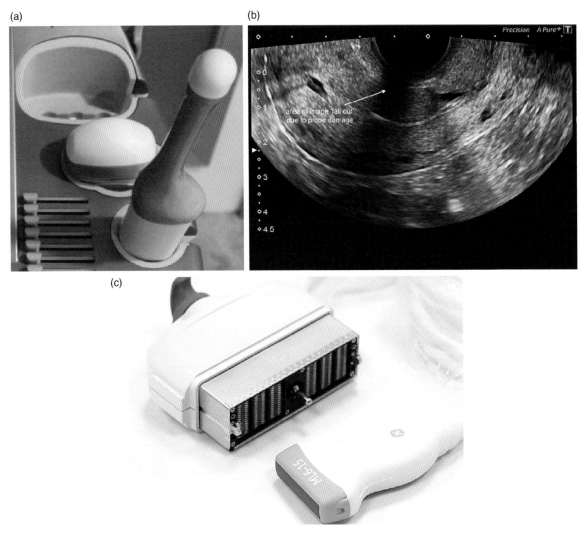

(c)

Figure 2.8 (a) Transducers correctly stowed. (b) Ultrasound image showing 'crystal drop-out' (fall-out) resulting in black line (arrow) in the image due to crystals not firing. (c) Connector 'pins' which must be inserted into the docking port without force to avoid damage.

and skills and can recognise the need for more expert help, to ensure patient safeguarding.

> *The most significant risk of any ultrasound examination is posed by the operator.* Poor technique, wrong interpretation of findings and so on may indirectly cause harm to a patient from inappropriate diagnosis and management.

2.1.6 Know Your System and Its Controls ('Knobology')

Ultrasound is a very operator-dependent imaging technique. It is essential that you develop the knowledge and skills to operate your ultrasound system well;

adaptability and technical competence are pivotal to your diagnostic confidence, and that is highly dependent on being able to utilise the ultrasound system optimally. Many operators rely heavily on pre-set default settings. These are programmed **baseline** settings for specific applications (for example, gynaecology, obstetrics) that provide a starting point and a reasonable image on a patient with 'average' BMI. However, the operator must have the knowledge and skills to adjust the controls beyond the pre-set to **optimise** image quality. Poorly adjusted system controls can create artefacts, mimic pathology or lead to pathology being missed.

Certain controls are common to all ultrasound systems and should always be utilised to achieve the

(a)   (b)

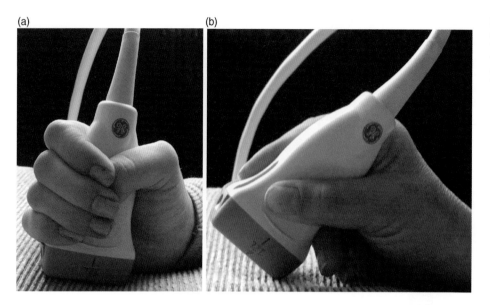

Figure 2.9 Photographs showing (a) correct 'power' grip for holding transducer; compared to (b) poor technique using 'pincer' grip.

optimum image. A number of individual controls influence image quality; however they do not operate in isolation. Instead, they interplay so that when one parameter is changed, it affects others. It is helpful to be familiar with each control by scanning a phantom or consented volunteer to ensure you understand how these controls operate and interplay to ensure that you can optimise your images.[1]

System 'Boot Up'

Prior to switching the system on, you should undertake a visual inspection of the main cart, keyboard, leads and the transducers for any sign of damage (Figure 2.10). When the ultrasound system is switched on, it goes through a boot up procedure, which initialises the system and performs internal control checks. Be aware of your machines' normal 'behaviour' during boot up; look out for unusual noises/error messages/smells, which may indicate a fault.

Enter Patient Demographics

Always ensure that the previous examination has been ended prior to new patient data entry so that images for a previous patient are stored. New patient details must be entered accurately, including the patient's full name, date of birth, gender and any unique identification numbers. In community settings and in some clinics, there is no computerised work list and so you must be able to enter the 'new patient' data to the screen at the start of every examination (Figure 2.11).

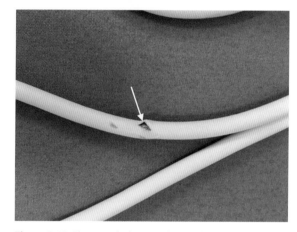

Figure 2.10 Photograph showing damaged transducer cable (arrow).

Always check with the patient that the details are correct.

2.1.7 System Pre-sets

Early ultrasound systems did not have pre-sets and were set up by the operator. As systems became more complex, manufacturers incorporated pre-sets into modern systems. Pre-sets are default baseline settings which facilitate diagnostic ultrasound use by non-expert operators to produce reasonable quality images. They are set up for a patient with an 'average' BMI. However, patients are clearly not all of 'average' BMI and it is important to understand how the system

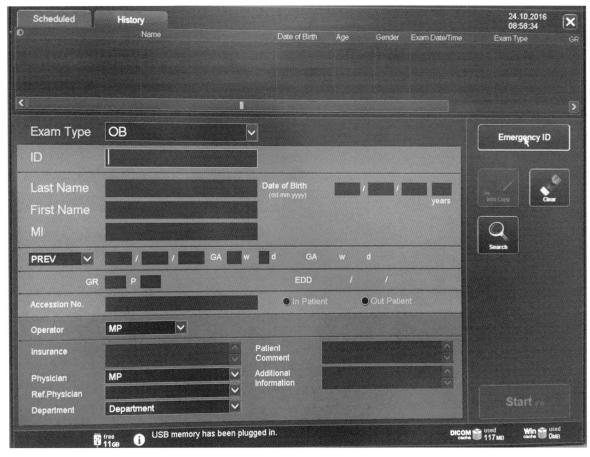

Figure 2.11 The patient data entry screen to be completed accurately prior to commencing any ultrasound examination.

controls work. There are often adaptations to common machine controls which can be made by the operator to over-ride the pre-set effectively that will enhance the image quality, for example, frequency, gain, TGC, depth and power.[1]

The factory pre-sets that are programmed into new ultrasound systems are not always optimum to every clinical setting. It is prudent to request that an application specialist attends a session with the scanning clinician to make appropriate local adjustments to the pre-sets.

Pre-sets are also assigned for a particular examination such as obstetrics, first trimester, gynaecology (transabdominal or transvaginal). They are often a default setting when a particular transducer is connected, although the operator can also select them. Always check that the correct application pre-set for the current patient examination is active before starting a scan (Figures 2.12a, b, c).

2.1.8 The Transducer

Transducers[1] consist of a transducer head, a connecting cable and a connector device that connects the transducer to the ultrasound machine (Figure 2.13). The transducer head has a footprint region (Figures 2.14a, b) where the sound waves leave and return to the transducer, and this is in contact with the patient. There is typically a position marker located next to the head of the transducer to help orientation (Figures 2.15a, b).

Transducers are broadly classified as:

1. transcutaneous (applied to the skin). Examples include linear and curved array.
2. endocavity. Examples include transvaginal, transrectal, oesophageal. (Figure 2.16).

They are further subdivided depending on their shape and resultant image format (Figure 2.17).

15

(a)

(b)

(c)

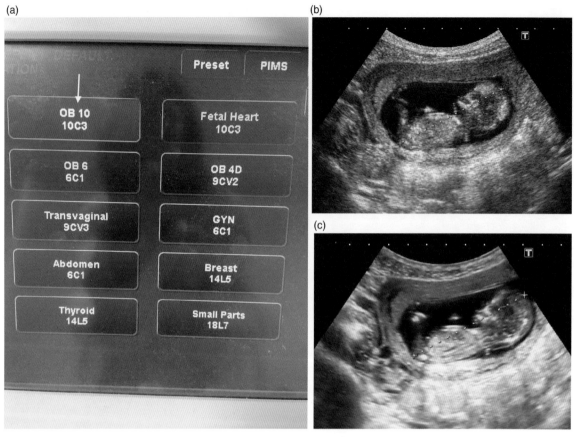

Figure 2.12 (a) Ultrasound image with the system pre-set highlighted (arrow). (b) and (c) The impact of incorrect pre-set and correct pre-set respectively in a first trimester scan.

2.1.8.1 Linear Array Transducer

The footprint is linear as opposed to curved, which means the scan lines run in parallel and remain close together throughout the entire depth of the image. This is preferable for imaging superficial structures, for example, sub-dermal implants. These transducers operate over a relatively high frequency range (typically 12–18 MHz) and are available in varying lengths depending on the application.

2.1.8.2 Curved Array Transducer

A curved array transducer is well suited for transabdominal scanning of the female pelvis and typically operate at frequencies between 2 and 7 MHz. This transducer has a curved front face, which is in contact with the skin, 'the footprint'. Such transducers require the operator to apply continued gentle physical pressure on the skin surface to maintain contact,

otherwise there is loss of contact at the edges of the image, resultant in dark lines at the edges of the image. However, the shape of the FOV, an inverted fan shape, is suited for imaging the female pelvic organs, where a narrow FOV close to the transducer encompasses the bladder as an acoustic window, and thereafter widens deeper in the body to encompass the female pelvic structures as shown in transabdominal pelvic ultrasound image (Figure 2.17).

Transducers come in a range of sizes. When choosing a curved array transducer, be aware of the footprint size (Figure 2.14a). It can be difficult to maintain contact when navigating the bony pelvis with a long footprint, particularly in thin patients where a shorter footprint might help. Applying additional pressure will be required to retain edge contact, potentially causing musculoskeletal strain on the operator and discomfort for the patient.

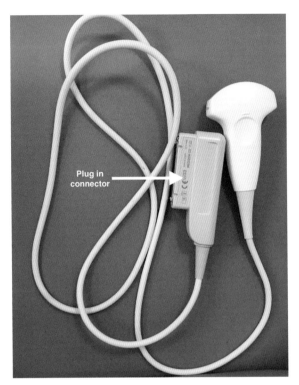

Figure 2.13 Photograph of ultrasound transducer, cable and connector.

2.1.8.3 Image Formation and Field of View

The ultrasound image is made up from a series of scan lines, and their orientation varies between linear and curved transducers. Figure 2.17 shows that the shape of the on-screen image from a linear array transducer is rectangular, being as wide superficially as it is at depth. This makes it suited to imaging superficial structures and the commonest application in SRH is in the assessment of sub-dermal implants. In addition, the shape of the image from a curved array transducer is shown as an inverted fan shape and gets wider with increasing depth. This is useful for TAUS imaging of the female pelvis where the urinary bladder occupies the narrower FOV close to the transducer, but is wider at the depth where the uterus lies.

Figure 2.17 also shows the orientation and spacing of the scan lines from each transducer. In a linear array, they are vertical, parallel and equally spaced, whilst in a curved array they are close together near to the transducer but fan out and become wider apart with increasing depth in the body. When scan lines are wider apart, the image resolution is poorer than when they are closer together. The circle (a) (Figure 2.17) shows a structure correctly positioned in the centre of the FOV and close to the transducer, where in a curved linear transducer the scan lines are closer

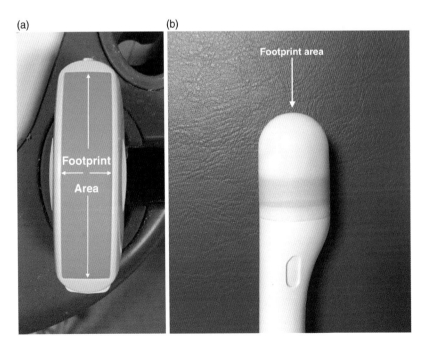

Figure 2.14 Footprint area highlighted: (a) Curved array transducer. (b) Transvaginal transducer.

(a) (b)

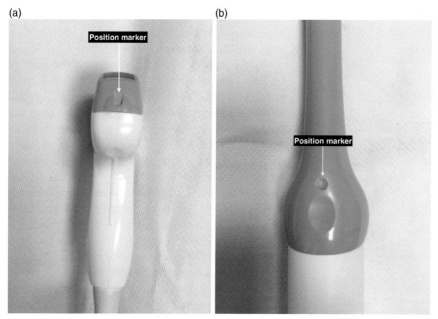

Figure 2.15 Position marker on transabdominal curved array transducer (a) and transvaginal transducer (b) which assists in correct orientation of the transducer relative to the anatomical plane. This is important to identify and use correctly to ensure correct orientation of anatomical planes on screen.

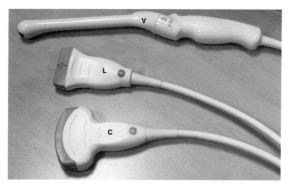

Figure 2.16 A range of ultrasound transducers: linear array (L), curved array (C) and transvaginal (v).

and image resolution is better. Figure 2.17b shows the same structure incorrectly positioned, located at the edge of the FOV and distant from the transducer. Here, the scan lines are wide apart and image resolution is undesirably reduced.

Table 2.1 summarises the applications, merits and limitations of both transducer types.

> **Practical Tip**
>
> Try to ensure that the region of interest is centred to the FOV and adapt your scanning technique so that the structure is as close to the transducer as practicable.

Table 2.1 Applications, Merits and Limitations of Linear versus Curved Array Transducer

Linear Array	Curved Array
Suited to: Vascular/superficial imaging.	Suited to: Most applications: obstetrics/transabdominal gynaecology, abdomen.
Linear/flat footprint, useful for maintaining contact where there are limited surface curves in the area being scanned.	Curved footprint, which can make contact difficult, particularly in patients with high BMI, or on extremely curved body surfaces. Contact can be maintained in some cases by the operator applying greater manual pressure with the probe (graded compression).
Scan lines are parallel and equally spaced throughout all the image.	Scan lines are closer together near to the surface of the transducer and get wider with increasing depth in the body. Also, the scan lines are closer together in the centre of the field of view than at the edges of the FOV. Where the scan lines are closer together, the image resolution is better.

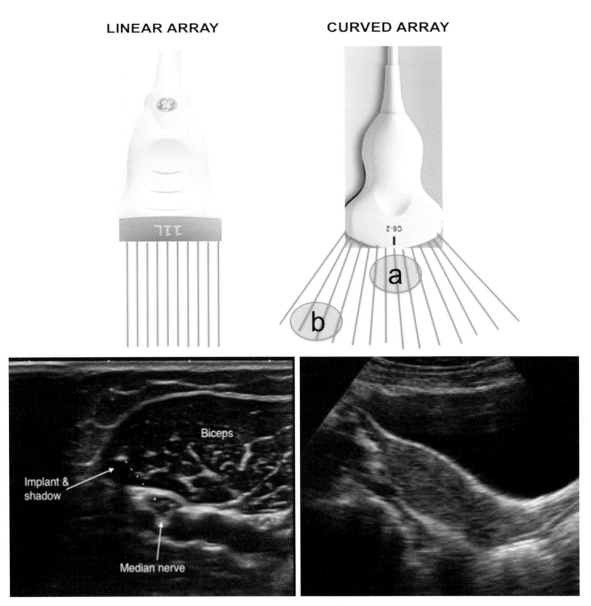

Figure 2.17 Transducer shape and resultant image format for linear and curved array transducers. For a linear array transducer the image format is rectangular, that is, as wide at the skin surface as at depth. For a curved array transducer, the image format is fan shaped, getting wider with increasing depth. This is useful as shown here for encompassing the uterus at depth in TAUS when the bladder is distended. The variation in the orientation and spacing of the scan lines is shown. The region of interest should be located in the centre of the FOV (circled area (a)). This is of particular importance when using a curved array transducer as scan lines are closer together and image quality is better. The circled area (b) is the same structure incorrectly located to the edge of the frame where the scan lines are further apart and image resolution is therefore reduced.

2.1.8.4 TVUS Transducer

This is now recognised as the first line imaging in many cases for the examination of the female pelvis, but appropriate patient consent must be obtained. TVUS produces higher resolution images compared to TAUS (Figure 2.19).

TVUS transducers, like other endocavity transducers, have a small footprint (Figures 2.14b and 2.16) and typically operate at frequencies in the range of 5–12 MHz.

19

Transducer Frequency

Transducer frequency determines how far the ultrasound beam will penetrate into the patient.

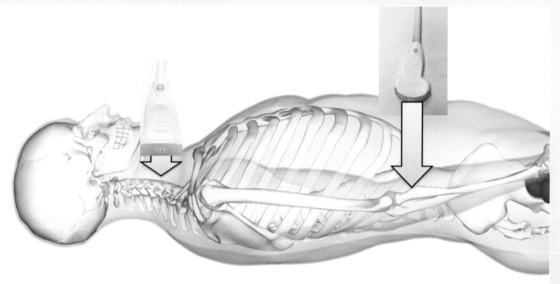

Increasing the frequency decreases beam penetration, but improves image quality.
Decreasing the frequency increases beam penetration, but reduces image quality (see Figure 2.18).

High frequency, linear array transducer. Designed for superficial imaging (e.g. thyroid, MSK).

Higher frequency = less depth penetration, but BETTER IMAGE QUALITY

Lower frequency, curved array transducer. Designed for general scanning (e.g. abdomen, obstetrics, gynaecology).

Lower frequency = greater depth penetration, but POORER IMAGE QUALITY

Figure 2.18 Schematic diagram showing relationship between frequency and depth of penetration.

Generally, higher frequency transducers are used for scanning superficial structures and intra-cavity scanning (for example, TVUS). Many systems now have multi-frequency or 'broadband' transducers where frequency can be selected on the console; alternatively the operator has to change the transducer manually to change frequency.

Different structures attenuate ultrasound by different amounts and the nature of tissue being scanned must be taken into account, when selecting frequency. For example, 10cm of solid liver tissue will attenuate the ultrasound beam more than 10cm of urine when scanning the pelvis TAUS. Hence, to scan to the same depth, it is usual to use a higher frequency when scanning through an adequately distended bladder, whereas a lower frequency, with resultant reduction in resolution, must be used for solid structures of similar depth (for example, liver).[1]

You should select the highest frequency that will permit adequate penetration to the posterior aspect of the ROI and vary the frequency throughout the ultrasound examination depending on the type of tissue and the depth you need to penetrate, to optimise image quality.

2.1.9 Common System Controls

Once the appropriate transducer and pre-set have been selected, the operator can often produce an enhanced image by adjusting only a small number of variables

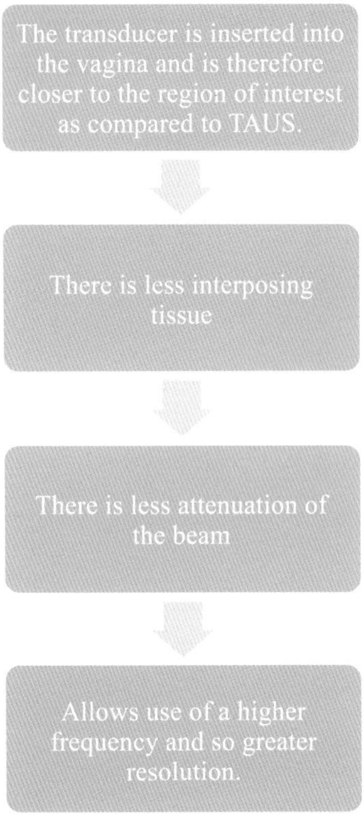

Figure 2.19 Flowchart showing principles underpinning why better image resolution (image quality) is achieved when using a transvaginal transducer.

(Figure 2.20). However, this will not necessarily produce an optimum image, and users are encouraged to develop in-depth knowledge and skills to optimise image quality.[1]

2.1.9.1 Overall Gain

Typically a dial that makes the *whole* image appear darker or brighter when turned anticlockwise/clockwise respectively (Figures 2.21a, b).

2.1.9.2 TGC

Usually slider buttons (6–8 in number) enable image brightness to be varied at different tissue depths. Moving a slider to the right will increase the brightness of the image at that depth, whilst moving slider to the left will make the image darker at that depth (Figures 2.22). The TGC controls need to be adjusted to produce a 'balanced' image at all depths (Figure 2.23).

2.1.9.3 Depth

The depth control determines the maximum depth of the anatomy displayed on the screen. It should be

adjusted to ensure that deep, irrelevant structures are not displayed (Figures 2.24 and 2.25).

2.1.9.4 Zoom

This function magnifies a selected area of the screen allowing it to be inspected in more detail.

2.1.9.5 Focus

The focus should be set to encompass the region of interest as this will improve the image resolution. The focal zones are usually shown as small arrow (>) at the edge of each image (Figure 2.26a). It is possible to switch in more focal zones to improve the resolution of larger structures. However, increasing the number of focal zones will result in a lower frame rate, which is suited to scanning static structures such as the uterus, but is less desirable for scanning a moving structure, such as a second trimester fetus (Figures 2.26b and 2.7).

2.1.9.6 Freeze

Freezing the image stores a number of recent frames in the memory (often hundreds) and displays the last frame. While the image is frozen, measurements can be made and annotations added to images can be archived.

2.1.9.7 Cineloop

Most machines have a cineloop function that is usually operated from a track ball when the image has been frozen. Multiple frames of the images are stored (>1000) which enables the operator to scroll back through frames stored after freezing the image to select the best image for measuring, archiving and so on. This is particularly useful when scanning a moving subject such as a fetus or the heart when it is difficult to freeze an image precisely and storing the actual cineloop can be useful when reviewing a moving structure, for example, fetal heart.

2.1.9.8 Power

Ultrasound is absorbed as it travels through tissues and the amount of absorption is tissue and depth dependent. It is also affected by BMI, with a higher power output typically being required for patients with high BMI. The power control has a similar impact on the image as the overall gain: increasing the power results in the entire image becoming brighter; decreasing the power results in the entire image becoming darker.

Yet, the power control is often not very evident on the control panel and is frequently overlooked. However,

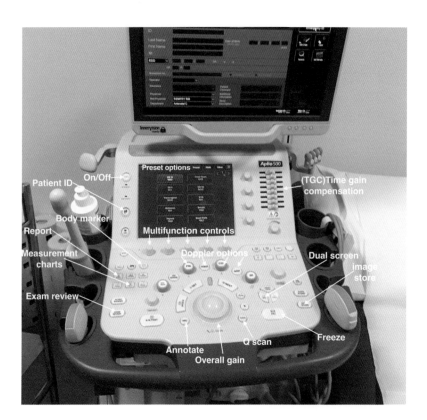

Figure 2.20 Control panel highlighting common controls used in basic conventional two-dimensional grey scale imaging.

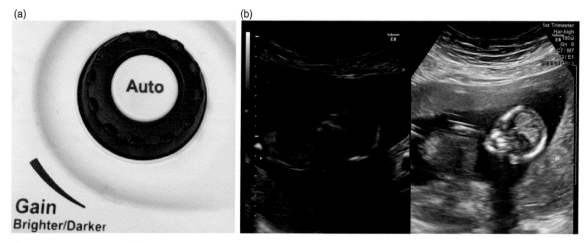

Figure 2.21 (a) Gain control. (b) Split screen image with gain set too low resulting in excessively dark image throughout (left) and gain set too high resulting in excessively bright image throughout (right).

power is an important factor in ultrasound safety and has an effect on the image quality (Section 2.1.3).

2.1.10 Operational Modes

Ultrasound systems can operate in a variety of modes; the more common ones are discussed briefly in the sections that follow.

2.1.10.1 Two-Dimensional (2D)/B-Mode Imaging

B-mode imaging stands for brightness-modulated imaging and is a rather dated term which relates to the image made up from a series of dots of differing brightness. This term has been superseded more recently by 2D imaging, where the on-screen image has two dimensions – width and height

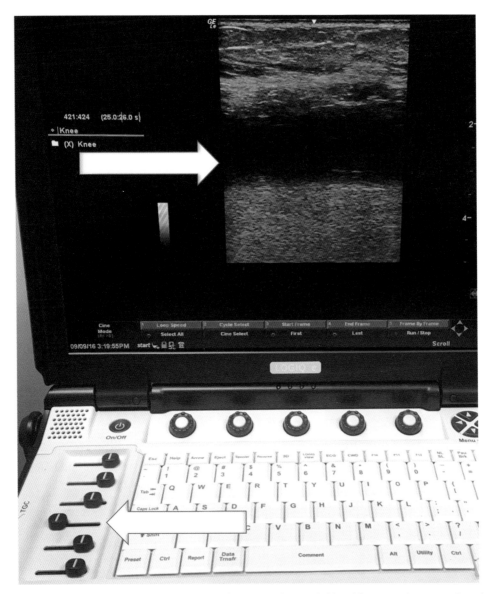

Figure 2.22 Effect of reducing the TGC at a specific depth resulting in dark band (large arrow) on image. Note the position of the errant slider control (large arrow) causing this effect (banding artefact).

which represents a cross-section of the body determined by the transducer position and is made up from a series of grey shades which reflect the nature of the tissue being scanned (Figure 2.3a, b and Figure 2.27).

2.1.10.2 M-Mode

This stands for 'motion-mode' and is used to demonstrate the movement of structures such as the heart. In SRH applications, it can be useful for documenting

the presence/absence of an embryonic/fetal heartbeat during pregnancy (Figure 2.28).

In addition, the use of M-mode negates the use of Doppler, which is not recommended in early pregnancy due to the risk of potential harm.[2]

2.1.10.3 Doppler

Doppler ultrasound is useful for detecting and measuring blood flow.[1] There are many types of Doppler available currently. However, the science, technique, optimum use and safety issues are outside the scope of this book.[1] The basic terms are introduced in the section that follows to allow recognition of the different Doppler modes and the relevant system controls. Be aware that manufacturers do not all use the same terminology; the more commonly used terms are used here.

Accessing Doppler Modes, Pre-sets, Common Errors

Optimising Doppler 'images' is a complex technique and there are many parameters that can influence the quality. Poorly optimised Doppler settings can have adverse effects on patient management. Whilst it is recognised that most ultrasound systems have Doppler settings incorporated into their pre-sets that are a reasonable scanning starting point, it is important that the operator pursues specific Doppler training to avoid mistakes.

For example, the rate at which ultrasound pulses are transmitted into the patient in Doppler is known as the pulse repetition frequency (PRF). Adjusting the PRF is different on different machines. Simply, having this parameter set incorrectly can make a structure appear wrongly highly vascular or avascular. This will likely have an adverse impact on the patient management and may wrongly assign a patient to a high/low-risk group, simply by having a system control set incorrectly.

2.1.10.4 PW or Spectral Doppler

PW or Spectral Doppler are alternate terms. PW/ Spectral Doppler uses the Doppler principle to collect signals arising from a specific position in the body. This is determined by selecting the PW control (Figure 2.29) that generates a moveable line on the screen which overlays the conventional 2D grey shade image. This PW Doppler line is broken by a 'box shaped' structure, the sample volume. The size and position of the sample volume and the position of the PW line can be adjusted. The benefit of this is that the operator can use the 2D basic image to identify anatomical structures and reliably position the sample volume (Figure 2.30). In general, the sample

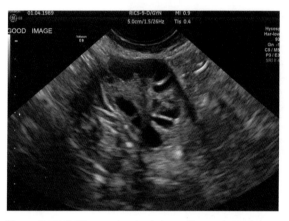

Figure 2.23 TVUS ovary showing balanced image due to the correct setting of gain and TGC.

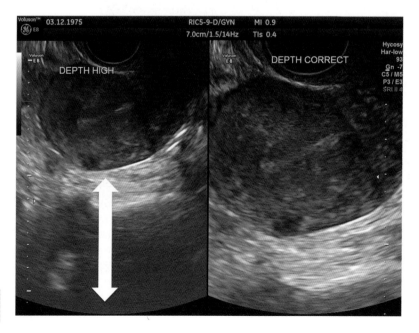

Figure 2.24 TVUS uterus. Split screen image with depth set correctly, with the posterior aspect of the region of interest (uterus) shown (right). Depth control set too great so that significant area deep (arrow) to the region of interest (uterus) is shown (left).

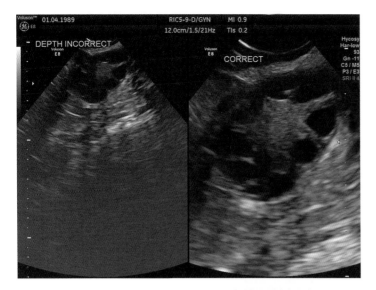

Figure 2.25 TVUS Ovary. Small structure (ovary with incorrect depth, no zoom applied), poor technique (left). Use of appropriate depth and zoom ensures that the region of interest (ovary) occupies the field of view on the monitor (right). Note – ovary is also centred to the FOV and is close to the transducer, thereby improving image quality as scan lines closer together.

(a)

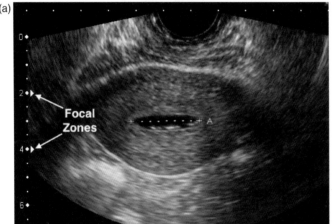

(b)

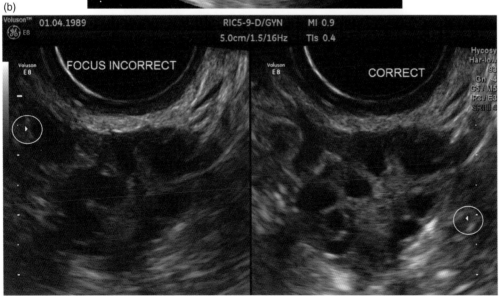

Figure 2.26 (a) Shows notation that indicates focal zones. (b) TVUS image of an ovary with the focus incorrectly set too close to the probe (left), compared to the correct focus position (right). Note – right-hand image with correct focus is much sharper than the same ovary with incorrect focus. This clearly demonstrates the need for the region of interest to be 'in focus'.

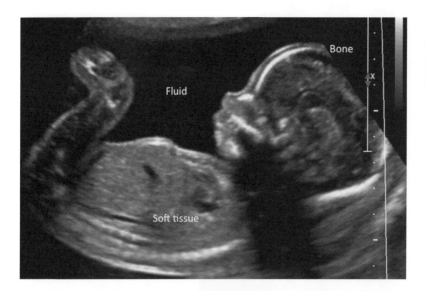

Figure 2.27 Conventional 2D ultrasound image of a fetus. Note areas which strongly reflect ultrasound appear white and clear fluid (amniotic fluid) appears black and soft tissue structures as varying shades of grey dependent on the nature of tissue.

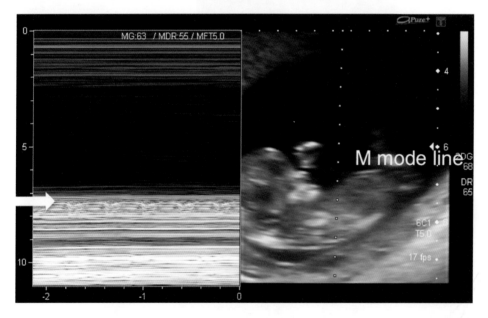

Figure 2.28 M-mode showing fetal heartbeat pattern (arrow).

volume should be similar to the size of the vessel being sampled and the angle should also be adjusted to be in line with the vessel direction to maximise the Doppler shift. When perpendicular to the vessel there will be no Doppler shift. Whilst PW has important applications in obstetrics to obtain quantified measurements, to date, it has minimal application in SRH.

2.1.10.5 Colour Flow Imaging

This uses the Doppler principle to generate a 2D colour image which is superimposed on the conventional grey shade 2D image and shows the velocity and direction of blood flow. Traditionally, blood flow towards the transducer is depicted as red and blood flow away from the transducer is blue (Figure 2.31a). This is a valuable resource for reviewing blood flow over large anatomical areas.

CFI is usually push button operated (Figure 2.29) and a box is generated which can be varied in size, position and angle. The conventional grey scale 2D image is used to identify the structure to be interrogated with Doppler (Figure 2.31b).

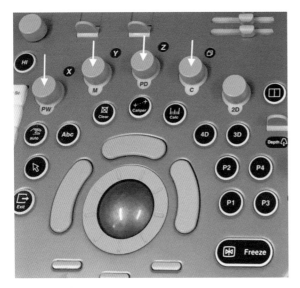

Figure 2.29 Demonstrates the common Doppler and M-mode controls (arrows) on the keyboard.

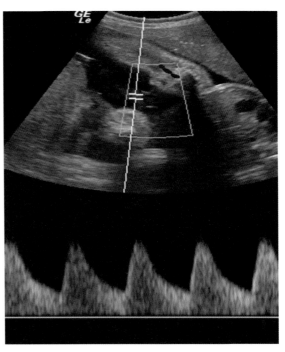

Figure 2.30 PW/Spectral Doppler applied to the fetal umbilical artery. The sample volume is shown as two horizontal parallel lines and the resultant Doppler trace is shown underneath.

(a)   (b)

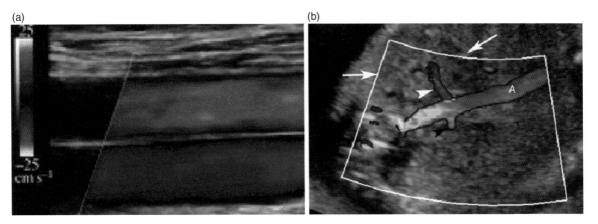

Figure 2.31 (a) Colour flow image of carotid neck vessels showing flow towards the transducer (red) and away from the transducer (blue). (b) Shows the colour box which can be varied in size, shape, angle and orientation applied to a fetal aorta (A) and renal arteries (arrow head).

2.1.10.6 Power Doppler

Power Doppler shows the strength of the signal in colour, often using a yellow–orange scale. It is particularly sensitive and is useful for the detection of flow in small blood vessels and those with low-velocity flow, for example, neovascularisation in tumours (Figure 2.32).

PART 2: CLINICAL CASES

These clinical cases are a useful way to demonstrate the added value of Doppler in SRH clinics. There are many additional examples of this throughout this book.

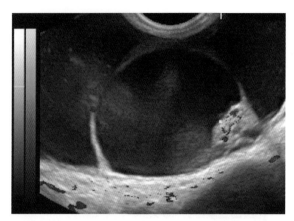

Figure 2.32 Adnexal cystic mass, with small solid area, which shows evidence of flow when Power Doppler is applied, raising the level of suspicion.

Case 2.1 Doppler in the Diagnosis of a Fibroid

This lady was referred due to a mass noted on pelvic examination prior to a planned IUS fitting to treat menorrhagia. Power Doppler shows vascularity in the solid area in the left of the uterus on TVUS, typical of a subserosal fibroid, notably with peripheral/circumferential flow (Figure 2.33).

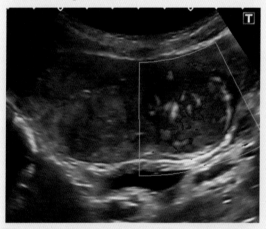

Figure 2.33 TVUS Power Doppler image showing circumferential/peripheral flow in a solid intra-uterine lesion, rather than centrally located. Appearances are consistent with a fibroid.

Case 2.2 Doppler in the Diagnosis of a Corpus Luteum

The blood flow distribution in the TVUS image (Figure 2.34) clarifies that the left ovary is normally positioned adjacent to the iliac vessels and that the

small cyst is a CL with high peripheral blood flow. The flow in an active CL is greater than a maturing follicle.

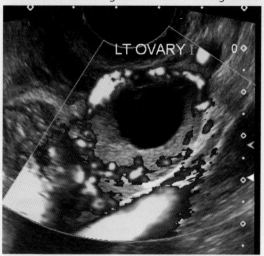

Figure 2.34 TVUS Power Doppler image showing high flow around a simple adnexal cyst. This is greater than expected for a maturing follicle and is consistent with a corpus luteum.

Case 2.3 Doppler in the Diagnosis of Retained Products

This lady presented with continued bleeding and positive PT seven weeks after medical termination of a six-week pregnancy. 2D TVUS of her uterus shows a small central area (13 × 9.5 mm, A-B callipers) of tissue

(a)

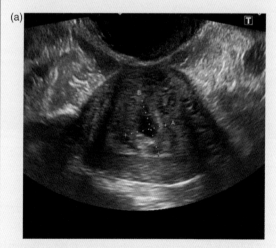

that could be retained products or resolving blood clot (Figure 2.35a).

(b)

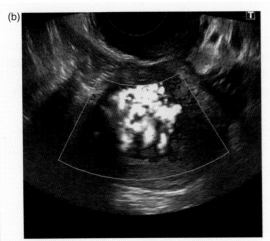

Figure 2.35 Conventional 2D TVUS ultrasound image showing small hypoechoic area in the centre of the uterus (a). Differentials included blood clot or RPCs, post-termination. Application of Power Doppler (b) confirmed high flow throughout the myometrium consistent with RPCs.

Colour Doppler in the same view shows high flow throughout the myometrium and this is consistent with retained products (Figure 2.35b).

Case 2.4 Doppler in the Diagnosis of Uterine Clot, in Contrast to RPCs

This lady had a similar history of protracted bleeding six weeks after surgical termination, and on 2D TVUS imaging a central area of possible tissue or resolving clot was found in the uterus. The use of Power Doppler shows no flow within the contents of the cavity, consistent with blood clot as opposed to RPCs (Figure 2.36).

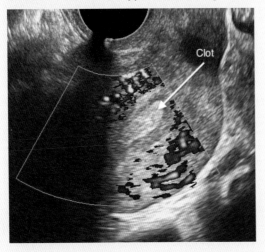

Figure 2.36 Conventional 2D TVUS image with Power Doppler showing no flow within the uterine cavity, only in the surrounding myometrium. Appearances consistent with clot in the cavity.

Case 2.5 Doppler in the Diagnosis of Malignant Pelvic Disease

This 45-year-old woman was referred for removal of a coil with missing threads. (a) On TVUS the coil was visible (Figure 2.37a). Figures 2.37b, c, d show the use of Power Doppler confirming a fibroid and solid projections (arrows) projecting into free fluid in the pelvis. After further investigations, a diagnosis of stage 3 epithelial cancer was subsequently made.

(a)

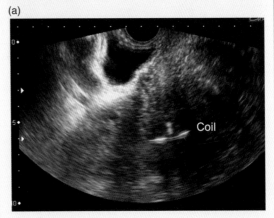

Figure 2.37a TVUS showing a coil.

(b)

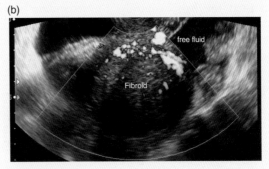

Figure 2.37b This image superior to the coil shows an intramural fibroid with peripheral flow and also some free pelvic fluid.

(c)

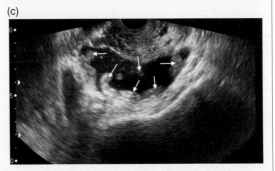

Figure 2.37c Free fluid was noted superior to the uterus, indicating on subjective assessment more than a 'normal' amount. On assessing the free fluid, solid projections were present (arrows).

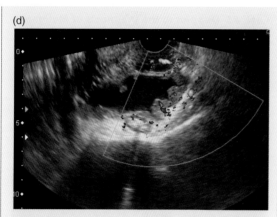

(d)

Figure 2.37d The use of Power Doppler shows blood flow within the 'papillae' confirming these are tissues and consistent with malignant ascites. Her Ca 125 was greater than 1,000 and subsequent treatment clarified stage 3 ovarian epithelial cancer.

Cases provided by Dr Mary Pillai

PART 3: SYSTEM OPTIMISATION/ ENHANCING THE IMAGE

Use of the ultrasound system is not a static process. It does not stop after you have selected a pre-set and adjusted the basic controls. Understanding some basic science and more advanced system settings is essential to optimising and subsequent correct interpretation of the image, thereby enhancing your diagnostic capability and safe and effective use of the equipment.

2.2 Ultrasound Image Formation

The basic stages involved in the formation of a conventional 2D ultrasound image are shown in Figure 2.38.

2.2.1 Transducer, Generation of Ultrasound, Acoustic Gel, Reception of Echoes

To produce a 2D, grey shade ultrasound image, the transducer has to produce short pulses of ultrasound which form the beam which passes along a narrow directional corridor into the tissue. In this respect, the transducer is analogous to a torch, and the position of the transducer by the operator determines the direction the ultrasound beam passes into the patient (Figure 2.2).

The transducer has three main functions, notably to:

1. generate the ultrasound beam;
2. receive the echoes from the patient and convert these into electrical signals; and

3. allow the operator to direct the beam into the patient to obtain the correct anatomical section.

The scientific definition of a transducer is *an electrical device that converts energy from one form to another.* One of the key components of the transducer is the PE array of elements. These are located behind the front face of the transducer (Figure 2.4b).[1]

2.2.1.1 Generation of Ultrasound

The 2D ultrasound image is formed by coupling the transducer to the skin using acoustic transmission gel. After unfreezing the system, the transducer becomes active and the crystal elements are fired.

The pulse-echo effect is utilised (Figure 2.39). The transducer PE elements/plate produce a short **pulse** of ultrasound which passes into the body. Then it does not transmit ultrasound temporarily (it pauses), whilst it acts as a receiver to listen to the **echoes** returning from the patient. Only 1 per cent of operating time is spent emitting ultrasound; the remainder is spent listening for returning echoes. It is rather like 'shouting and listening' for an echo in audible sound. The ultrasound system has advanced software which measures the length of time it takes between a transmit pulse being sent from the transducer and the time at which echoes from a specific depth are received back at the transducer; this is the PERT. Simplistically, the system acts like an expensive timer to measure the PERT and it then runs an algorithm to calculate the depth of structures and ensure that they are accurately spatially located at the correct depth in the final image.[1]

2.2.1.2 Production of a Frame

In practice, the transducer elements do not fire separately, but typically fire in groups; the latter is required to achieve image-enhancing options such as focusing. Figures 2.40a, b show diagrammatically how the frame of an image is produced simplistically using example of elements firing singly. The elements at one end of the array become active and fire an ultrasound pulse into the body. After attenuation (interaction) processes occur, echoes are received by the transducer element. The first scan line corresponds with the transducer orientation marker – red dot. Each scan line is produced by one pulse-echo sequence. Elements across the array fire in turn, each producing a scan line, until the last one in the array is fired at the right-hand edge of transducer and then the frame is complete. The frame is built up rapidly line by line. The more lines there are per frame (line density), the

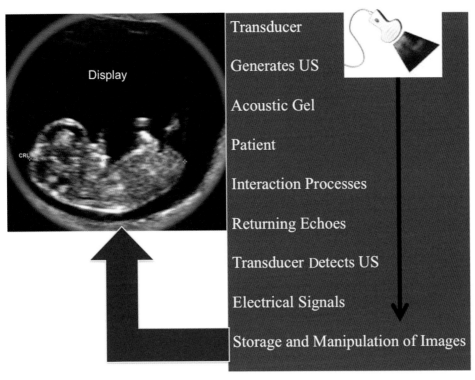

Figure 2.38 Block diagram showing basic stages in the formation of a 2D grey scale ultrasound image.

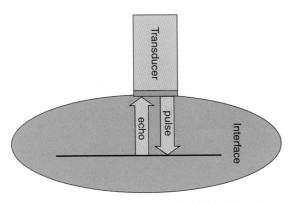

Figure 2.39 Diagrammatic representation of the pulse-echo effect.

closer they are together and this means that the image resolution is better. Where scan lines are further apart, the image resolution is poorer.

Then the composition of the next frame starts, with the element firing recommencing from the left-hand side. For real-time imaging, a frame rate > 25 frames/second is required. The frame rate is usually shown on the screen (Figure 2.40c) and you should be aware of this.

High/rapid frame rates are required for imaging rapidly moving structures (for example, fetal heart), whereas lower frame rates can be used for static structures (for example, uterus). If the FR is too low for fetal heart imaging (for example, 12 frames/second) there will be a 'lag' in the image. Crudely speaking, the ultrasound system cannot keep pace with the movement of the FH and the image appears 'jerky'.

There is no frame rate button on an ultrasound system; the frame rate is affected by many other factors (see Sections 2.2.7, 2.2.8, 2.2.9).

Practical Tip

Use higher frame rate for imaging rapidly moving structures (for example, fetal heart).

Can use lower frame rate for imaging static structures (for example, uterus/ovaries).

2.2.1.3 Interaction Processes within the Patient

Ultrasound interacts within the tissues of the patient by a number of mechanisms to produce the image. These include reflection, scattering, refraction, absorption and wave front divergence. All of these

(a)

The real-time 2D image is built up line by line..........

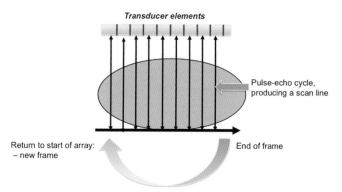

Transducer elements

Pulse-echo cycle, producing a scan line

Return to start of array: – new frame

End of frame

Figure 2.40 (a) Diagrammatic representation of the construction of a single frame of a 2D ultrasound image.

(b) Construction of an actual 2D ultrasound image (sub-dermal implant) from a linear array transducer, made up of a series of equally spaced, parallel lines. When the transducer is activated by pressing the freeze button, the elements closest to the left-hand side of the scan image start to fire (indicated by orientation red dot).

(c) The numerical value of the FR is shown on the screen display.

(b)

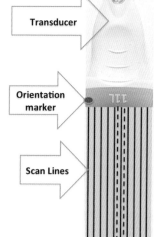

Transducer

Orientation marker

Scan Lines

The number of lines per frame = the LINE DENSITY.

The more lines there are per frame, the greater is the line density and simplistically, the better the resolution, as the scan lines are closer together. Imagine, doubling the number of lines using the same transducer shown here. There will be more scan lines, closer together, improved resolution.(See effect of hashed lines).

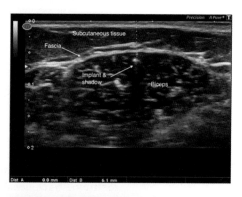

Subcutaneous tissue
Fascia
Implant & shadow
Biceps

(c)

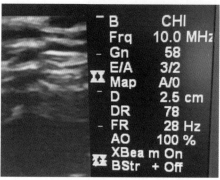

(a)

(b)

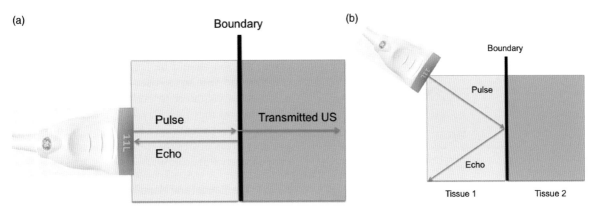

Figure 2.41 (a) Diagrammatic representation of reflection. If the ultrasound beam is directed at a boundary between two tissues with different values of acoustic impedance, some of the beam will be reflected back to the transducer (reflected), whilst some will continue into the body to image deeper structures (transmitted). (b) Shows the reflection that occurs at an equal and opposite angle when the ultrasound beam is at an angle to a boundary, resultant in weaker/no echoes detected by the transducer.

processes result in a reduction in the overall ultrasound beam intensity as it passes through the patient (i.e. the beam typically gets weaker). Here we are going to consider three basic processes – reflection, scattering and refraction (Section 2.3.3).

Reflection

Each tissue has a property (**acoustic impedance**), which is important in image formation. It is a different value for different tissues. When the ultrasound beam hits a boundary where there is a difference in acoustic impedance, reflection occurs generating an echo which normally goes back to the transducer. It is not the actual value of acoustic impedance that matters, rather the difference in values in acoustic impedance between two tissue types on either side of a boundary. Reflection occurs where there is a large anatomical boundary (for example, uterine cavity echo).

The strongest echo will be produced when the ultrasound beam hits the boundary at 90 degrees (Figure 2.41a). If the beam is *not* perpendicular to the interface, some of the reflected ultrasound energy will not be directly returned to the transducer and the echo will be weaker than expected or will not be received (Figure 2.41b). A good example of this is demonstrated in Chapter 4, in Figure 4.4 of an axial uterus. This TVUS image is of very poor quality due to the beam being almost parallel to the tissue boundaries, and it is impossible to obtain a suitable angle of insonation when the uterus is axial in orientation.

> **Practical Tips**
>
> Try to manipulate the transducer to ensure that the ultrasound beam hits a boundary at 90 degrees to get maximum strength echo at a boundary (for example, cavity echo/endometrium).
>
> Where the ultrasound beam is parallel to a boundary, *no* echo will be received.
>
> If the ultrasound beam hits a boundary at an angle, it will be reflected at an equal and opposite angle and will be weaker than expected or not detected at all.

Scattering

Scattering occurs when ultrasound interacts with very small targets. These are typically found in parenchyma such as liver, kidney, ovarian stroma and uterine myometrium. Such small reflectors reflect ultrasound differently to large boundaries. Here, the ultrasound is reflected in multiple different directions, over a wide angle (Figure 2.42a). Consequently, the echoes received from such structures are weaker than from a boundary (Figure 2.42b).

Of interest, RBC are very small structures and it is scattering of the ultrasound by the RBCs that contributes to Doppler ultrasound.

> **Practical Tip**
>
> Practically, the strength of the echoes produced by scattering is not affected as much by the transducer angle as compared to large boundaries. The echoes look similar in appearance irrespective of angle.

(a)

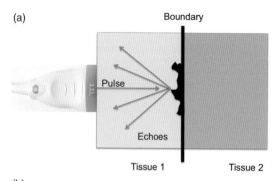

(b)

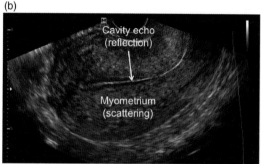

Figure 2.42 (a) Diagrammatic representation of scattering resulting in weak echoes which may not be detected by the transducer. (b) Clinical example – uterus with cavity echo produced by reflection and myometrium produced by scattering.

Received Echoes

US echoes are detected by the transducer. The magnitude of the echo will depend upon a number of factors one of which is the acoustic nature of the tissues which have been insonated. The echoes are converted into an electrical signal within the PE elements/plate of the transducer and these signals can then pass via the cable, through the transducer port and into the main ultrasound system for signal manipulation and processing.

Signal Processing

Ultrasound systems have complex real-time processors which play an important part in the construction of the digital ultrasound image. This involves rapid processing of the electrical signals, their digitisation and manipulation to form the on-screen image displayed. It also allows the manipulation of the digital image, for example, freeze frame, zoom and use of colour tints and so on.

2.2.2 Optimising the Image – Know Your System Controls!

Everyone who uses ultrasound in diagnostics has a duty of care to the patient to produce high quality images. Poor system settings can make structures look pathological, when in fact they are normal, and suboptimal imaging can result in a missed or incorrect diagnosis. You should be familiar with your system controls and you are advised to scan a phantom or a consented volunteer to evaluate what each control does and how they interplay with other.[2,3] The impact of such adverse events have been highlighted recently in many areas of healthcare in 'Human Factors and Patient Safety Publications'.[6]

2.2.2.1 The Manual and Manufacturers' Support

Each ultrasound system has a manual (online tool or paper based) which is an important reference tool for enhancing your use of the ultrasound system. Remember, your role is to obtain OPTIMUM images to inform clinical patient management. Some self-directed learning time, working through the manual to better understand the functions on your system, is time well spent. Do not be frightened of the machine and its complex looking buttons; find out what each does and the impact it has on the image.

In addition, the company applications specialists typically offer excellent support and are generally very willing to attend on site to give support on how to get the best out of your ultrasound system. Many companies run training courses to help purchasers get the best out of their equipment.

2.2.2.2 Power

Increasing the power setting increases the ultrasound beam intensity and that causes the entire image to appear uniformly brighter throughout the image. Also, the beam will penetrate further into the body for the same tissue type (Figure 2.43a, b – images with high and low power and impact on MI and TI). Reducing the power reduces the beam intensity and the image will become darker throughout.

The power control should be set so that the ultrasound beam just penetrates to the back of the region of interest. However, the power setting is usually an integral part of a pre-set and it is sometimes difficult to identify how to adjust this as the control is not always as overt as other controls (Figure 2.43a).

Power is important in influencing the MI and TI. As power increases, the MI and TI increase and vice versa (Figure 2.43b). To better understand this, scan the same structure with higher and lower power settings and compare the values of MI and TI on-screen. Aim to use the minimum power that provides a

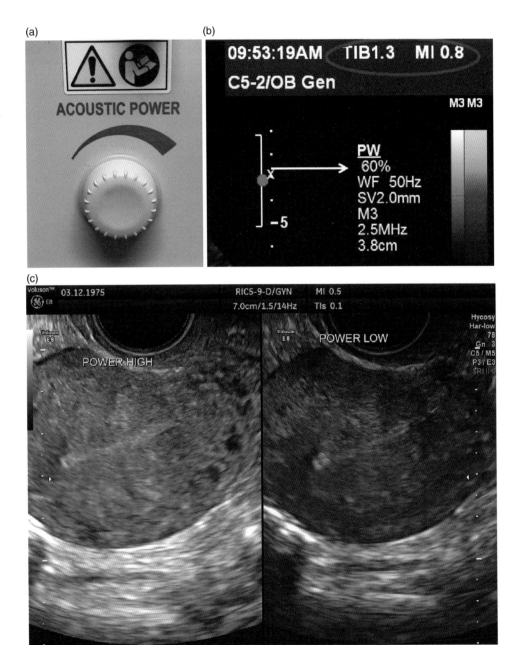

Figure 2.43 (a) Overt power control, easily accessible to user. (b) MI and TI (on-screen indices) and the per cent output power, in this case 60 per cent (arrow). (C) TVUS image of uterus with high power setting (left). Same patient, reduced power resulting in darker image (right). Note that in the latter, the soft tissue resolution of the endometrium is poorer. Power setting must be adequate to maintain a high-quality image.

diagnostic image to keep the 'dose' to a minimum – ALARA principle.[2,3]

Figure 2.43c shows the impact of high and low power setting on TVUS uterus (same patient). Although the use of lowest power is advocated, there is a danger that if the power is too low, that useful information in the image is lost.

In fact, many systems default to a very high power setting in the pre-set (for example = 100%), the rationale for this being that it improves image quality.

35

2.2.2.4 Overall Gain

The echoes returned to the transducer from structures within the patient are weak in amplitude. When they interact with the PE elements/plate in the transducer, they are converted into corresponding small voltages. These are also very weak and must be amplified so they can be processed for image formation. The overall gain controls the amount of amplification applied to all the returning echoes from all depths and amplifies them all uniformly.

The gain control is usually a dial which increases the amplification of all echoes when rotated clockwise and reduces amplification of all echoes when rotated anticlockwise.

High overall gain increases the amplification of echoes at all depths and renders the overall image brighter. Conversely, low overall gain decreases amplification of echoes at all depths and renders the overall image darker. In either case, there is a loss of valuable diagnostic information (Figure 2.21a, b).

The aim is to ensure that the echoes displayed are not too bright or too weak/dark, but the image looks balanced.

2.2.2.5 Interplay between Gain and Power

The gain and power controls similarly affect the image display and are somewhat interchangeable; increasing the value of both parameters uniformly increases the brightness of the entire image and vice versa. It is good practice to always use minimum power and higher overall gain where possible to reduce 'dose', compliant with the ALARA principle. In addition, you should only change to a lower imaging frequency when the power and gain controls are set to maximum as reducing frequency reduces diagnostic image quality.[1-3]

There are no absolute or correct settings and adjustment is required for each individual patient and the structure being examined to optimise the image.

2.2.2.6 TGC

The ultrasound beam is attenuated when the beam passes from the transducer through tissues and as the echoes return to the transducer. The echoes returning from deep within a patient would be weaker than those from superficial structures if the same degree of amplification were applied to all echoes from different depths. In the absence of pathology, echoes from different depths in same tissue should be of same grey shade. The TGC controls enable echoes from greater depths to be amplified to a greater extent than those from superficial structures to balance the image. Incorrect setting of the TGC can cause artefacts, loss of information, misinformation, any of which could result in incorrect diagnosis.

Moving one of these controls to the left decreases the brightness of the image at that specific depth due to reduced amplification of those echoes producing a dark band in the image at a specific depth (Figure 2.22). Conversely, a bright band would be evident if the control was moved to the right.

2.2.2.7 FOV/Sector Angle

It is possible for the operator to alter the size of the field of view from left to right on the image. A small sector angle is useful when studying a small anatomical area, for example, the ovary. A narrow field of view improves visual acuity as distraction or extraneous ultrasound signals from surrounding structures are removed (pinhole camera effect). This also improves the image resolution, since the scan lines in the distal field are closer together towards the middle of a sector compared to those occupying the lateral part of a wide sector. Increasing the line density increases spatial resolution. Reducing the sector angle without changing other system controls may also increase the frame rate as it refreshes more often (Figure 2.44).

2.2.2.8 Depth

The depth control determines the maximum depth of the tissue displayed. It does not alter how far the ultrasound beam travels into the body. The depth control needs to be altered to ensure that areas much deeper to the region of interest are not shown (Figures 2.24 and 2.25). Decreasing the depth ensures the region of interest fills the screen and irrelevant structures are not included.

Typically, the greater the depth shown on the screen, the lower is the system frame rate; the lower the depth, the higher is the frame rate. Lower frame rates are not suitable for imaging rapidly moving structures, whilst high frame rates are better for imaging rapidly moving structures.

> **Practical Tip**
>
> You should always use the depth control prior to using the zoom control.

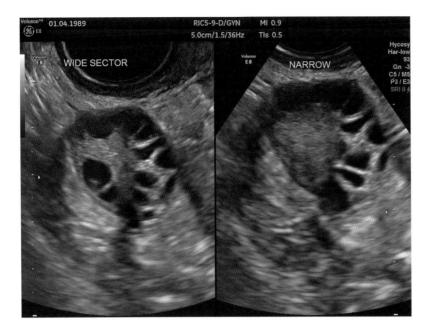

Figure 2.44 Split screen TVUS image of the ovary with wide sector angle (left) and narrower sector angle (right). In the latter, the ovary is centred to the FOV and use of narrow sector eliminates irrelevant surrounding structures, allowing operator to better concentrate on the ovary.

2.2.2.9 Focus

The focus control is rather like the focusing control on a normal camera; you would not want a photograph that is out of focus and so you need to ensure that you can use your ultrasound system focusing controls to optimise your image quality. The ultrasound beam which emerges from the ultrasound transducer has a finite width. The image quality is improved where the beam width is kept narrow. This is the function of the focus control. When you switch in one focal zone, the ultrasound beam is narrowed in that region and the image resolution is improved in that limited region. Beyond the focal region, the beam gets wider and the resolution is poorer (Figure 2.45a). Note – the position of the focus indicator varies between manufacturers. Some require you to place this in the centre of the ROI (Figure 2.45b), whilst others require the focus to be placed just level to the back of the ROI. In some systems, a bar is shown which makes the placement of the focusing from the front to the back of the ROI helpful (Figure 2.45c).

Increasing the number of focal zones in use concurrently is commonly referred to as multiple zone focusing. The benefit of this is that there is a narrow ultrasound beam over a greater depth of tissue. Consequently, the image resolution is better over a greater depth. This is important when scanning large structures such as the kidney/liver, but is not so important in typical SRH applications where the size of structures such as the uterus and ovaries are normally smaller. Generally, the depth and range of focusing you set, should encompass from the front to the back of the ROI (Figure 2.45c) to improve image resolution.

Increasing the number of focal zones typically comes with a penalty – a reduction in frame rate – since it takes longer to generate a single image frame and therefore there are less frames per second (reduced/slower FR). Slower FR is not suited to the imaging of rapidly moving structures (for example, fetal heart) since the system cannot 'keep up' and the image appears 'jerky'. However, for imaging large structures (for example, liver), this is not a problem since the liver is a relatively static structure on breath-hold. For imaging of small structures in the female pelvis (for example, uterus and ovaries), it is usual to limit the number of focal zones to ensure the beam is narrow over the ROI, whilst maintaining the FR and enhancing image quality. Clearly, in early pregnancy scanning this is important as a faster FR is required for imaging the heartbeat.

2.2.2.10 Zoom

You are probably familiar with the zoom control on a camera which is used to ensure that the ROI is magnified in the frame. The principle is the same in ultrasound imaging. Zooming the image is important when the region of interest is small and needs to be made

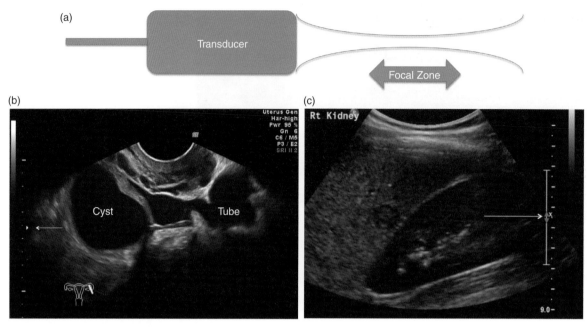

Figure 2.45 (a) Diagrammatic representation of narrowing of ultrasound beam in focal region. (b) Focal point (arrow) correctly positioned to the centre of an ovarian cyst and hydrosalpinx. (c) Focus 'bar' centred to the ROI (kidney).

bigger on-screen for more detailed assessment and to remove irrelevant areas from the image, improving visual acuity. There are two types of zoom – write and read.

Write Zoom

The operator selects the zoom control during live scanning and this generates a box on the screen, the size and position of which can be varied by the operator to concentrate on the ROI. Simplistically, the ultrasound system ignores any echoes returning to the transducer except those within the write zoom box. Write zoom has the advantage over read zoom since it magnifies during live scanning, in real-time and typically provides better image quality than the read zoom. It may result in a higher frame rate (valuable in early pregnancy).

Read Zoom

Like write zoom, the operator also selects the area to magnify using an on-screen box which can be varied in size and position. However, this control just magnifies the selected area on a frozen image. It is useful to magnify areas for image storage and measurement. The box can also be moved round the frozen image to magnify different areas as required. However,

over-magnification can result in pixels becoming visible in the image, reducing image quality.

2.2.2.11 Harmonics

This control is also incorporated into a pre-set. The underpinning physics is complex and will not be considered here. Harmonics can be switched on or off and when on, there are usually variable levels that can be selected (Figure 2.46). The benefits to the operator include:

- Improved resolution in patients with high BMI, due to increased penetration without a loss of detail. Clearer images are achieved at depth with significantly less compromise to the image quality seen when using lower frequencies.
- Reduction in noise/image clutter, which is valuable when scanning simple cysts.
- Reduction in some artefacts (for example, reverberation).

2.2.2.12 Interplay between System Controls

Many system controls interplay with others and changing one will usually have an effect on another. You must familiarise yourself with the impact of changing parameters on other settings to optimise image

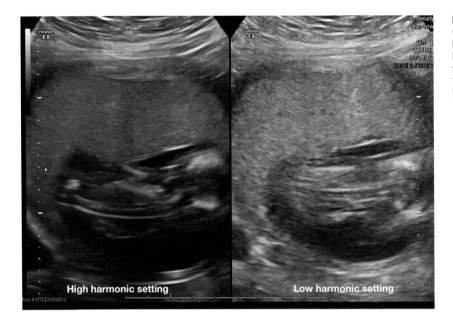

Figure 2.46 Image of a sixteen-week fetus in a woman with high BMI and an anterior placenta. The left image with the high harmonic setting is considerably. clearer than the same view with the low harmonic setting (right side).

quality. Common ones that interplay are depth, sector angle, frame rate and line density.

> Increasing the depth in isolation typically reduces the frame rate as it takes longer to produce a frame and vice versa.
>
> Increasing the sector angle in isolation typically reduces the frame rate as it takes longer to produce a frame and vice versa.
>
> For a given depth, narrowing the sector angle *may* result in a higher line density *in some systems*.
>
> When adjusting several controls (for example, depth and sector angle), there will be an impact on FR and line density. Can you work it out?

2.2.2.13 3D Imaging

Three-dimensional TVUS is becoming established as core imaging for assessment of the female pelvis. Unfortunately, many SRH clinics do not have access to this technology. However, Figures 2.47a, b show some common pathologies seen in SRH using 3D ultrasound. In 3D, ultrasound, a special 3D probe is used and this collects ultrasound data from a volume of tissue rather than just a slice as in 2D imaging. The 3D volume can then be interrogated and images produced in specific imaging planes (x, y, z planes) as well as 3D reconstructions.[1] This technology also allows the operator to scroll through different sections of pelvic structures after the scan has been completed: a

form of 'off-line' image review. This has the potential to reduce scan time and allow a thorough inspection of structures in multiple planes, after the examination is complete, to aid clinical decision making.

2.3 Artefacts

Artefacts are parts of the image that are not a true representation of the actual tissues scanned within the body. They are more likely to occur with older and simpler ultrasound equipment. It is important for an operator to be able to recognise an artefact and be aware of its impact on the image. Some artefacts have diagnostic benefits whilst others are a nuisance in ultrasound imaging, such as bowel gas which strongly reflects ultrasound producing a bright echo with a deeper shadow which leads to the inability of the beam to penetrate and image deeper pelvic structures (Figure 2.48).

There are many artefacts in diagnostic ultrasound.[1] Here we will address those which are more prevalent in SRH applications. However, some artefacts have diagnostic benefits which aid clinical decision making (Table 2.2).

2.3.1 Acoustic Shadowing

This occurs due to two processes:

1. Reflection
2. Absorption

(a)

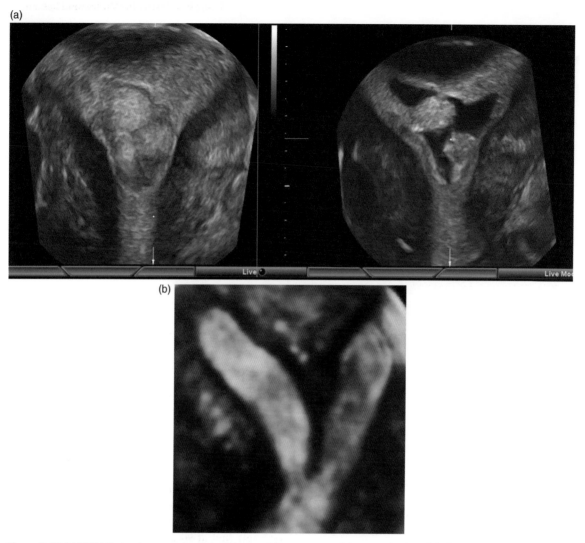

Figure 2.47 (a) 3D TVUS, showing coronal grey shade image of the uterus containing several polyps (left), better outlined with saline instillation (right). (b) 3D TVUS showing a septate uterus.

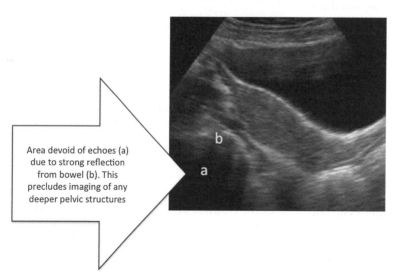

Area devoid of echoes (a) due to strong reflection from bowel (b). This precludes imaging of any deeper pelvic structures

Figure 2.48 TAUS pelvis showing bowel gas which strongly reflects ultrasound producing a bright echo with a deeper shadow which leads to the inability of the beam to penetrate and image deeper pelvic structures.

Table 2.2 Common Artefacts in SRH Ultrasound and Their Diagnostic Benefits

Artefact	Simple Description	Examples of Diagnostic Benefits
Acoustic shadowing	Shadow found deep to a structure.	Deep to: • an intrauterine system. • a sub-dermal implant. • a dermoid 'cyst'.
Post-cystic Enhancement	A bright area seen deep to a clear, simple fluid collection. Often called 'bright up'.	Urinary bladder used as an acoustic window in transabdominal scanning. Confirmation of a simple cyst.
Edge shadows, refraction	Shadows at the postero-lateral edge(s) of simple fluid-filled structures such as a cyst.	Can help in confirmation of a simple cyst as opposed to collection of blood (for example, endometrioma), no edge shadows.
Reverberation	Series of equally spaced parallel lines.	Deep to an intrauterine system.

As an operator, you must be able to recognise them and understand how they arise as your knowledge and understanding of artefacts will affect your diagnostic decision making.

Reflection

Acoustic shadowing is seen deep to a strong reflector such as gas, bone, calculi, IUS, sub-dermal implant (Figures 2.49a, b, c, d). The ultrasound beam interacts at the surface of a strong reflector generating a strong echo back to the transducer (green arrows). There is no/little transmission of ultrasound deep to the reflecting surface and so the area deep to this appears devoid of echoes and is dark/black on the image.

Absorption

When the ultrasound beam travels through a tissue which absorbs ultrasound, such as a dermoid, the beam is reduced in intensity as it passes deeper through the lesion. Consequently, it looks darker towards the deeper aspect of the dermoid, and if it is highly absorbing, it can result in an acoustic shadow (Figure 2.49d).

For an operator, shadowing can be a nuisance as it may obscure deeper structures.

Practical Tip

Scan from multiple different angles/directions in an attempt to 'see around' the bone/gas.

2.3.2 Post Cystic Enhancement (PCE)

PCE occurs deep to fluid-filled structures which do not absorb ultrasound, for example – a simple cyst. TGC settings are set to compensate for solid tissue on either side of the cyst. Consequently, the intensity of ultrasound deep to the cyst is greater than in the solid tissue on either side at the same depth. This results in a bright area deep to the fluid – PCE ('bright-up'). This effect is used to advantage in transabdominal scanning of the pelvis using the urinary bladder as an acoustic window.

This can be useful diagnostically in confirming a fluid-filled (cystic) structure (Figures 2.50a, b).

2.3.3 Refraction/Edge Shadowing Artefact

You are probably familiar with refraction relating to light where an object is displaced from its correct position (Figure 2.51a). This can also happen in ultrasound imaging when ultrasound hits a boundary at an angle (not at 90 degrees), across which there is a change in the speed of sound (Figure 2.51b). The speed that ultrasound travels through different tissue varies slightly. When refraction occurs, there is a change in the direction of the ultrasound beam and it travels along a direction not expected and the ultrasound system assumes the echoes are returning from a straight beam. Consequently, a structure is displaced on the image from its true position.

This can give rise to an edge shadowing artefact which is often seen towards the deeper edges of a cystic structure (Figure 2.51c).

Practical Tip

The presence of edge shadows can help in establishing that a cystic structure contains 'serous type' fluid as opposed to blood, for example, latter not seen at the edge of endometrioma (Figure 2.51d).

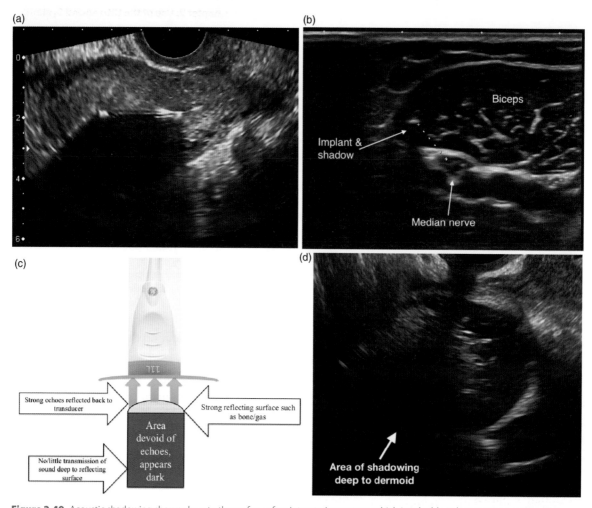

Figure 2.49 Acoustic shadowing shown deep to the surface of an intrauterine system, which is valuable in locating its exact position (a) and a sub-dermal implant (b). Diagrammatic representation of acoustic shadowing formation (c). (d) TVUS showing a dermoid 'cyst' which absorbs ultrasound on both transmit and receive. Consequently, as the beam gets deeper into the lesion it becomes weaker and appears darker distally, shadowing (arrow).

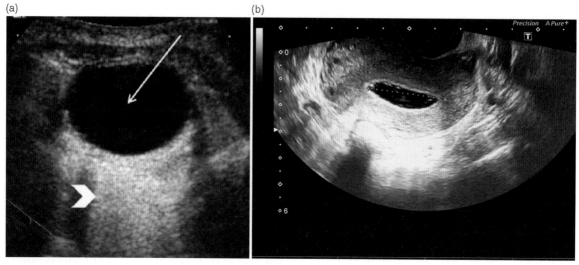

Figure 2.50 (a) PCE distal to simple cyst. (b) Gel contrast within the endometrial cavity demonstrating echo enhancement resulting in a brighter image beyond the fluid (PCE).

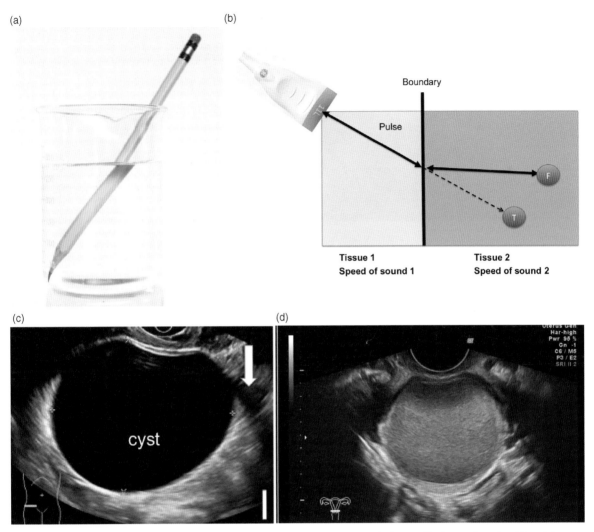

Figure 2.51 (a) Refraction shown by pencil in water. (b) Diagrammatic representation of refraction. T is the true/actual position of the reflector in the tissue. Due to refraction, the US beam is deviated from its true course resulting in an echo being generated from a false position (F). (c) Edge shadowing due to refraction effect at the edge of cystic structure. (d) Endometrioma which has no edge shadowing as blood-filled structure.

2.3.4 Reverberation

Reverberations are a series of equally spaced multiple reflections that occur when strong reflectors are insonated at 90 degrees; that is, they lie parallel to the transducer face. They are more common at shallow depths. They are often seen deep to an IUS in its long axis (Figure 2.52).

2.3 Summary

This chapter has covered the basic principles of ultrasound imaging for a non-expert user. As you become more proficient in your use of the ultrasound equipment, you should refer to a dedicated ultrasound science and equipment text.[1]

This chapter has shown you the importance of knowing how to use the equipment properly and how both incorrect system settings and artefacts can affect your clinical decision making. Structures can be made to look abnormal if the system controls are wrongly set. Never forget that the greatest risk to the patient is the operator. Be aware of your limitations and always be prepared to seek more expert help as required.

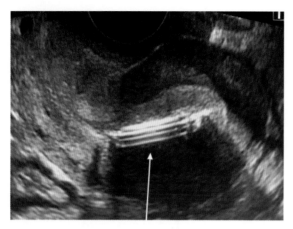

Figure 2.52 Reverberation deep to an IUS shown as equally spaced white lines due to multiple reflection.

References

1. Hoskins PR, Martin K, Thrush A. *Diagnostic Ultrasound: Physics and Equipment*. 2nd edn. Cambridge: Cambridge University Press, 2010.

2. BMUS statement on the safe use, and potential hazards of diagnostic ultrasound. June 2000, reconfirmed by BMUS, March 2012.

3. BMUS guidelines for the safe use of diagnostic ultrasound equipment (Created by BMUS 2010, adopted by EFSUMB Board of Directors, 2011)

4. Monnington SC, Dodd-Hughes K, Milnes E, Ahmad Y. Risk management of musculoskeletal disorders in sonography work. *HSE*, 23 March 2012.

5. Work related musculo-skeletal disorders (sonographers). www.sor.org/learning/document-library/work-related-musculo-skeletal-disorders-sonographers

6. Human factors in healthcare: a concordat from the national quality board. www.england.nhs.uk/wp-content/.../nqb-hum-fact-concord.pdf

Chapter

3

Communication Skills in Ultrasound Assessment

Karen Easton

3.1 Introduction 45
3.2 Communication 45

3.3 Dealing with a Possible Diagnosis 47
3.4 Summary 48

3.1 Introduction

Ultrasound has become the standard investigation for many abdominal and pelvic conditions, which is often offered with little notice to patients. Transvaginal scanning is an invasive procedure. Whilst the value of clearer definition is obvious to the healthcare professional, for some women it is a daunting prospect that may cause them to refuse this type of examination if the advantages are not communicated well.

Communication is not an exciting study topic for most, borne out by the limited research into the subject compared to vast sums spent on the development of ultrasound equipment and interpretation of findings. However, as any experienced healthcare professional will know, if we get it wrong we damage the therapeutic relationship with our patients and possibly also relationships with other healthcare professionals. Often, patients arrive in the ultrasound room with no idea of what the examination comprises and the potential findings. Although leaflets can be given to explain the procedure, nothing prepares a patient for an unexpected or abnormal result.

Preparation of the patient is the time where the clinician can begin a relationship with a patient that will be the foundation for any potential diagnosis. This has to take place in a very short time, but is of paramount importance to begin to prepare the way for any news to be given. In a sexual and reproductive health setting, ultrasound is often used to support a 'one stop shop' model of care. This can give rise to difficulties in the event of an unexpected finding, for example, gynaecological cancer. However, the availability of ultrasound as a clinical tool supports improved clinical care, with patient involvement.

Immediate feedback, although sometimes distressing, ultimately enhances the patient's journey.

3.2 Communication

Not all news given during an ultrasound appointment is bad news, but sonographers cannot assume they know what will be bad or good news for an individual patient. A viable pregnancy is not good news for every woman, just as a diagnosis of suspected cancer is not necessarily bad news for a patient who has been attending medical professionals for some time with no treatment or diagnosis made – at least with a potential diagnosis, progress can be made in dealing with a problem.

Giving potential diagnoses can be stressful, especially for the inexperienced sonographer. Patients given the same news can react in many different ways. Preparation is key for helping us to do this well.

Walter Baile et al.[1] have developed a six-step protocol for breaking bad news in cancer care which can be easily adapted to the ultrasound examination.

3.2.1 Practising Giving Diagnoses

Rehearsal of giving diagnoses helps when faced with the actual task. Important preparation includes ensuring:

- Privacy, including ensuring that any person who comes into the room with the patient is appropriate. Involving a significant other during the investigation can be an important asset or detriment to communication with the patient.
- That the patient is emotionally prepared for the examination and possible outcomes, so that the

45

clinician can gauge to an extent what the impact of good or bad news will be for that patient.

- Sensitivity to the patient's body language and demeanour. This may give an indication of likely reactions to possible results, and wishes for the outcome of the pregnancy the patient may have. This might be helpful when attempting to mitigate an adverse reaction.
- Eye contact. It can be difficult to maintain this during an investigation that involves looking at the screen. It is important to place the screen so that an easy turn of one's head can facilitate looking at the patient during the assessment when findings are becoming clear.

3.2.2 Finding Out How the Patient Perceives Her Condition

The saying 'before you tell – ask' is important here. For example, not every pregnancy is good news. Not every mass is a surprise. Open-ended questions at the beginning of the consultation can give clues and hints about how to break news and how much information to include, both pictorial from the screen and verbal before the patient leaves the room at the end of the examination. Checking what outcomes are expected is an important part of the preparation for giving news. For example, not showing a woman the screen if she plans to terminate a pregnancy can reduce the psychological sequelae for her after the event, so positioning the screen away from her line of sight prior to her entering the room will be helpful. However, no assumption should be made. You should always sensitively ask her wishes regarding seeing the screen, and if she is uncertain, then ask whether seeing or not seeing can help her in the decision-making process.

3.2.3 Giving Results

The amount of information disclosed is a patient choice. Whilst some wish full disclosure of findings, for others this may exacerbate anxiety to a level they find difficult to cope with, especially those who are to be referred on to another healthcare professional for further management of any problem found. For some, shunning information is a coping strategy. Questions such as 'would you like me to tell you the outcome of the scan, or would you like to wait until the doctor/specialist explains what your treatment options may be?' can give the patient permission to moderate any news they are told.

3.2.4 Getting to Know the Patient

Chatting during the investigation can give the clinician an opportunity, if necessary, to prepare a patient for potential bad news to lessen the impact at the end of the examination. This will be influenced by the type of language used. It is good practice to avoid lots of medical terminology and jargon, which takes practice to achieve (see Section 3.1). The skill to split one's concentration between the examination and the patient is difficult but remains an important part of any consultation to ensure that the patient feels valued and included in the investigation. If there are parts of the examination where this is difficult, an explanation should be given: 'I will be quiet for a few minutes now, but will explain things to you after that'. This can ease the patient's anxiety, whilst ensuring the clinician can concentrate on vital parts of the investigation. Sometimes it becomes apparent that certain diagnoses should be given without a second person being present, for example, the patient's mother in the case of an unexpected pregnancy. Although this approach can be difficult to achieve in practice, patient confidentiality and welfare must be the first priority.

3.2.5 Dealing with the Emotional Response

Any investigation and diagnosis can cause very different emotional responses from patients and their supporters. There may be shock, anger, sadness, disbelief, relief or denial. Dealing with these can be stressful, particularly if they come out of the blue, even with the preparation in step 1. Sometimes, a few minutes to digest the news without further information being given can give patients time to restore their equilibrium. This can be difficult to allow in a tight timetable of a clinic list, but is an important step in helping patients to deal with any news they receive.

3.2.6 Formulate a Treatment or Follow-Up Plan

The next step may be to formulate a treatment plan or refer to another healthcare practitioner for on-going management. It is important that the clinician explains what the next steps may involve, so that further anxiety can be mitigated. Lack of information only adds to anxiety. Referring back to step 2 and using what one knows about the patient's perceptions and expectations can help with planning and checking that the news given has been heard. Allowing the patient to summarise what she has been told can be a valid way of ensuring that their perception of the findings is accurate and will help ensure that expectations are allied. This is important, as giving and receiving information can be very difficult depending on the individual patient and not all information given will be retained. Repeating the reassurance that findings will be acted upon, and even in the situation of advanced cancer palliative care will be available, is important.[1,2]

3.3 Dealing with a Possible Diagnosis

3.3.1 Unexpected Pregnancy Loss

Ultrasound in pregnancy is a common assessment tool used for both planned and unplanned pregnancies. The news that a pregnancy is non-viable can be devastating to a woman or a couple, even when the pregnancy is unwanted. This may be surprising, but feelings of guilt about not wishing to carry on with the pregnancy can occur at the time of the scan or indeed, many years later. Miscarriage, especially in the absence of any signs, is a shock when found on ultrasound. The sonographer is the first person to face the woman in this situation. It may be at a routine antenatal scan, and the woman's partner may also be present and his or her feelings will need to be considered. It is important to take time to gently prepare the woman or couple for this possibility as the scan progresses. It is wise to have a check scan performed by another clinician if possible. Leaving the room to go and ask for someone else to come and confirm the findings can give a couple time to assimilate the news and prepare for it. News of a failing pregnancy can be devastating. Revealing this diagnosis should be as gentle but as honest as possible. The woman may require a further scan, either by another sonographer immediately, or at a later date to confirm any findings. The option of a further scan in a few days is recommended in the *NICE Guidance on Pain and Bleeding in Early Pregnancy*.[3] This gives the woman and her family time to come to terms with the diagnosis before management options are discussed with her.

The sonographer in a pregnancy advisory clinic scanning to plan for a potential termination may find a failed or failing pregnancy. In this circumstance, the woman may have terrible feelings of guilt, thinking she may have caused this by not wishing to continue with the pregnancy. This is a paradox which can haunt the woman for many years afterwards. It is important to be open and honest that this would have occurred whatever her wishes. Limiting emotional morbidity surrounding the potential termination of a pregnancy with honest reassurance is of great importance as depression and difficulties with anxiety are common after termination of pregnancy.

Contraception failure may result in a viable intra-uterine pregnancy with an intrauterine device in situ. Where possible, the device should be removed without delay, since the threads may become inaccessible with further advancement of the pregnancy. It should be explained that removal of the device, where possible, has a better pregnancy outcome than when the pregnancy continues with a device left in situ.

3.3.2 Sub-optimally Placed IUC

Ultrasound is often used to assess the placement of an IUC (see also Chapter 10).

Misplacement can lead to the failure of the device. IUC threads not being visible on speculum examination is a relatively common problem. It is recommended that the woman is advised of this and provided with alternative contraception until the position of the device can be clarified with ultrasound. In most cases, an ultrasound scan will show the device remains correctly positioned and the patient can be reassured that it can be left in place while this method is desired. It is unnecessary to remove or change a correctly placed device simply because the threads have retracted, and attempts to retrieve the threads may result in misplacement.

A woman can be reassured that when IUC change or removal is desired, this can very simply be performed in most cases.

If a device appears misplaced or embedded, the patient can be referred to a specialist clinic where removal and/or replacement can be performed in the outpatient setting, usually with ultrasound guidance.

If ultrasound fails to locate the device, a plain X-ray of the abdomen and pelvis is recommended (Chapter 10). If the device is not detected on X-ray, it can be presumed expelled and it can either be replaced or another preferred method of contraception initiated or continued. Counselling during this process can reassure the woman that this is a rare consequence and can maintain her confidence. Expulsion or misplacement of an IUC can cause distress or fear and put the woman off the method of contraception. Occasionally it can contribute to relationship difficulties. Support and gentle reassurance can help avoid these difficulties occurring.

3.3.3 Ovarian Pathology

Ovaries containing several cysts are a common physiological finding. This should not be confused with a diagnosis of PCOS (Chapter 12). The normality of ovarian cysts can be difficult to convey to women who often have no knowledge that the function of ovaries is to produce cysts during a monthly cycle, and sometimes these cysts do not resolve for several months. The diagnosis of PCOS is covered in Chapter 12.

Some ovarian cysts are abnormal and have readily recognisable ultrasound characteristics (or descriptors – Chapter 6). These include:

- Haemorrhagic – these are usually corpus luteum cysts which have bled internally and will resolve over several weeks (Figure 6.32a–d).
- Infective – tubo-ovarian collections of pus or fluid in chronic pelvic inflammatory disease. This may require further management, either antibiotics, if acute, or surgery/further investigation and referral to a gynaecologist (Figure 6.36a–c).
- Dermoid – typically containing fat, hair and occasionally teeth. They can become large and sometimes require surgical removal (Figure 6.42a–d).
- Endometriomas (chocolate cysts), which can cause pain, especially around the time of menstruation and can lead to pelvic adhesions, ovulatory dysfunction and subfertility (Figure 6.34a–d).
- Cystadenomas – typically fluid filled with low level echoes. These can become very large (Figure 6.31).

Other benign and malignant adnexal masses are not readily recognisable and require further forms of assessment including Ca125 and CEA and a Risk of Malignancy Index or IOTA ADNEX classification (Chapters 6 and 15). The result of these further tests will determine whether the mass should be referred to a gynaecological oncology service.

The finding of an adnexal mass can be frightening for the woman and her family. It may be obvious that a cyst is malignant (for example, the presence of ascites), but in many cases the nature of the mass is unclear. It is often difficult to achieve a fine balance of communicating the urgency of further referral without causing panic, and this is stressful for both patient and clinician. Assessing how much the woman wishes to know and how to phrase the potential diagnosis takes considerable skill. Information should be honest, but not so blunt as to cause panic and deter her from taking up the option of specialist referral. Time taken with the woman at this point is vital, but can be difficult to achieve in the middle of a busy list or clinic.

3.4 Summary

Communication and the early development of a therapeutic relationship are vital skills. Communication has a profound effect on the patient's response, ability to cope with the information given and compliance with any treatment options presented. Kind, caring and calm relaying of information with the use of repetition and positive body language (engaging by visual contact, leaning slightly towards her and including anyone supporting her in the conversation) are all important skills to develop. Using simple language that you are comfortable with helps to engage and hold the attention of anxious women in vulnerable situations. Listening and watching their cues give clues to how the information is being received, but checking with them what they understand and backing findings up with written information where possible improve outcomes for patient care.

References

1. Baile WF, Buckman R, Lenzi R, Glober G, Beale EA, Kudelkab A. SPIKES – A six-step protocol for delivering bad news: application to the patient with cancer. http://theoncologist.alphamedpress.org, 16 April 2016.

2. Sep MSC, van Osch M, van Vliet LM, Smets EMA, Bensing JM. The power of clinicians' affective communication: How reassurance about non-abandonment can reduce patients' physiological arousal and increase information recall in bad news consultations. An experimental study using analogue patients. *Patient Education and Counseling.* 2014;95:45–52.

3. National Institute of Clinical Excellence. Ectopic pregnancy and miscarriage: diagnosis and initial management. *NICE guidelines* [CG154], December 2012.

Ultrasound of Pelvic Anatomy Scanning Techniques and 'Normal' Findings

Mary Pillai and Julie-Michelle Bridson

4.1   Introduction   49

4.2   Indications for Pelvic Ultrasound   49

4.3   Systematic Examination   50

4.4   Transabdominal Pelvic Assessment – Bladder Distension   52

4.5   Transvaginal Pelvic Assessment   55

4.6   Adnexal Imaging, Including the Ovaries and Fallopian Tubes   58

4.7   The Uterus   58

4.8   The Pre-menopausal Endometrium   61

4.9   The Post-menopausal Endometrium   63

4.10   Uterine Vascularity   66

4.11   The Normal Ovary   67

4.12   The Recto-Uterine Space   70

4.13   Accuracy and Reproducibility of Measurements   70

4.14   Conclusion   72

4.1 Introduction

A well-performed ultrasound examination of the female pelvis requires good communication skills and a practitioner with a sound understanding of expected pelvic anatomy, including age and cycle-related changes, the range of normal variation and the impact of medications on the ultrasound appearances. All ultrasound practitioners should adopt a systematic scanning technique and an ability to utilise the ultrasound machine to optimise the image (Chapter 2). Given the intimate nature of the examination, informed consent must be obtained.[1]

A full medical history is essential for the correct interpretation of the scan findings. Ultrasound should complement and follow the principles of clinical examination. For example, transvaginal (TV) ultrasound can be used to pinpoint pelvic pain or assess mobility of structures by applying gentle pressure with the ultrasound probe while using the free (left) hand to palpate suprapubically.

Potential sources of error arise when a scan is performed by someone with inadequate knowledge of reproductive anatomy, physiology and pathology. Errors also occur when findings are interpreted or reported without relevant information about the presenting history, the menstrual cycle, relevant medical treatments or menopausal status. Findings should be reported clearly and in a consistent manner to ensure that another clinician continuing care of the patient can interpret the findings appropriately. Equally, operators should be mindful of their own technical and diagnostic capability and seek more expert help when required to safeguard patients.

4.2 Indications for Pelvic Ultrasound

The common indications for pelvic ultrasound relevant to SRH work include, but are not limited to,

1. Evaluation of pelvic pain, including severe dysmenorrhoea.
2. Evaluation of abnormal bleeding.
3. Evaluation of a pelvic mass.
4. Evaluation of primary or secondary amenorrhoea.
5. Follow-up of a previously detected abnormality.
6. Pregnancy (routine dating and early pregnancy problems).
7. Evaluation of suspected pelvic infection.
8. Evaluation of a congenital uterine anomaly or variant.
9. Locating intrauterine devices with missing threads.
10. Evaluating pain associated with the use of IUC.

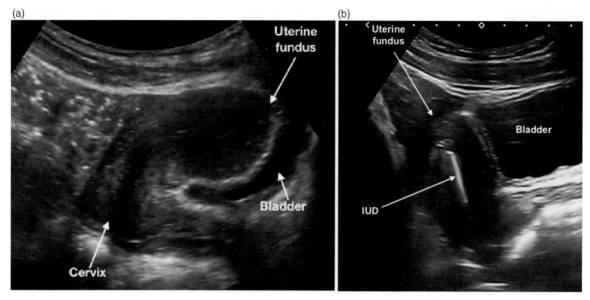

Figure 4.1 TA long axis/sagittal images of uterine anteversion. In (a) the bladder is almost empty, but owing to the anteversion the fundus lies close to the abdominal wall and there is normal abdominal wall fat. Hence bladder filling is unnecessary to enable visualisation. In (b) a copper IUD is shown in the uterus.

11. Ultrasound guidance to assist a difficult IUC fitting.
12. Ultrasound guidance to assist difficulty dilating the cervix and to minimise the risk of creating a false passage or perforating the uterus at surgical termination.
13. Evaluation of complications following termination of pregnancy.

4.3 Systematic Examination

The female pelvis consists of the bladder, the ureters, the uterus, the adenexae, the vagina and the rectum. It is important to adopt a system to ensure that all of the pelvis is imaged in at least two anatomical planes, both to build confidence about the range of normality and to aid recognition of the abnormal from the range of normal. Transabdominal (TA) and TV ultrasound are complimentary, and a systematic approach is important to ensure thorough evaluation of the pelvic structures.

Evaluation should include:

- The uterus: its size, shape, outline, position/ orientation, the textural appearance of the myometrium and endometrium.
- The adenexal regions.
- Presence of any free fluid. If present, whether it is normal or abnormal in volume, and

whether it appears to be serous (hypoechoic, for example, ascites), or consistent with fresh blood (containing solid reticular areas of clot). The appearance of clot may be variable, dependent on the stage of clot resolution. Rapid hydration of patients can create the transient appearance of a small volume of fluid in the recto-uterine pouch.

- Points of tenderness.
- Whether the pelvic organs move freely ('sliding sign' – when gentle pressure is applied by the TV probe) or appear adherent to adjacent organs, as may occur with endometriosis or inflammatory conditions.

The uterosacral ligaments fix the position of the cervix in the upper vagina. The uterine corpus, however, is relatively mobile and may lie 'anteverted' with the fundus directed towards the bladder and anterior abdominal wall (Figure 4.1a,b), or 'retroverted' with the fundus directed away from the bladder towards the rectum (Figure 4.2a,b). The position of the uterus should be recorded. In addition to the term 'version' the term 'flexion' may be used to describe the orientation of the uterine axis to the cervix. Flexion is the bending forwards or backwards of the uterus on itself, so when there is an acute angle between 90 and 180 degrees between the cervix and the fundus, the uterus may more appropriately be described as anteflexed.

(a)   (b)

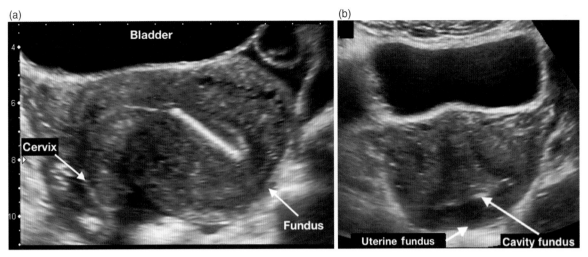

Figure 4.2 TA images of uterine retroversion. (a) TA longitudinal image of a uterus containing an IUD. The view is through a full bladder showing the fundus directed posteriorly in the same direction as the cervix (arrows). (b) A transverse TA image of a retroverted uterus. The distended bladder enhances the imaging of the uterus by displacing the bowel out of the field of view. It is notable the fundus of the uterus lies posterior to the endometrial cavity clarifying the position is retroverted.

(a)   (b)

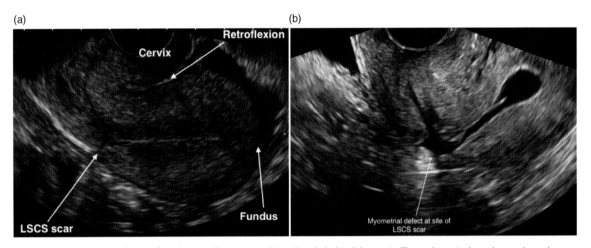

Figure 4.3 (a) TV image of a retroflexed uterus. The corpus is lying directly behind the cervix. The endocervical canal turns through an acute angle at the cervico-isthmic junction, which in this patient also corresponds with the site of a caesarean scar. (b) Gel contrast has been introduced filling the cavity, which helps demonstrate the acute angle of retroflexion between the cervix and the endometrial canal, and also shows a myometrial defect at the site of the caesarean scar.

When the fundus is bent backwards at an angle of 180–270 degrees, it is retroflexed (Figure 4.3a,b). If there is minimal angulation between the cervix and the corpus, the uterus is more appropriately described in terms of version so the entire uterus lies forwards (anteverted) or backwards (retroverted). Where the axis is horizontal such that there is no angle between the cervix and the corpus, the uterus is described as

axial (Figure 4.4). The axial uterus is difficult to scan and may give poor quality images due to the distance from the probe to the corpus on both TA and TV scanning.

The uterus is more often anteverted or anteflexed than axial or retroverted/retroflexed. However, these positions should be considered normal variation and not synonymous with pathology.

51

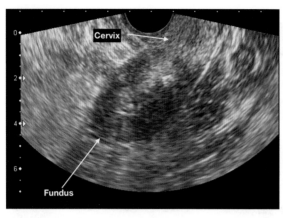

Figure 4.4 TV image of an axial uterus demonstrating poor image quality as it is not possible to obtain a good angle of insonation.

4.4 Transabdominal Pelvic Assessment – Bladder Distension

Assessment of the pelvis via the transabdominal route, using a relatively low frequency (2–6 MHz) curved array transducer, is often considered convenient and avoids an intimate examination for the patient. It is customary to ask the patient to attend with an adequately distended bladder, which may be essential for the visualisation of a retroverted/flexed uterus. Distension of the bladder helps to displace the bowel and acts as an acoustic window to access the deeper pelvic structures (Figure 4.5a). However, excessive distension such that the patient is uncomfortable during the examination is unhelpful to the examination and reduces patient comfort and tolerance. It can also cause technical examination issues as the pelvic structures can be displaced further from the transducer, reducing image quality. With an anteverted/flexed uterus, it may be unnecessary to have a distended bladder.

The transabdominal image quality may be impaired in women with a high BMI, although the quality of transvaginal imaging is much less impaired by high BMI. In the former, applying gentle pressure to the anterior abdominal wall (graded compression) can reduce the thickness of adipose tissue by displacement and can improve image quality.

4.4.1 Systematic Approach to Scanning – Initial Survey

It is good practice to start all pelvic examinations (TAUS and TVUS) with an initial pelvic survey ensuring that the pelvis is scanned thoroughly in at least two planes. Commence in the midline, immediately above the symphysis pubis to obtain a sagittal section through the pelvis (Figure 4.5a,c) and then move and angle the transducer to the right and left of the midline to ensure all the parts of the pelvis have been imaged, right out to the lateral pelvic walls (indicated by the iliac vessels – Figure 4.5b). The transducer is then rotated through 90 degrees and the procedure repeated to image the entire pelvis in the second (transverse) plane (may be coronal in TVUS).

During the initial survey, the depth control is set initially to ensure that the operator images to the posterior wall of the pelvis (Figure 4.6a). This will allow the operator to get an overall impression of the pelvic anatomy and is also useful in directing the rest of the scan. This facilitates identification of structures, their position relative to other structures and any obvious gross abnormality.

The pelvic structures (uterus, ovaries, pregnancy, etc.) are then examined separately in more detail by ensuring they are centred to the field of view (FOV), reducing the depth and then magnifying them as required using the zoom control for detailed inspection (Figure 4.6b). It is important to sweep through every structure in its entirety to ensure it has been thoroughly assessed in two planes. There can be a tendency to freeze a good quality image rather than 'sweeping through', and this can lead to pathology being missed.

Whilst scanning is taking place, the system settings should be adjusted – particularly frequency, image depth, magnification/zoom, focus, power, gain and time gain compensation (TGC) – to optimise the image quality.

4.4.2 Uterus

The uterus is then scanned in detail in a minimum of two anatomical planes – long axis (longitudinal, Figures 4.5a,c) and short axis (transverse, Figure 4.5d).

The uterus is identified in its midline sagittal plane and the system settings adjusted to optimise image quality. Once the true long axis of the uterus is found (fundus–cervix/vagina) then the transducer is angled right to left to sweep through the entire uterus.

Short axis (transverse/coronal) imaging of the uterus should then be undertaken by turning the probe anticlockwise (towards yourself) through 90 degrees and moved/angled from the fundus down through the cornua and cervix. On short axis sections, the ovaries may be seen lateral to the uterus around

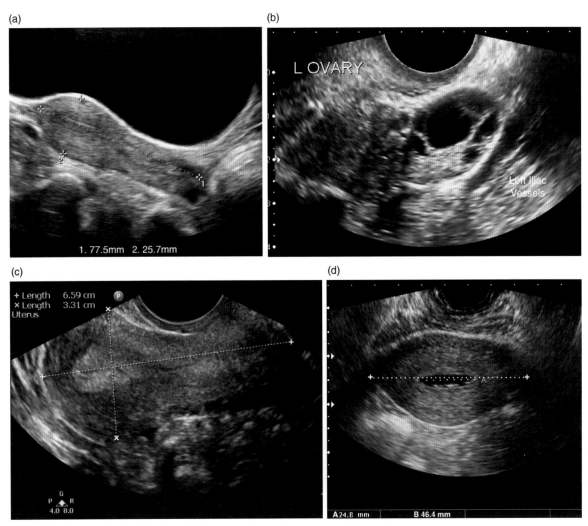

(a)

1. 77.5mm 2. 25.7mm

(b)

L OVARY

Left Iliac
Vessels

(c)

+ Length   6.59 cm
× Length   3.31 cm
Uterus

G
P ◆ R
4.0 8.0

(d)

A 24.8 mm   B 46.4 mm

Figure 4.5 (a) TA long axis image of a normal anteverted uterus imaged through a distended bladder. The callipers demonstrate the long axis and AP measurements. (b) TV long axis image. The transducer has been moved laterally to image the left adnexal region and left pelvic sidewall lateral to the uterus. The ovary medial to an iliac vessel is demonstrated. (c) TV image showing the long axis section of the uterus with callipers demonstrating the long axis and AP measurements. The bladder has been completely emptied for this examination. (d) A TV transverse section demonstrated by turning the transducer through 90 degrees anticlockwise from the long axis. The transverse uterine measurement is demonstrated.

the level of the fundus (Figure 4.7). Occasionally the ovaries are lower and more posterior.

4.4.3 Measuring the Uterus

1. **Long axis and AP diameter** – uterine measurements (when performed) are made on a midline long axis (sagittal) section, with the callipers placed from fundus to cervix (to the external os where this can be identified). On the same section, callipers are placed on the outer edge of the anterior and posterior wall of uterus, at the widest point, and at 90 degrees to the long axis measurement (Figures 4.5a, c).

2. **Maximum transverse diameter** – this is measured by placing the callipers across the widest part of the uterus from outer edge on the right to outer edge on left on a short axis section (Figure 4.5d).

3. The normal length of the uterus in women during reproductive years is from 6.5 to 8.5 cms and may be slightly longer in multiparous women. However, in women who are amenorrhoeic and hypoestrogenic (for example, lactational

(a)

(b)

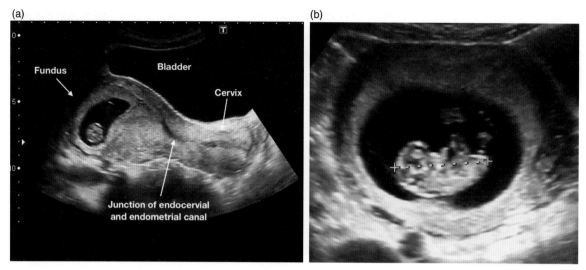

Figure 4.6 (a) TA overview of pelvis showing the whole uterus in long axis with an early pregnancy, imaged through a full bladder. The endocervical–endometrial canal can be followed to a gestation sac positioned at the fundus of the endometrial cavity. (b) The region of interest (the pregnancy) has been magnified to enable more accurate fetal measurement for dating.

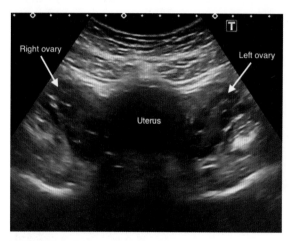

Figure 4.7 TA Transverse overview of uterus in the midline showing the ovaries in the adenexae at the same level as the uterine fundus.

amenorrhoea, long-term Depo provera, GnRH analogue use or hypothalamic/weight-related amenorrhoea), the uterus is likely to be small.

4. Where pelvic structures appear normal, there is no particular benefit to measuring them; rather they should just be reported as they 'appear normal in size'. Where measurements are appropriate (for example, suspected abnormal size), it is appropriate to measure the structure in at least two planes (Figures 4.5a,c). Where a volume calculation is required, then three planes

are required (long axis, short axis and maximum transverse diameter – Figure 4.5c,d). These measurements are used by the ultrasound system to compute the estimated volume of a structure. Volume estimates are notoriously unreliable due to measurement error and also assumption of the shape of a structure.

4.4.4 Endometrial Assessment

Assessing and measuring the endometrium on a TAUS is not recommended. TVUS is the preferred method as it provides greater image quality (see Section 4.9.1).

4.4.5 Imaging the Ovaries

The ovaries are often best identified in the midline short axis section, where they are often located postero-lateral to the uterus (Figure 4.7). The bladder can be used as an acoustic window to image the ovaries using a contra-lateral approach, where the transducer is moved to the left side of the patient and angled through the bladder to image the right ovary in short axis/transverse section (TS) and vice versa (Figure 4.8).

During imaging of the ovary, it is also essential that the ovary is located in the centre of the screen and the depth and magnification/zoom adjusted to ensure the ovary is shown optimally (Figure 4.9a,b). The transducer is then angled cranio-caudally to image the entire ovary in this section. This is then repeated for the other ovary.

The transducer is then rotated through 90 degrees and the process repeated to image both ovaries in their long axis (longitudinal) section. Imaging out as far as the internal iliac vein and artery by angling

steeply towards the lateral pelvic wall provides a useful landmark, as a normally positioned ovary will lie immediately medial to these vessels at about the level of the uterine fundus (Figure 4.5b).

4.5 Transvaginal Pelvic Assessment

Since the probe is located in the vagina, it is much closer to pelvic structures as compared to transabdominal route. This allows the use of higher frequency ultrasound, which improves the image resolution (Chapter 2). The frequency range of a transvaginal transducer is typically in the 5–12 MHz range, which gives high resolution imaging at a range of up to 7–10 cms. Unless the pelvic structures have been clearly and adequately visualised by the transabdominal route, and the region of interest adequately imaged, it is appropriate to seek consent to undertake a TV scan. Before commencing the TVUS, the patient should be asked to empty her bladder completely, which will facilitate obtaining the best transvaginal images and is more comfortable for the patient. If the bladder is not completely empty, the image quality tends to be compromised.

If pregnancy is a possibility and this has not been confirmed transabdominally, it is good practice in any

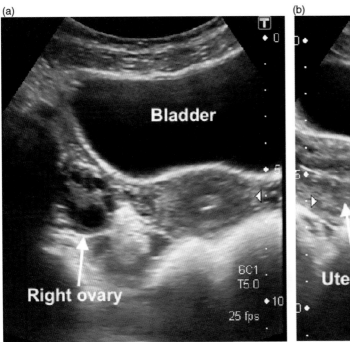

Figure 4.8 A diagram illustrating the transducer applied in a transverse plane to the left side of the lower abdomen and angled so the beam points towards the right pelvic sidewall. The distended bladder displaces other pelvic contents and enhances the imaging of the right ovary. (Artwork courtesy of Mark Pountney, University of Liverpool.)

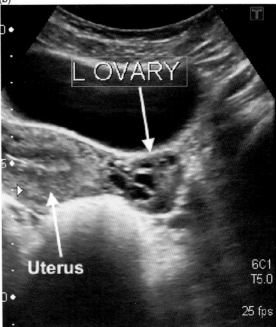

Figure 4.9 (a) TA transverse image with the beam directed through the bladder to the right adenexal region showing the right ovary. (b) TA transverse image with the beam directed to the left adenexal region showing the left ovary.

SRH clinic to ask the woman to collect a urine sample when emptying her bladder. If the possibility of pregnancy still needs clarification after completing the transvaginal scan, a urine pregnancy test can then be performed.

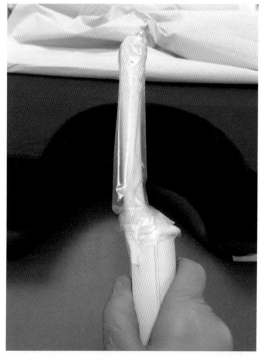

Figure 4.10 Image of gloved hand holding a TV probe with a wedge in position.

It is mandatory to wear gloves (on both hands) and to clean and cover the probe with an appropriate cleansing agent and protector for each examination (Figure 4.10). The probe should be carefully introduced to achieve a long axis section through the pelvis (with the reference notch or mark at the 12 o'clock position) whilst the operator is watching the screen. The cervix should readily come into view. The orientation can be with the probe at the top of the screen with structures appearing upside down, or this can be inverted so the probe appears at the bottom of the screen depending on the preference of the operator (Figure 4.11a,b).

Depending on the degree of anteflexion of the uterus, it may be necessary to use a wedge or other object (for example, the patient's own fists, a folded pillow/blanket or dedicated TV support) under the pelvis to allow sufficient posterior movement of the probe handle to bring the fundus into the field of view (Figure 4.12). The best access to TV imaging of an anteflexed uterus will be afforded by the use of a lithotomy couch. However, the lithotomy position is more intrusive for women and so its routine use is questionable, given that it will be unnecessary in the majority of pelvic scans.

Where difficulty is encountered inserting the probe, the operator should enquire whether the woman would prefer to insert it herself. Whether to offer and attempt a TV examination in women who have not been sexually active requires careful consideration. If a woman is comfortable using tampons, then the concept of a TV scan may be acceptable to

(a)

(b)

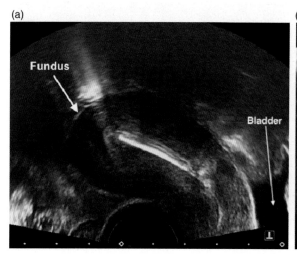
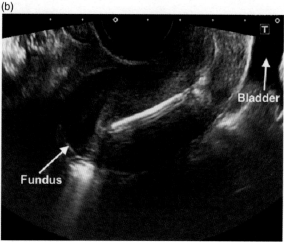

Figure 4.11 (a) TV image orientation from the bottom of the screen. (b) TV image orientation from the top of the screen.

her, but extra care must be taken when inserting the probe. Asking the patient to breathe out as the probe is inserted can assist. If there is any significant resistance then it is appropriate to discontinue and reassure the patient about alternative interventions. For women who are not sexually active or not comfortable using tampons, then TV imaging is not appropriate. Where

transvaginal imaging is not possible, the transrectal or translabial approach can be considered, but this analysis is beyond the scope of this chapter.

As with abdominal imaging, TVUS requires a systematic approach to the examination:

1. The probe is inserted with the orientation notch at the 12 o'clock position so as to obtain a long axis (longitudinal/sagittal) section of the uterus. On this image, the endometrium should appear as a thin stripe (Figure 4.13a) or a thicker layered tissue (Figure 4.13b). To be measurable, there must be a distinct endometrial–myometrial border. The probe is moved from right to left and back through the whole uterus, ensuring the entire uterus has been imaged in this plane. The operator should be mindful of SSOTMO (see Box 4.1). The appearance outside as well as within the uterus should be noted.

2. The midline long axis of the uterus is located and then the probe turned counter clockwise through 90 degrees to obtain a transverse/coronal view (Figure 4.14a,b). Tilting the probe inferiorly down to the cervix and superiorly up to the fundus will ensure the entire uterus is imaged in this plane.

3. Any points of tenderness elicited by the examination should be noted.

4. The operator can apply gentle pressure on the transducer while using his or her free hand on the abdomen to exert counter pressure, which may help to elicit symptoms in the presence of pain. This may also allow assessing for uterine mobility.

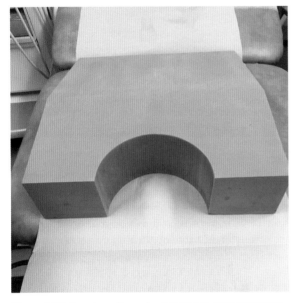

Figure 4.12 A wedge with a cut out section to assist positioning for TV scanning. Elevation of the pelvis is needed where the uterus is anteverted but may be unnecessary and even unhelpful where the uterus is retroverted.

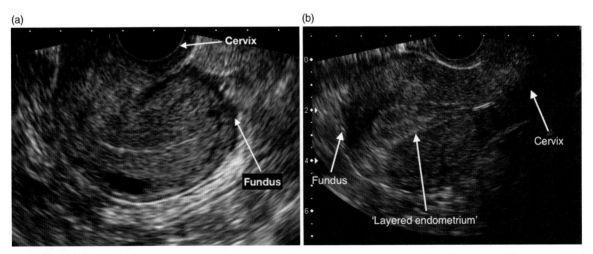

Figure 4.13 (a) TV long axis image demonstrating a thin endometrial stripe (day 5/post-menses) in a retroflexed uterus (the cervix at the top of the screen is directly above the corpus). (b) TV long axis image demonstrating the endometrial appearance in early proliferative phase, thicker and beginning to show the layered appearance

(a)   (b)

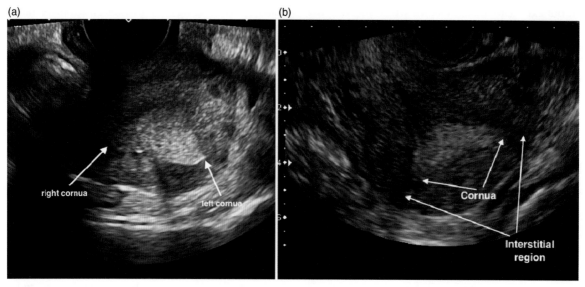

Figure 4.14 (a and b) TV transverse coronal images showing the cornual and interstitial areas (arrows).

4.6 Adnexal Imaging, Including the Ovaries and Fallopian Tubes

The optimal approach for visualising the adenexal regions is transvaginal ultrasound. At the level of the fundus, the cornua on the right side and the interstitial area where the fallopian tube runs through the cornual myometrium should be identified (Figure 4.14b). The transducer is angled to direct the beam towards the right pelvic sidewall to visualise the adenexa and the iliac vessels, and this is then repeated on the left side. Where the ovaries do not readily come into view, repeat the steps of finding the long axis (longitudinal) midline section of the uterus, then rotate the transducer 90 degrees to obtain a transverse section, moving to the level of the fundus and then angling the probe to the right, looking for the ovary and iliac vessels (Figures 4.5b and 4.15). This will usually reveal the right ovary. Repeating the same manoeuvre on the left will usually enable identification of the left ovary.

When the uterus is being scanned transversely from the cervix to the uterine fundus, moving laterally at the fundus, the interstitial portion of the tubes should be identified (Figure 4.14b). From the interstitial/cornual region, directing the beam laterally should follow the fallopian tube and image outwards to the pelvic sidewall. Normal fallopian tubes are not visible on routine pelvic ultrasound, although they may be demonstrated by instilling positive contrast into the endometrial cavity (HyCoSy, see Chapter 11).

The ovary should come into view just before reaching the iliac vessels on the pelvic sidewall (see section 4.5). In women of reproductive age, normal ovaries are readily identifiable by their characteristic appearance (Figure 4.16).

4.6.1 Assessing Structures on Ultrasound

During scanning, it is useful to think about the SSOTMO acronym (Box 4.1) to help you assess particular structures, for example, the uterus. Remember, in the SRH context, the appearances will be affected by the reproductive status, age and hormonal medications.

4.7 The Uterus

The central location, size and distinctive pear shape of the uterus makes it a relatively easy landmark to identify with ultrasound. When examining the uterus the following should be evaluated;

1. The uterine size, shape, outline (smooth, irregular, local distortion, etc.) and texture.
2. Uterine orientation (ante/retroverted, axial or ante/retroflexed).
3. The endometrium.
4. The myometrium.
5. The cervix.

Sonographically, the cervix has the same consistency as the myometrium and it is not affected by cyclical hormonal changes, although it can sometimes be

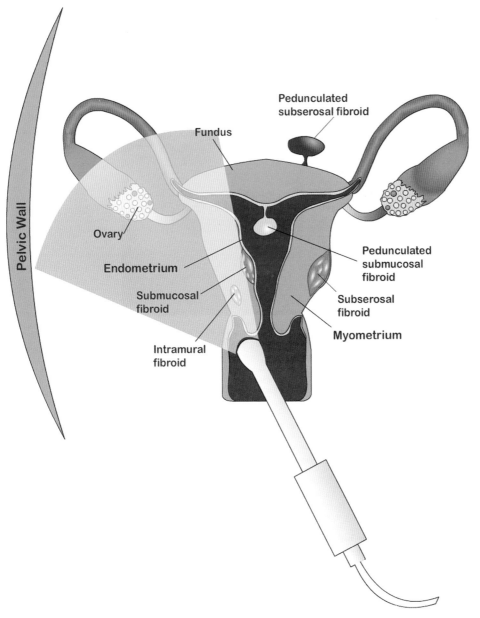

Figure 4.15 Diagram showing TV imaging of the right pelvic sidewall (artwork courtesy of Mark Pountney, Liverpool University.)

possible to see mucus in the cervix mid-cycle. It is common to see mucus retention cysts (Nabothian follicles) in the cervix, commonly measuring around 10 mm. These are a normal finding (Figure 4.17).

4.7.1 Uterine Measurements

There is no particular value to measuring the uterine dimensions routinely, but this may be helpful in some circumstances including;

- Primary or secondary amenorrhoea (as a guide to oestrogen status).
- Where the woman has experienced pain with a correctly sited IUS, small dimensions of the endometrial cavity in a hypoestrogenic woman may be a cause of pain (Chapter 10).
- To evaluate a uterine abnormality or pelvic mass, to help guide appropriate management (Chapter 6).

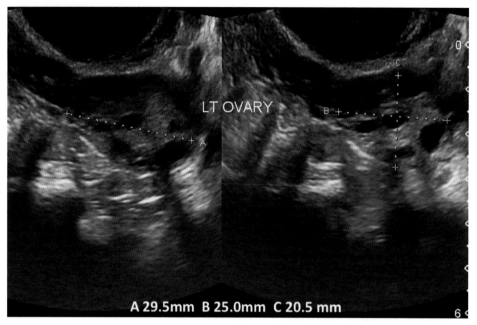

Figure 4.16 A normal ovary measured in three perpendicular planes. The volume in ml³ is calculated by multiplying the three diameters by π/6 (0.523). This gives a volume of 7.9 ml (normal). Modern machines will do the calculation automatically.

Box 4.1 Acronym for Assessing Ultrasound Appearances

This is dependent on pattern recognition skills and experience.

S	Size	Does the structure look normal in size, large or small compared to expectations? (Subjective assessment of size).
S	Shape	Is the shape of the structure as you expect it would be? For example, is the uterus a 'pear' shape?
O	Outline	Is the outline of the structure as you expect? Typically, smooth, with no 'lumps/bumps' or indentations?
T	Texture	Is the texture of the structure what you expect in a 'normal' case, in the absence of pathology?
M	Measurements	Any measurements should be accurate and also set into the clinical context. Is the measurement within the normal range? This is important information for a clinician who may not know what the 'normal' or 'abnormal' acceptable measurements of the pelvic organs should be.
O	Origin	If there is pathology evident, try to work out the origin. Where is it arising from? It can help narrow the differentials.

The uterus varies in size with the menstrual cycle. However, this variation is small and not clinically significant. Conversely, the normal endometrial cyclical changes are important.

The myometrium and cervix should be evaluated for contour and textural changes, echogenic masses and cysts. Masses that may require follow-up or treatment should be measured in at least two dimensions. (For abnormal findings see Chapter 6.)

4.7.2 Prepuberty

Prepubertal children are not normally represented in SRH work, but it is appropriate that clinicians have an understanding of developmental changes in pelvic anatomy. Ultrasound is the imaging modality of choice for evaluating the paediatric female pelvis and may be indicated to assess oestrogen/pubertal status in a girl with prepubertal bleeding, delayed puberty/primary amenorrhoea or to evaluate pain.

The size of the uterus and vagina is highly oestrogen dependent. Following birth, the uterus undergoes involution during the first four years of life and remains very small until the onset of puberty. The average prepubertal uterus measures around 2.5 × 1.0 × 0.8 cm or volume 1–2 cc (Figure 4.18) compared with a post-pubertal volume of around 60

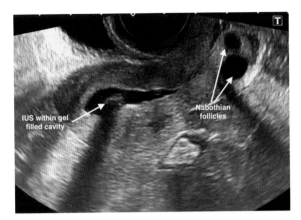

Figure 4.17 A TV long axis image of the uterus. The cavity has been filled with gel to assist retrieval of an IUS with retracted threads. The cervix has two Nabothian cysts (arrowed – also called Nabothian follicles).

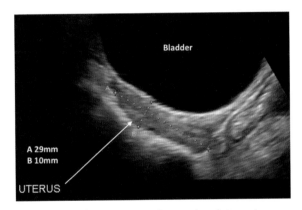

Figure 4.18 TA long axis image of a prepubertal uterus via a distended bladder. The uterine measurements were indicated to investigate an episode of prepubertal bleeding. The dimensions and appearance (no visible endometrium and cervix the same diameter as the corpus) are consistent with prepuberty.

cc. The prepubertal uterus appears very thin with a corpus equal in size to the cervix. A midline echo may be seen up to the age of six months but then will not be seen until puberty stimulates growth of the endometrium.

During scanning of the pelvis of a prepubertal girl, it is essential to be aware that in some girls the uterus is so thin that it can be difficult to identify with certainty using ultrasound. Failure to understand this has occasionally led to misdiagnosis of uterine agenesis with considerable distress and unnecessary further investigation with MRI. In a prepubertal child, placing any object on or through the extremely sensitive hymen is unacceptable, so TVUS is not an option.

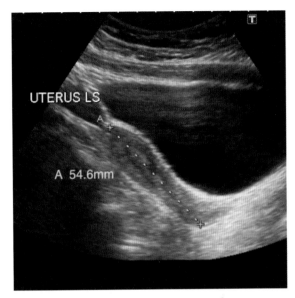

Figure 4.19 A post-menopausal uterus with a long axis measurement.

Unlike uterine size, ovarian volume increases exponentially from birth to puberty.

4.7.3 Post-menopause

The uterus, endometrium, vagina and ovaries are all smaller in post-menopausal women compared to during reproductive years.[2] After the menopause, the uterus may reduce to around 5.0 × 2.0 × 1.5 cm. (Figure 4.19). This can sometimes account for difficulty and pain when removing an IUC after the menopause. This is important to bear in mind if planning to fit an IUS for use with HRT, as the frame may be too big for the cavity where the woman is hypoestrogenic. In some circumstances it may be appropriate to consider giving a short course of systemic estrogen before coil fitting or removal.

4.8 The Pre-menopausal Endometrium

During reproductive years, the appearance and thickness of the endometrium are dependent on the stage of the menstrual cycle.

During menstruation, blood maybe seen in the uterine cavity. Towards the end and immediately after menstruation, the endometrium is thin (often <5 mm – Figure 4.20a). During the follicular phase it proliferates, becoming thicker under the influence

61

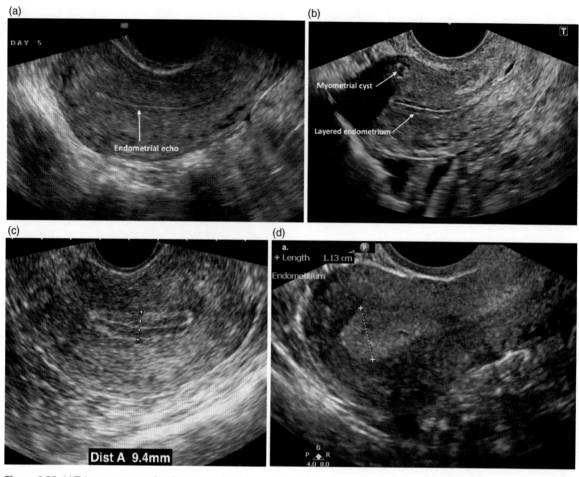

Figure 4.20 (a) Thin post-menstrual endometrium. (b) Mid-cycle 'trilaminar' endometrium. (c) Transverse section of mid-cycle endometrium (the myometrial junction is clear, but this is not the recommended long axis view for endometrial measurement). (d) Luteal phase endometrium showing thickening but absence of layering. The correct section for endometrial measurement is demonstrated, across the widest part on a long axis image.

of rising oestrogen and this manifests as a three layer or 'trilaminar' appearance, particularly around ovulation (Figure 4.20b,c). Typically in the luteal phase the midline looses definition so the layered or 'trilaminar' appearance is lost (Figure 4.20d). The endometrial midline may appear linear or non-linear (Figure 4.21a,b). Both the midline and the endometrial–myometrial junction are usually regular but it can be irregular, interrupted or not defined (Figure 4.22a,b). Compared with the myometrium the endometrium may appear hyperechogenic, hypoechogenic or isoechogenic (Figure 4.23a,b,c). When the endometrial–myometrial junction is poorly defined and when the endometrium is isoechogenic it may be impossible to define the borders and therefore it is unsuitable for measurement (Figure 4.22a,b).

Where assessment is clinically indicated, hysteroscopy is recommended unless instillation of contrast enhances the image sufficiently to allow assessment (Figure 4.24a,b).

The endometrial thickness is maximal around five days after the pre-ovulatory LH peak and averages 10–14 mm in AP diameter (Figure 4.20d). After ovulation, production of progesterone by the corpus luteum changes the endometrium to secretory type, which becomes homogenous so the layered appearance is no longer obvious. Drugs with oestrogenic or progestogenic activity will also influence the endometrial appearance on ultrasound. There may be cystic areas in the endometrium, which should be noted particularly if the endometrium appears thick (Figure 4.25a,b). They have been associated with a

(a)

(b)

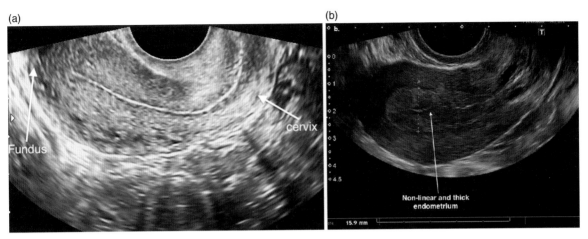

Figure 4.21 Appearances of the endometrial midline. (a) Linear thin endometrium. (b) Non-linear thick endometrium.

(a)

(b)

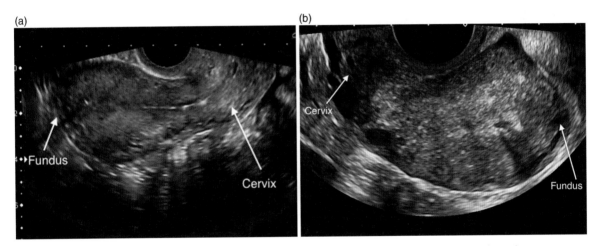

Figure 4.22 (a and b) Non-defined or indistinct endometrial midline and no visible endometrial–myometrial border. In these cases endometrial measurement is not possible. Loss of a clear endometrial outline can occur with adenomyosis and with endometrial cancer.

prolonged proliferative phase (for example, PCOS with anovulation) and with use of Tamoxifen. They may increase the likelihood that there will be hyperplasia on biopsy.

In women taking cyclical hormonal medication, the appearance of the endometrium will change depending on the hormone combination being taken at the time of the scan.

Synechiae are tissue adhesions obliterating the endometrial cavity. They may appear as strands of tissue crossing the endometrium, but are revealed much more clearly where there is fluid or a gestation sac filling the cavity (Figure 4.26).

Fluid may be present naturally within the cavity, and in this situation the use of contrast is not indicated.

The fluid may be hypoechoic (Figure 4.27) or hyperechoic with a 'ground glass' appearance (Chapter 13, Figure 13.9c).

4.9 The Post-menopausal Endometrium

The endometrial appearance on ultrasound – particularly the thickness, regularity and to a lesser extent the blood flow – correlates with the likelihood of endometrial pathology.

During the past 25 years, ultrasound has become the primary screening tool in women who present with symptoms of endometrial pathology, particularly PMB.

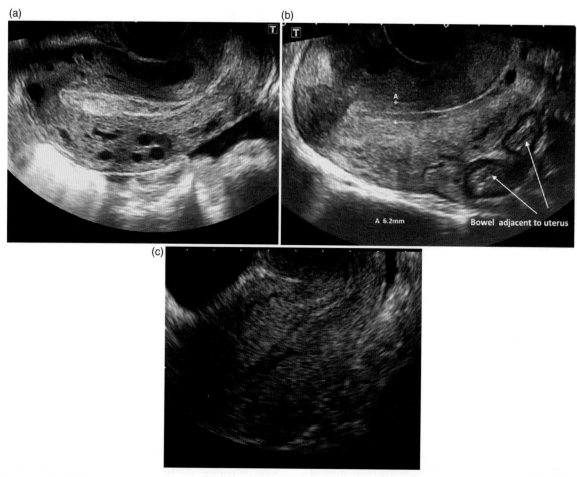

Figure 4.23 (a) Hyperechoic endometrium. (b) Isoechoic endometrium. (c) Hypoechoic endometrium – unsuitable for measurement where there is no distinct endometrial–myometrial junction.

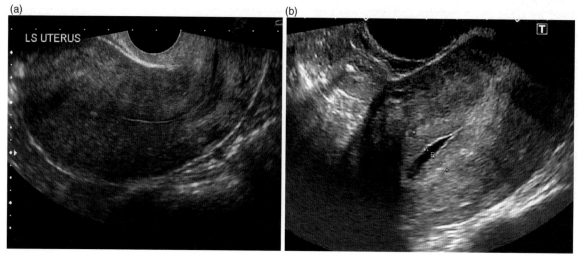

Figure 4.24 (a) Indistinct endometrium. (b) Endometrium clarified with gel contrast, defining the endometrial margins both against the myometrium and the cavity.

(a)   (b)

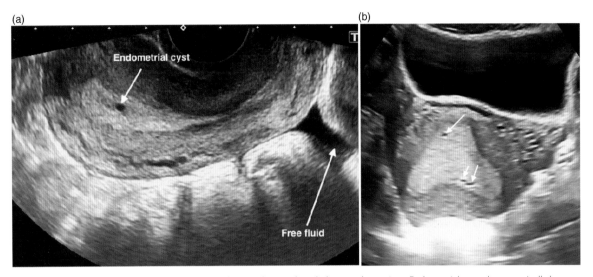

Figure 4.25 (a) TV long axis image showing an endometrial cyst in luteal phase endometrium. Endometrial cysts do not typically have the bright surrounding 'ring' that would be expected with an early pregnancy implantation sac. A small amount of free fluid demonstrated is a normal finding during reproductive age, especially during the post-ovulatory phase. Some free fluid is also very common during early pregnancy. (b) A TA transverse image of a retroverted uterus imaged through a distended bladder, showing several endometrial cysts and an arcuate shaped cavity.

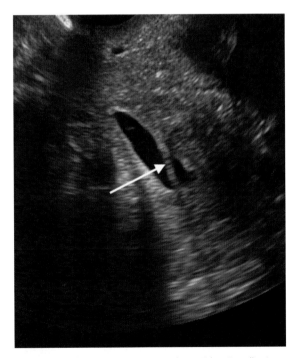

Figure 4.26 The arrow points to a endometrial cavity adhesion (synechia) revealed by instillation of gel contrast. The woman had a history of morbidly adherent placenta requiring manual removal at her last delivery.

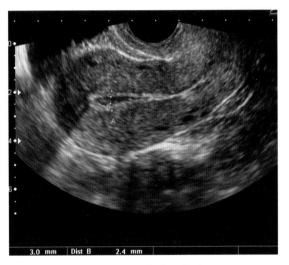

Figure 4.27 A long axis image of a fluid-filled cavity. Measurement of the endometrium when there is fluid in the cavity should not include the fluid measurement. The two individual endometrial measurements should be added (or the fluid thickness subtracted from a measurement including the double endometrium and fluid).

4.9.1 Measurement of Endometrial Thickness

The IETA group (2010) produced a consensus paper on how to perform ultrasound examination of the endometrium and endometrial cavity and the definitions to be used when reporting the findings.[3] The agreed convention is that measurement is made on a long axis (longitudinal) view and includes the double thickness (made from the outer edge or endometrial–myometrial border on one side to that on the other side) and is made where the thickness appears the greatest (Figures 4.20d, 4.21b and 4.28). It is essential that the whole cavity is evaluated and any area of focal thickening is regarded as an indication for further assessment. A thin regular endometrial line measuring less than 4 mm (Figures 4.20a, 4.21a and 4.29) is very reliable for the exclusion of endometrial cancer, and obviates the need for further investigation such as hysteroscopy or biopsy, unless abnormal bleeding persists. The incomplete visualisation or the presence of a focal lesion results in endometrium that cannot be clearly measured and should be regarded as abnormal and requiring further evaluation (Figure 4.22). This may occur where the endometrium has almost the same echogenicity as the myometrium or where there are fibroids or overlying calcification. Sometimes it may be possible to clarify the endometrial thickness by the instillation of negative contrast (Figure 4.24). Endometrial sampling disrupts the endometrium so measurement should be made before and not after endometrial sampling.

Where the endometrium cannot be measured, fluid instillation will more clearly outline the cavity and give acoustic enhancement that enables reliable measurement (Chapter 5). Where intracavity fluid (or contrast) is present, the thickness of both single layers should be measured and added (Figures 4.24b and 4.27) so the fluid thickness is not included in the measurement.

To be regarded as normal, the post-menopausal endometrial double thickness must be less than 4 mm, regular and clearly visible throughout the totality of the endometrial cavity. For women on HRT there is no agreed cut off for endometrial thickness. Sequential HRT will have a variable effect on the endometrium, which will be maximal towards the end of the combination phase and thinnest following endometrial shedding when the progestogen is withdrawn. It is therefore most appropriate to measure the endometrium around day 5–7 with sequential therapy. It is generally agreed that a thickness of 8 mm or more in a woman with abnormal bleeding using HRT requires further investigation; however, between 4 and 7.9 mm there is no consensus.

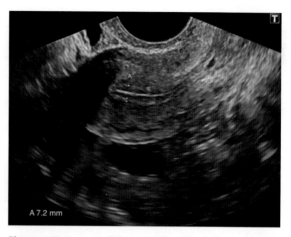

Figure 4.28 Long axis TV image with endometrial measurement. The trilaminar appearance is consistent with mid-cycle and the measurement is normal.

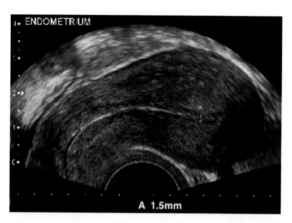

Figure 4.29 A long axis TV image showing thin regular endometrium.

4.10 Uterine Vascularity

The majority of blood flow to the uterus comes from the uterine arteries with a minor contribution from the ovarian arteries. The main uterine arteries can be visualised laterally at the level of the cervix. They give rise to the arcuate arteries, which are orientated circumferentially and may be seen in the outer third of the myometrium (Figure 4.30a,b). These vessels give rise to radial arteries, which run perpendicular to

(a)

(b)

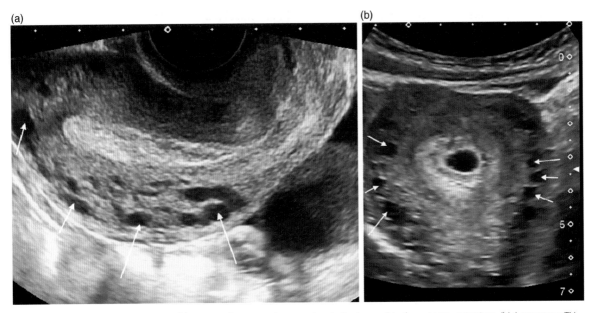

Figure 4.30 (a) A long axis TV image of the uterus demonstrating arcuate arteries (arrows) in the outer myometrium. (b) A transverse TV image with early gestation sac also demonstrating the arcuate arteries (arrows) in the outer myometrium.

the muscle fibres in the inner two-thirds of the myometrium and terminate in short basal arteries which supply the basal layer of endometrium (Figure 4.31). When the uterus is enlarged due to adenomyosis, the blood flow pattern within the myometrium retains its normal appearance whereas fibroids typically have circumferential blood vessels in or around the periphery of the fibroid (Chapter 6, Figures 6.8b, 6.9b). Blood vessels do not normally cross the myometrial–endometrial border. However, with endometrial shedding there may appear to be flow across this junction on Colour Doppler. It is important to be aware that Doppler findings in benign and malignant endometrial pathology are inconsistent and therefore their value in differentiating endometrial cancer is limited. Endometrial thickness is the only differentiating parameter on ultrasound.

4.11 The Normal Ovary

The ovary appears ovoid in shape and typically contains a number of sonographically visible antral follicles (2–9 mm size) in women of reproductive age (Figure 4.32). Antral follicle counts are included in the assessment of ovarian reserve. During reproductive years, around ten primary oocytes begin to mature each cycle, giving the appearance of small echolucent cysts within each ovary. Usually, only one follicle

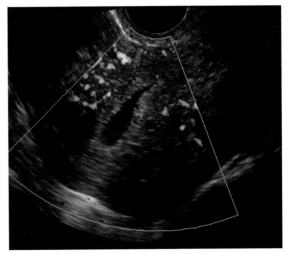

Figure 4.31 A transverse TV image of the uterus demonstrating radial arteries running perpendicular to the myometrial muscle fibres to small basal arteries at the myometrial–endometrial junction.

dominates and grows to around 20 mm by mid-cycle when it ruptures at ovulation (Figure 4.33a,b). The cyclical follicular development may be tracked with ultrasound as a means of surveillance during fertility treatment (Chapter 11). This characteristic appearance of follicles, and the presence of a corpus luteum during the luteal phase, enables differentiation of

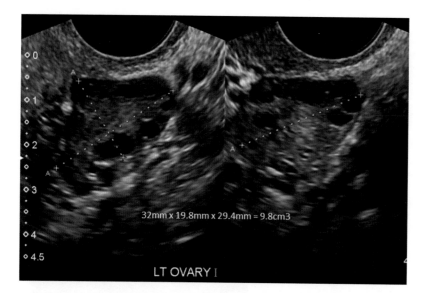

Figure 4.32 Ovarian appearance during reproductive years. A volume calculation is demonstrated – 3 perpendicular diameters multiplied by 0.523. The appearance is consistent with polycystic morphology (relatively large but just <10 cc³; however > 12 antral follicles).

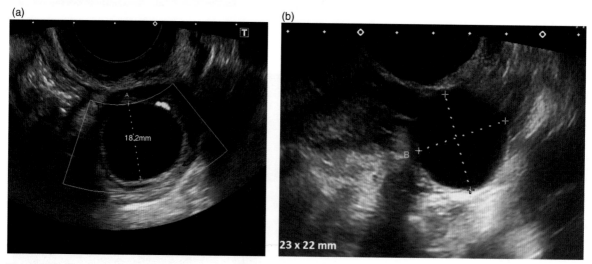

Figure 4.33 (a) An ovulatory follicle demonstrating peripheral circumferential flow with Colour Doppler. This is not as prominent as the colour flow in a corpus luteum. (b) An ovulatory follicle demonstrating the 'full' appearance and size on the day of ovulation.

the ovary from other pelvic structures. Where there is uncertainty, bowel peristalsis helps distinguish between bowel and the ovaries, which are static. The position of a normally sited ovary, medial to the iliac vein, further helps identification (Figure 4.34a,b). The size and appearance of a 'functional' normal ovary will vary with the time of the menstrual cycle. The appearance will also change with age. When a volume calculation is required, ovarian size is measured in three perpendicular planes (Figure 4.32). These values are then multiplied and the result multiplied by π/6 or (0.523) to give the volume of an elliptical

shaped structure. The population average ovarian volume is 0.7 cc at two years, rising to a peak of 7.7 cc in teenage years and then declining to 2.8 cc at menopausal age.

Owing to the small ovarian size and lack of follicles in women of peri or post-menopausal status, normal ovaries frequently cannot be identified unless there are residual small simple cysts. Residual cysts are observed in up to 20 per cent of women more than five years into the menopause. The ovaries may also be difficult to identify in women with significant fibroid enlargement of the uterus.

(a)   (b)

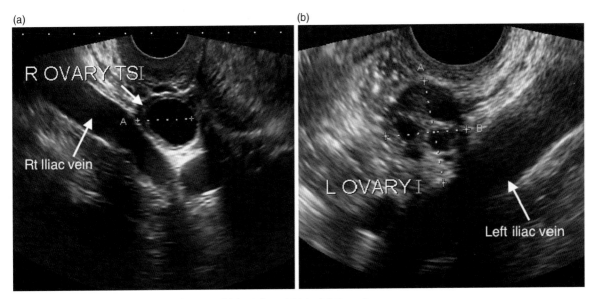

Figure 4.34 Normal ovarian position adjacent to (a) the right and (b) the left iliac veins.

(a)   (b)

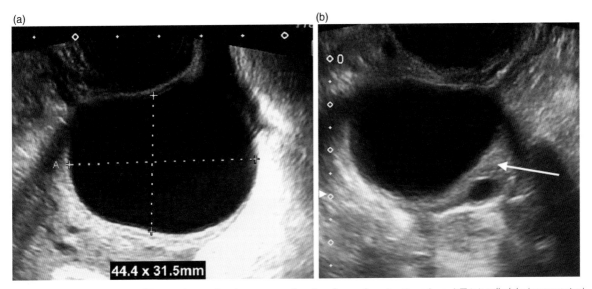

Figure 4.35 (a) A simple cyst. (b) A simple cyst showing a surrounding rim of normal ovarian tissue (arrow). This is called the 'crescent sign' and is considered a benign or 'B' feature.

Simple cysts are frequently noted on pelvic ultrasound, particularly among women using a Levonorgestrel IUS where they are thought to be due to delayed atresia of a developing follicle (Figure 4.35a,b). These cysts mostly do not cause symptoms and naturally resolve within one or two cycles. Provided a simple cyst is under 5 cm diameter and fulfils the 'simple' criteria, it can be regarded as non-specific and does not require any follow-up. A 'simple' cyst is defined as anechoic (that is, appears black internally consistent with a content of clear fluid), is a single locule, with a thin walled capsule, no septations and no irregularity of the cyst wall. There is also post-cystic enhancement, an area of brightness, directly deep to the cyst (Chapter 2). The presence of recognisable ovarian tissue around the cyst wall (crescent sign – Figure 4.35b) is a further sign of benignity. The presence of septations and papillary projections

(> 3 mm) into the cyst lumen increases the possibility of malignancy and should be referred for further assessment (Chapters 6 and 15).

4.11.1 The Corpus Luteum

After ovulatory rupture and collapse of the dominant follicle, the granulosa cells proliferate and blood vessels invade the ruptured follicle forming the corpus luteum, and driving production of progesterone. The corpus luteum has a characteristic ultrasound appearance (Figure 4.36a), typically demonstrating a high peripheral blood flow, which gives a characteristic vascular pattern (Figure 4.36b) often referred to as the 'ring of fire'. Very commonly areas of haemorrhage are seen within the corpus luteum (Figure 4.37a,b) and occasionally these form large haemorrhagic cysts (Chapter 6, Figure 6.32a). Very rarely spontaneous intraperitoneal bleeding may arise from a highly vascular corpus luteum.

4.12 The Recto-Uterine Space

This is the space between the uterus and the rectosigmoid colon (also called the Cul-de-sac or Pouch of Douglas) and is the most dependent area in the peritoneal cavity; hence any free peritoneal fluid will tend to firstly accumulate here, under the influence of gravity. This space, posterior to the uterus, should be evaluated for the presence of fluid or a mass (Figure 4.38a,b). It is important to distinguish fluid and faeces in bowel from free fluid, and a normal amount of free fluid from an abnormal amount.

4.12.1 Fluid

A small amount of fluid in the pelvis is not significant in women of reproductive age. It is a normal finding that is very common around the time of ovulation (Figure 4.38a). Where fluid fills the utero-vesical space (anterior cul-de-sac), this indicates that the volume is more than would be consistent with normal physiology. If fluid covers the uterine fundus, then this is excessive in amount and should be regarded as indicating pathology (Figure 4.38b). In post-menopausal women, fluid is not normally found in the pelvis and any amount should be regarded as suspicious of pathology.

It should be remembered that rapid hydration can result in small volumes of fluid in this area and this is not abnormal.

4.13 Accuracy and Reproducibility of Measurements

Where measurements are made during an ultrasound scan, it is essential the measurements are accurate and reproducible. To achieve this there must be;

1. A clearly defined anatomical plane that will allow all operators to freeze the same anatomical section.

(a)

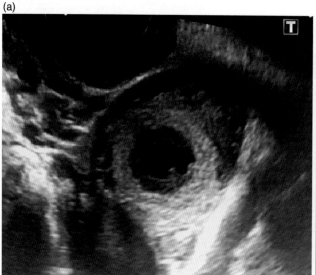

(b)

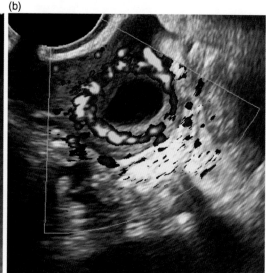

Figure 4.36 A corpus luteum (a) without and (b) with Colour Doppler demonstrating high flow.

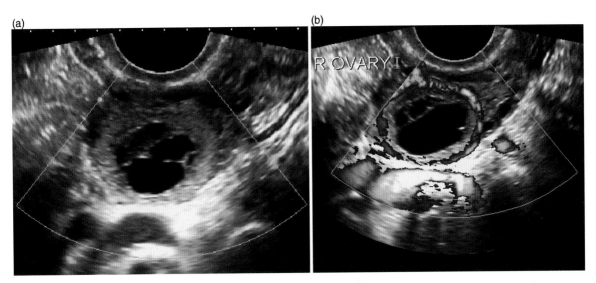

Figure 4.37 A haemorrhagic corpus luteum (a) without and (b) with Colour Doppler.

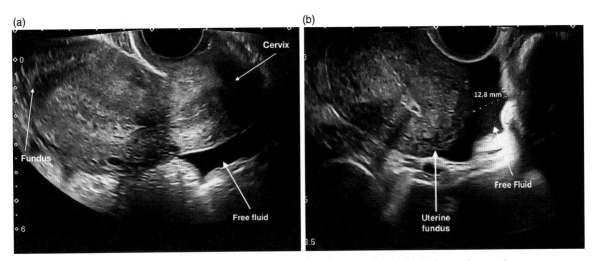

Figure 4.38 (a) Fluid in cul-de-sac (normal amount). (b) Fluid surrounding the uterine fundus (likely abnormal amount).

2. Prescribed end points for positioning the callipers, so that all operators will place the callipers in the same position.

In reality, this is difficult when imaging pelvic structures since:

Uterus – whilst it might be fairly simple for a variety of operators to obtain a similar midline section through the uterus, it is very difficult to prescribe the calliper positioning, particularly in the region of the cervix. Consequently, the placement of the callipers can be subjective and variable between operators, thereby contributing to measurement inconsistency.

Ovary – an ovary is a walnut shaped structure and is rather amorphous, lacking landmarks which will assist the operator in identifying the mid-long axis (longitudinal) plane. This makes reproduction of the scan plane very difficult between operators, which is further compounded as it is not possible to prescribe exact calliper placement. The size and appearance of the ovaries will also change throughout the cycle in women of reproductive age.

Where measurements are to be used to inform clinical decisions, it is essential that they are audited and that intra-operator (within one operator) and inter-operator (between different operators) errors are investigated (Chapter 17).

4.14 Conclusion

Ultrasound provides a convenient, low-cost, non-invasive tool for investigation and management of a range of gynaecological symptoms and signs, including problems with long acting contraception. The transabdominal and transvaginal routes of imaging are complimentary with different information potentially available from each. Knowledge of the normal range of findings is essential to the correct interpretation of abnormal findings, and when provided in conjunction with clinical history, can assist accurate diagnosis and guide best patient management. Measurements should be used cautiously.

References

1. Intimate examinations and chaperones. *GMC*, March 2013.

2. Merz E, Miric-Tesanic D, Bahlmann F, Weber G, Wellek S. Sonographic size of uterus and ovaries in pre- and postmenopausal women. *Ultrasound Obstet Gynecol* 1996;7(1):38–42.

3. Leone FPG, Timmerman D, Bourne T, Valentin L, Epstein E, Goldstein S et al. Terms, definitions and measurements to describe the sonographic features of the endometrium and intrauterine lesions: a consensus opinion from the International Endometrial Tumor Analysis (IETA) group. *Ultrasound Obstet Gynecol* 2010;35:103–112.

5

Contrast Sonohysterography

Mary Pillai

5.1 Introduction 73
5.2 Technique 73
5.3 Imaging the Endometrium 75
5.4 Extent of Lesion 76

5.5 Fibroids 76
5.6 Cavity Dimensions 78
5.7 Imaging When an IUC Is In Situ 78
5.8 Summary 78

5.1 Introduction

An important limitation of standard sonographic diagnosis is that the endometrial cavity is a virtual space. Intracavitary pathology may be suspected where the endometrium appears thick, but may not be reliably demonstrated with transvaginal imaging alone. A lower thickness would be expected in the immediate post-menstrual phase, but there are practical limitations in asking women to return for repeat imaging timed to their cycle.

The addition of negative contrast or 'fluid infusion sonography' (FIS – Figure 5.1a,b) enhances the imaging in several ways;

- It detects 'focal endometrial pathology' and enables an estimate of its extent.
- It distinguishes intrauterine polyps from endometrium throughout the cycle.
- It enables assessment of the proportion of myoma protruding into the cavity, and hence more accurate FIGO staging and treatment planning.
- It estimates the cavity volume.
- Where an intrauterine device is in situ, it enables visualisation and measurement of the endometrium separate to the device.
- Where the endometrium is poorly defined and too indistinct for ultrasound assessment, it enhances the endometrial–myometrial junction which may enable satisfactory evaluation and measurement.
- It enhances visualisation of pelvic structures beyond the cavity through improving through transmission of the beam (analogous to filling the bladder for transabdominal pelvic scanning).

Contraindications include pregnancy or acute pelvic inflammatory disease. It is not indicated where there is spontaneous intracavitary fluid.

5.2 Technique

The required equipment is simple:

1. A speculum
2. Gel (GIS) or saline (SIS)
3. A quill or 2 mm catheter for gel or a balloon catheter for saline.

SIS has been used for sonohysterography, combining transvaginal ultrasound with simultaneous infusion of sterile saline through a balloon catheter into the endometrial cavity. The fluid acts as a negative contrast medium that distends the cavity, allowing display of its contours and contents. Use of gel was first described in 2007 (GIS) and was concluded to be a simple technique with minimal inconvenience for the patient, and an attractive alternative to saline infusion.[1] Its greater viscosity obviated the need for a balloon catheter. However, in addition to imaging, patients requiring ultrasound in an SRH setting are likely to require uterine instrumentation. A potential additional benefit to the use of Instillagel in this circumstance is that local absorption of the Lidocaine may reduce any discomfort with subsequent instrumentation of the cavity. Adequate filling of the cavity combined with a time elapse of several minutes during the scan may be sufficient to allow this. Use of gel has no influence on the histology of subsequent sampling.[2]

The author's preferred medium is Instillagel.[3] Each 100 g contains Lidocaine hydrochloride 2 g,

(a) (b)

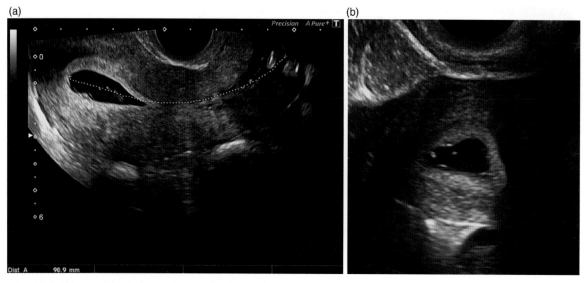

Figure 5.1 (a) Long axis/sagittal view of a normal endometrial cavity distended with gel. (b) Short axis/transverse view. The bright areas in the cavity are tiny air bubbles in the contrast.

Chlorhexidine gluconate solution (antiseptic) 0.25 g and small amounts of Methyl hydroxybenzoate (E218) and Propyl hydroxybenzoate (E216) as preservatives. The gel vehicle consists of Hydroxyethylcellulose, propylene glycol and purified water. It is available in 11 ml and 6 ml syringe sizes. There are 230 mg lidocaine in an 11 ml syringe and 125.4 mg in a 6 ml syringe. The maximum dose of Lidocaine that should be administered by tissue infiltration is 200 mg, but the Summary of Product Characteristics describes doses of up to 800 mg instilled into the urethra producing low circulating levels that are below the level of toxicity. The Gel has some useful physical properties; it offers the same negative contrast as saline but its viscosity is much higher than saline resulting in less backflow through the cervix and more stable filling of the uterine cavity, obviating the need for a more expensive balloon catheter. It is important to flush any air bubbles out of the gel as ultrasound will not transmit through air, so any air will result in bright areas in the image with reduced definition of intracavitary contents.

The method of instillation with Instillaquill® (CliniMed Ltd) is demonstrated in Figure 5.2 and aims to distend the endometrial cavity with gel (video clip of gel entering cavity). When the cavity reaches filled capacity the woman will usually experience cramping, and some return of gel around the quill will be noted. It is important to explain this before starting and introduce the contrast very slowly, stopping when

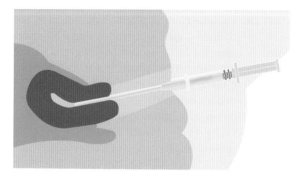

Figure 5.2 Installation set-up with quill inserted well into the cervical os.

the patient indicates the first cramping is experienced. The volume of gel inserted before any backflow gives a good estimate of the cavity volume. If backflow occurs as soon as gel insertion starts, then it is not entering the cavity and the positioning of the quill needs adjustment.

The quill for the introduction of the gel can be inserted into the external os during bimanual examination or during speculum examination. The author's preference is to use a speculum to ensure the cervix has been inspected. This also enables an estimate of the cavity volume and leaves the operator with one hand free to assist when needed with directing the transabdominal transducer to visualise the cavity during gel instillation. Anecdotally, the suprapubic pressure of applying the transabdominal probe seems to stimulate relaxation of the internal cervical os, enhancing successful filling of the cavity, and may distract the patient from any discomfort.

When the external os is narrow, holding the quill firmly over the opening and applying slight pressure to expel the gel will usually allow flow of gel into the cavity or this manoeuvre will itself hydro-dilate the os to enable insertion of the quill. If not, then stabilising the anterior lip of the cervix and inserting an Os Finder (Cory Bros, Shenley, UK) or small dilator permits introduction of the quill. In the author's practice, Lidocaine 10 per cent spray is applied to the cervix three minutes prior to any tenaculum or injection.

Sonohysterography can also be performed by introducing a catheter connected to a syringe of saline or gel that can be left in place while a transvaginal probe is introduced, allowing contrast instillation whilst imaging transvaginally. This has a further advantage that the gel can be aspirated into the syringe where biopsy is indicated, obviating the need for repeated passage of an endometrial sampler to empty the gel before tissue is obtained.

5.3 Imaging the Endometrium

It is important that the whole cavity is evaluated. From a sagittal midline view showing the endocervical and endometrial canal directing the beam laterally to the right moves through the cornua of the cavity and as the cornua disappears and the right adnexa comes into view. Then directing the beam back through the midline view, through the left cornua to the left adnexa will ensure the whole uterus has been imaged longitudinally. Following this, turn the transducer anticlockwise through 90 degrees to obtain a transverse view and follow this from the cervix to the uterine fundus. This ensures the whole uterus including the whole endometrium has been viewed transversely. Figure 5.3 illustrates how limited endometrial assessment is with TV ultrasound alone and Figure 5.4 shows how the assessment is enhanced with instillation of contrast. Figure 5.4 also shows how focal findings may be missed if the whole cavity is not systematically visualised. Where the endometrium appears thick or indistinct, the introduction of contrast enables differentiation of polyps (Figure 5.5) and focal areas of thick irregular endometrium (Figures 5.6 and 5.7).

When there is fluid in the cavity, the endometrium is measured separately on either side of the fluid where it appears thickest and the two single thicknesses added (Figure 5.8). If the endometrium is thickened asymmetrically, the anterior and posterior endometrial thicknesses should be reported separately.

(a)   (b)

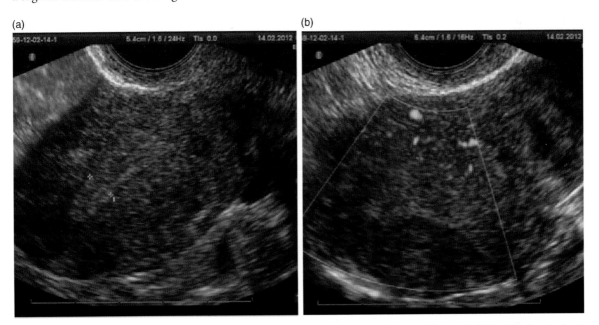

Figure 5.3 Case history: A 55-year-old pre/perimenopausal lady with intermenstrual bleeding. Her FSH was 38. (a) A midline longitudinal/sagittal view showing a normal endometrial thickness for pre-menopausal. (b) On this transverse view, the endometrial cavity outline can just be seen but is generally uninformative.

(a)

(b)

(c)

(d)

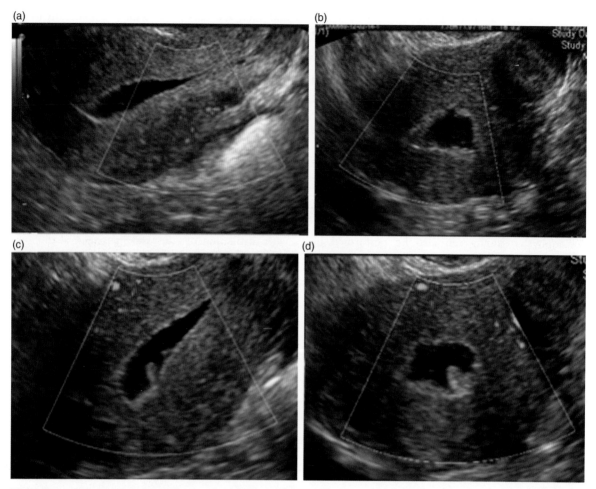

Figure 5.4 In the same case gel contrast has been introduced, giving much clearer definition of the endometrium and the myometrium. (a) Midline sagittal view and (b) Transverse view show a normal cavity and endometrium, and also a subserosal fibroid on the left side. (c) The sagittal view moving across the left side and (d) Transverse view at the level of the cornua. These views reveal some polys in the left cornual region. An endometrial biopsy was taken and a plan for medical curettage with progestogen, followed by review and IUS fitting. However, the biopsy revealed complex hyperplasia with atypia, so instead the patient was referred and underwent laparoscopic total hysterectomy and BSO. The histology contained severe endometrial atypia but no carcinoma. The ovaries contained luteal and follicular cysts.

Where the endometrium appears abnormal, then it can be helpful to examine with Colour Doppler. Usually no flow is demonstrated in the endometrium (colour score 1). A Colour Doppler score can be assigned where there is flow: mimimal colour: score 2, moderate colour: score 3 and abundant colour: score 4.

5.4 Extent of Lesion

Without fluid a polyp or lesion may be seen, but with the addition of fluid the extent of attachment of the lesion can be seen (Figures 5.9 and 5.10). The maximum diameter of the lesion against the maximum diameter for the base where attached to the uterus determines whether a lesion should be described as

sessile or pedunculated. Where the base of the lesion is attached to less than 25 per cent of the endometrial surface, it is described as 'localised' and where the base attaches to more than 25 per cent it is described as an 'extended' lesion. The type of localised lesion can be further subdivided into pedunculated (where the base attachment is narrow compared with the lesion diameter – Figures 5.9 and 5.10) or sessile (where the base is as wide or wider than the lesion – Figure 5.7).[3]

5.5 Fibroids

Where a fibroid is intracavity, the FIGO type (Chapter 6, Figure 6.3) should be determined together with the measurement of the lesion.

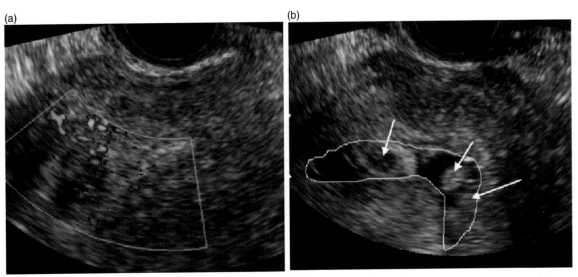

Figure 5.5 Case history: A 44-year-old lady referred after a failed IUS fitting. The lady requested this for heavy menstrual bleeding and intermenstrual bleeding. (a) A transvaginal image without contrast is uninformative as it is impossible to distinguish the endometrium and the cavity. (b) With instillation of gel contrast, at least four endometrial polyps are revealed (arrows).

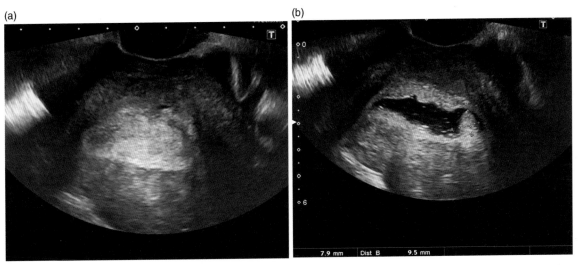

Figure 5.6 (a) This transverse TV vies indicates thick endometrium but the cavity is not defined. (b) Insertion of gel outlines a polypoid area of endometrium.

Grading of Submucus Fibroids

Grade 0 = 100 per cent intracavity
Grade 1 ≥ 50 per cent intracavity
Grade 2 < 50 per cent intracavity

Figures 5.10–5.14 illustrate examples of submucus fibroids in women referred for IUS fitting or investigation of unresolved bleeding problems. Instillation of gel better clarifies:

- The anatomical relationships with the extent of fibroid within the cavity.
- The extent of attachment to the cavity wall.
- The appearance of the endometrium throughout the cavity.

These issues clarify the suitability of the fibroid for hysteroscopic treatment.

In cases with multiple fibroids and/or large fibroids distorting the whole uterus, it may be impossible to

(a) (b)

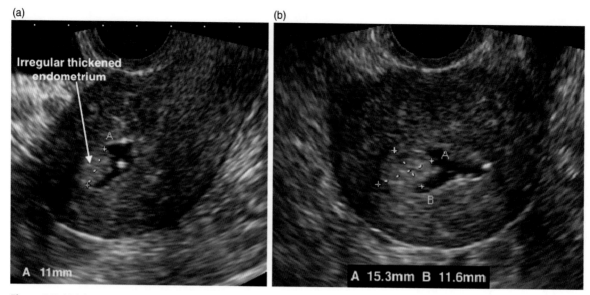

Figure 5.7 (a) A longitudinal TV view after instillation of gel shows an area of irregular endometrial thickening at the fundus of the cavity (arrow). (b) This transverse view of the same cavity shows the irregular thickened area in the right cornual region measuring 11 × 15.3 × 11.6 mm. The surface of the lesion appears irregular and it would be important to biopsy this area as elsewhere the endometrium appears thin and regular.

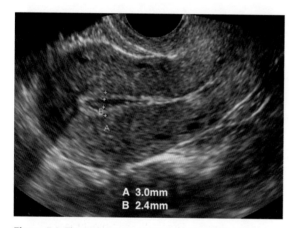

Figure 5.8 The endometrium has been enhanced by the instillation of gel. The two single endometrial thicknesses are measured on either side of the contrast/fluid giving a double thickness of 5.4 mm.

determine the shape and position of the endometrial cavity with ordinary transvaginal ultrasound. In these cases, instillation of gel enables determination of the position and size of the cavity, its relationship to any fibroids as well as the appearance and thickness of the endometrium (Figures 5.15 and 5.16).

5.6 Cavity Dimensions

Instillation of fluid enables more accurate assessment of the cavity size (Figure 5.17).

Smaller cavity dimensions are common when women are relatively hypoestrogenic, for example, during breastfeeding or whilst on Depo provera. Instillation of fluid also enables more accurate assessment of the myometrium and measurement of the myometrium prior to implanting GyneFix (Figure 5.18).

5.7 Imaging When an IUC Is In Situ

Introduction of contrast confers significant advantages where endometrial assessment is indicated in any woman with a coil in situ. Without contrast it can be impossible to assess the endometrium, but introduction of contrast readily demonstrates the endometrium separate to the IUC and enables thorough evaluation without the need to remove the IUC (Figures 5.19 and 5.20).

5.8 Summary

Sonohysterography introduces a fluid contrast which takes imaging a step further, by providing much more accurate assessment of the configuration and size of the endometrial cavity, possible endometrial pathology, intracavity lesions (fibroids and polyps) and assessment while an IUC is in situ. The improved transmission of the ultrasound beam through fluid

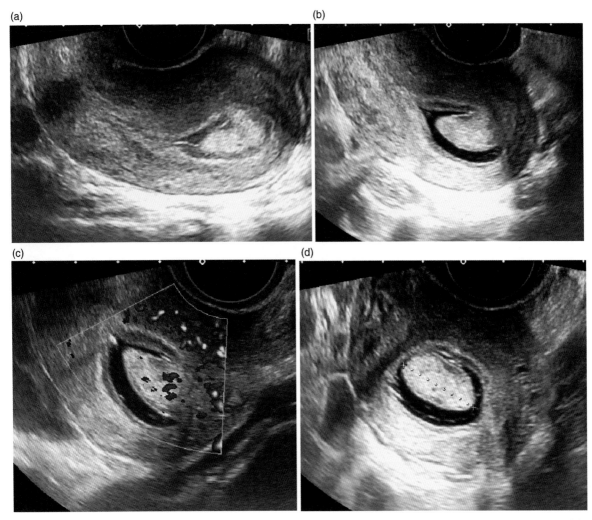

Figure 5.9 (a) Fibroid polyp (type 0) can be seen without contrast. (b–d) Instillation of contrast demonstrates it is pedunculated. The colour flow image c. demonstrates feeding vessels with a pattern more typical of a polyp than the circumferential flow pattern seen with fibroids.

may also enhance imaging the adenexal regions. The technique of gel sonohysterography is minimally invasive, easily learnt and requires no equipment beyond that used at a contraception clinic that already provides ultrasound.

References

1. Exalto N, Stappers C, van Raamsdonk LA, Emanuel MH. Gel instillation sonohysterography: first experience with a new technique. *Fertil Steril.* 2007;87:152–155.

2. Van den Bosch T, Domali E, Van Schoubroeck D, Timmerman D. The use of gel instillation hysterosonography in a single examiner setting. *Ultrasound Obstet Gynecol.* 2007;30: 413.

3. Pillai M, Shefras J. Experience with Instillagel * for hysterosonography and analgesia in a complex contraception clinic: a QIPP initiative. *J Fam Plann Reprod Health Care.* 2012;38(2):110–116.

(a)　　　　　　　　　　　　　　　　　　(b)

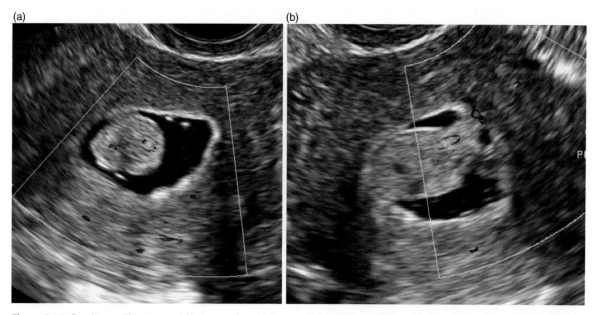

Figure 5.10　Case history: This 44-year-old lady was referred following a failed IUS fitting. She had requested the IUS for heavy menstrual bleeding. (a) Gel instillation clarifies there is a single polyp and the endometrium is thin and regular. (b) The extent of the base of the polyp is a small area in the left side of the cavity.

(a)　　　　　　　　　　　　　　　　　　(b)

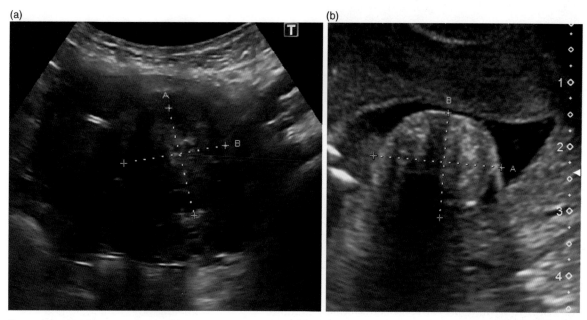

Figure 5.11　(a) A TA transverse view of the uterus. Without contrast a fibroid can be seen and measured, but its relationship to the endometrial cavity can only be evaluated when contrast is introduced (b), revealing a type 0 fibroid. The endometrium cannot be seen or evaluated without contrast but can readily be measured and seen throughout the cavity when contrast is introduced.

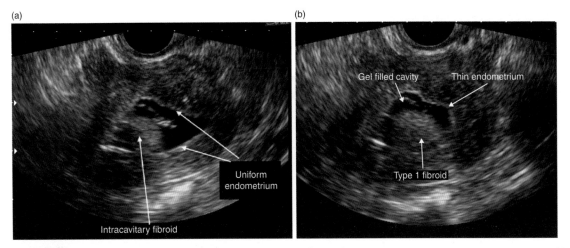

Figure 5.12 Case history: A 50-year-old lady referred for increasing bleeding despite an IUS. (a–b) Instillation of gel reveals a type 1 fibroid (> 50 per cent protruding into the cavity). Uniformly thin endometrium is demonstrated through the rest of the cavity.

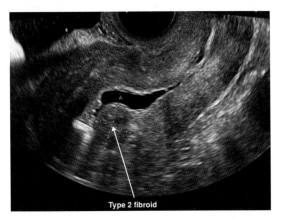

Figure 5.13 A small type 2 fibroid is demonstrated following instillation of gel. This may be suitable for resection as the depth of fibroid is no more than 50 per cent of the thickness of the myometrium.

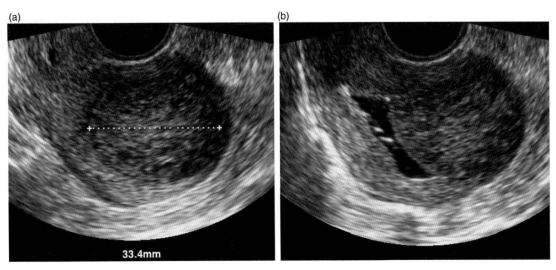

Figure 5.14 (a) Large type 2 fibroid. Its relationship to the cavity and myometrial depth is difficult to see, however, with instillation of gel. (b) The cavity and endometrium are outlined. It can also more clearly be seen that the fibroid extends through most of the myometrial thickness virtually to the serosa, making it unsuitable for resection.

(a)
(b)
(c)
(d)

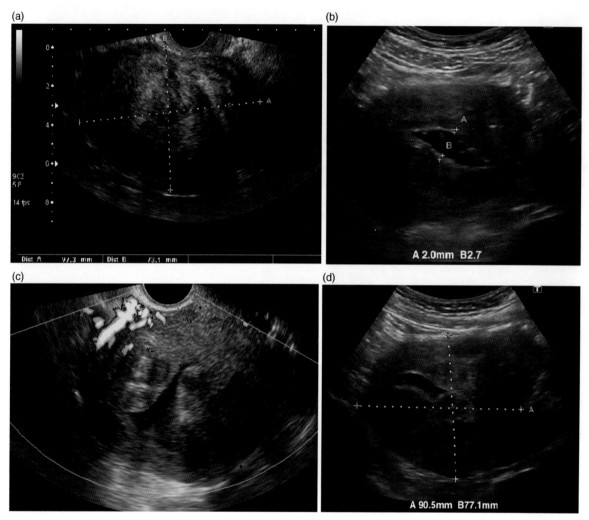

Figure 5.15 Case history: This 45-year-old lady requested an IUS for HMB and was referred when a pelvic mass was noted during the fitting. (a) Shows a TV sagittal view of a large fibroid uterus, but the position and shape of the cavity and appearance of the endometrium cannot be assessed. (b–d) TA and TV views following instillation of gel. They show the position and shape of the cavity as well as the appearance and thickness of the endometrium. The gel instillation also clarifies that the fibroids are intramural (type 3–5) rather than intracavitary.

(a) (b)

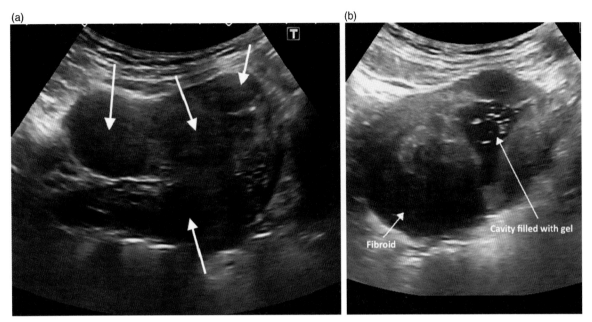

Figure 5.16 Case history: This 47-year-old lady was referred for an IUS for heavy menstrual bleeding after a failed fitting elsewhere. (a) A transabdominal midline longitudinal view of the pelvis shows a mass. The arrows point to several rounded hypoechoic 'tumours' consistent with fibroids. It is impossible to define the position or shape of the endometrial cavity or the relationship of the fibroids to the cavity. (b) A transverse TA view after gel has been introduced. It is now possible to see the outline of the endometrial cavity. The fibroids are not distorting the cavity but the cavity is enlarged (took 8 ml gel to fill).

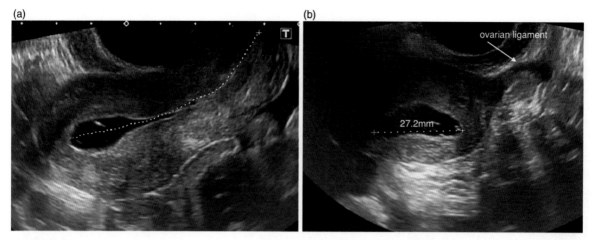

Figure 5.17 (a) A TV long axis or sagittal view. (b) a TV transverse view of the cavity outlined by gel with dimensions measured. The transverse view shows the left ovarian ligament (arrow), which can be followed laterally to help identify the ovary.

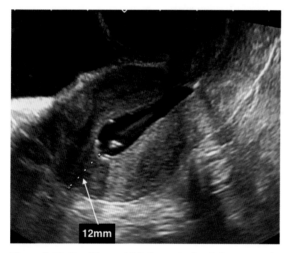

Figure 5.18 Case history: A fully breast feeding lady associated the onset of persitstent pelvic discomfort with postnatal placement of an IUD. She requested a frameless device. The gel contrast enhances measurement of the fundal myometrium (arrow) at the intended implantation site for the device. Absorption of the Lidocaine content may provide some local anaestheitic benefit provided it is left and retained for several minutes prior to the fitting.

(a)

(b)

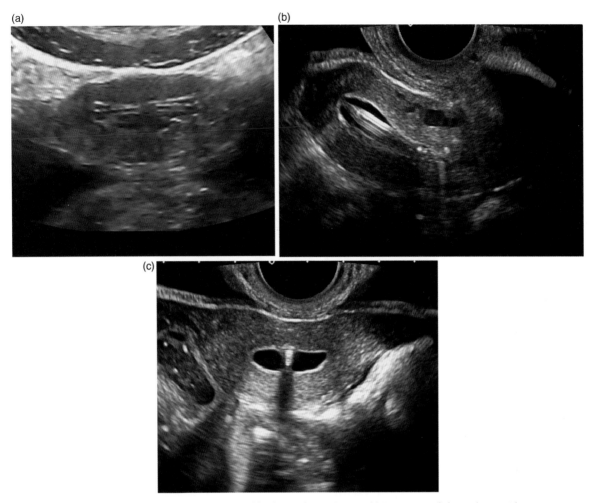

(c)

Figure 5.19 Case history: A lady referred with abnormal bleeding with an IUS in situ. (a) A transverse abdominal view without contrast. The arms of the IUS frame are visible but the endometrium cannot be assessed. (b) A transvaginal longitudinal view with gel contrast. (c) A transvaginal midline transverse view with gel contrast. Instilling the gel reveals regular thin endometrium that can be examined throughout the cavity.

(a)

(b)

(c)

(d)

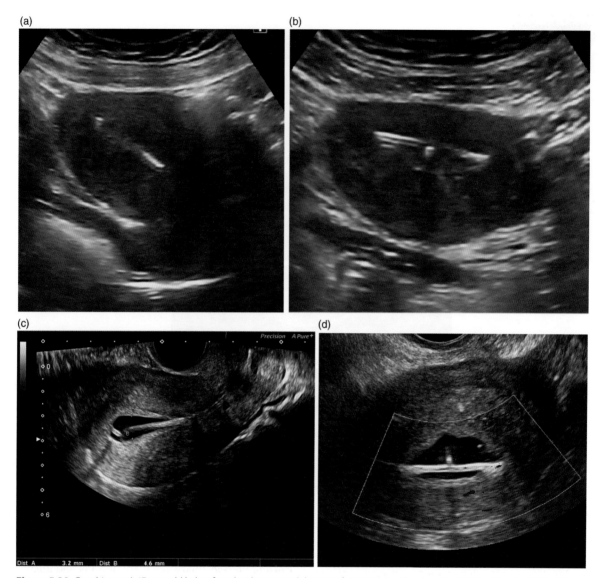

| Dist A | 3.2 mm | Dist B | 4.6 mm |

Figure 5.20 Case history: A 47-year-old lady referred with a 4-month history of intermenstrual and post coital bleeding. An IUD had been in situ for 4 years. (a, b) The figures are longitudinal and transverse TA views showing a normal size anteverted uterus with an IUD centrally situated. However, the endometrium cannot be visualised. (c, d) The figures show instillation of gel outlines regular normal thickness endometrium (can be measured) throughout the cavity with no polyps. A Pipelle biopsy contained malignant cells although not obviously endometrial. Subsequent investigation confirmed stage 1 B cervical cancer.

Ultrasound of Abnormal Pelvic Anatomy: Benign Pathology

Mary Pillai

6.1   Introduction   87
6.2   The Uterus – Myometrium   87
6.3   Fibroids – FIGO Classification   87
6.4   Myometrial Scars   89
6.5   Adenomyosis   91
6.6   Congenital Uterine Anomalies/Variants   93
6.7   The Endometrium   95
6.8   Synechiae   97
6.9   Adnexal Masses   98

6.10   Fallopian Tubes   102
6.11   Tubo-Ovarian Abscess   105
6.12   Cysts of the Parametrium and Peritoneal
        Inclusion Cysts   105
6.13   The Ovary: Differentiating Benign Adnexal
        Pathology from Malignancy   106
6.14   Benign Ovarian Masses   109
6.15   Adnexal Torsion   113
6.16   Follow-Up   113
6.17   Summary   114

6.1 Introduction

Ultrasound is the imaging of choice for any woman with a suspected pelvic pathology including any pelvic mass. It has good sensitivity and specificity for distinguishing benign conditions like fibroids, endometriomas and dermoid cysts, and for differentiating between benign and malignant ovarian pathology.

6.2 The Uterus – Myometrium

The most common pelvic masses are fibroids. Uterine fibroids (also called leiomyomas or myomas) are benign tumours of the uterus and are clinically apparent in around 50 per cent of Caucasian women by the time of completing reproductive age, and are more common among women of Afro-Caribbean race. A high proportion of fibroids are asymptomatic and may be found coincidentally when pelvic imaging is performed for an unrelated indication. Clinically fibroids present with a variety of symptoms including heavy menstrual bleeding, dysmenorrhoea and intermenstrual bleeding (see Chapter 13). When they are large there may be pressure symptoms such as a sensation of bloatedness or increased urinary frequency.

Where there is a large pelvic mass, transabdominal ultrasound will be essential to provide an adequate field of view to evaluate the mass (Figure 6.1a,b). Once a pelvic mass is greater than 6 cms in diameter it will usually lie beyond the range and focal region of a transvaginal probe (Figure 6.1c). In addition, it is important to assess the kidneys and bladder to report whether or not there is any evidence of ureteric obstruction/hydronephrosis due to pressure from a large pelvic mass (Figure 6.2a,b). Normally positioned kidneys are easily recognised when scanning in the right and left renal angles.

Apart from pregnancy, the two main conditions causing uterine enlargement are fibroids and adenomyosis. These conditions arise within the myometrium, which is best assessed with a combination of TA and TV ultrasound. Fibroids should be described according to their position, size (measured in three dimensions), shape, outline and texture. Traditionally they have been referred to as cervical, submucus, intramural, subserosal and pedunculated. These have been further described in the FIGO classification.

6.3 Fibroids – FIGO Classification

The FIGO classification describes fibroid types as 0–7, which are position dependent (Figure 6.3).[1]

Depending on the relationship to the cavity and myometrium, submucus fibroids are classified as

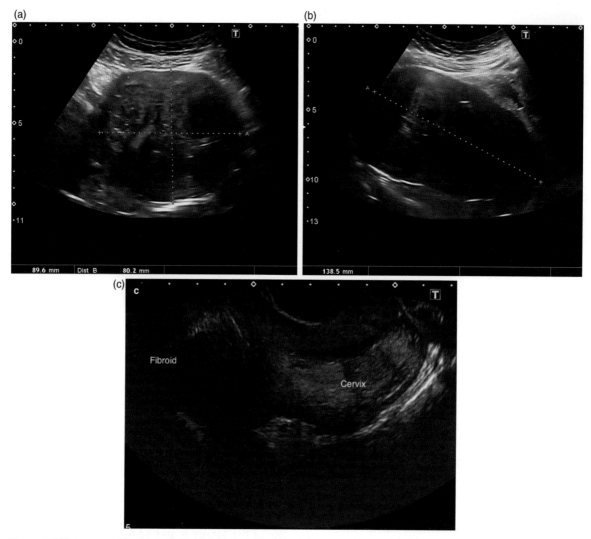

Figure 6.1 TA transverse (a) and longitudinal (b) ultrasound images of a large pelvic mass, found to be a large fibroid uterus (8.9 cm × 8.0 × 13.9 cm). (c) Longitudinal TV image of the uterus. The size of the mass is well beyond the field of view of a TV transducer so only the cervix below the mass can be imaged by the transvaginal route.

type 0, 1 or 2 (Figures 6.4a–c, 6.5a,b, 6.6). Intramural or interstitial fibroids are classified as type 3 (Figure 6.7) or type 4 (Figure 6.8a,b). In practice large intramural fibroids may extend from the endometrial border through the full thickness of myometrium to include a subserosal component (type 3–type 5 – Figure 6.9a,b). Subserous fibroids are classified as types 5, 6 or 7 with type 7 being attached to the serosa by a pedicle (Figures 6.10 and 6.11). In clinical practice the classification of submucus fibroids has greatest relevance since these are the fibroids that most likely cause symptoms, and their size and position will help determine the most appropriate treatment options.

The extent to which the cavity is distorted by fibroid(s) determines whether an IUS may be retained and successful at controlling HMB. The size and percentage of fibroid within the cavity determines its suitability for hysteroscopic fibroid resection. So in clinical practice categorising type 0, 1 and 2 fibroids has greatest importance in assessing the most appropriate treatment options.

Intracavitary lesions that are attached to the endometrium by a narrow stalk are classified as type 0 (also sometimes called fibroid polyps – Figure 6.4), whereas types 1 and 2 require a portion of the lesion to be intramural, with type 1 being less than

(a)

(b)

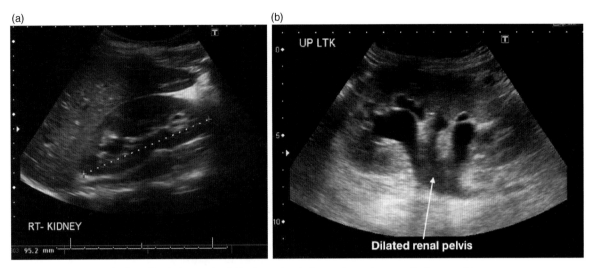

Figure 6.2 (a) A normal kidney. (b) A kidney with mild hydronephrosis due to obstructive uropathy from a pelvic mass.

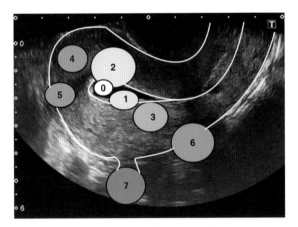

Figure 6.3 FIGO classification of fibroids. In addition to types 0–7 illustrated, fibroids may arise within the cervix or within the peritoneum in a rare condition called leiomyomatosis peritonei.

50 per cent intramural (Figure 6.5) and type 2 at least 50 per cent intramural (Figure 6.6). Type 3–7 fibroids are extracavitary and therefore unsuitable for hysteroscopic assessment or treatment. They are less likely to be associated with HMB, IUS expulsion or failure of the IUS to control HMB. Type 3 fibroids may just abut the endometrium (Figure 6.7), while type 4 lesions are intramural leiomyomas that are entirely within the myometrium, with no extension to the endometrial surface or to the serosa (Figure 6.8). Subserosal leiomyomas (types 5–7) represent the mirror image of the submucosal leiomyoma, with type 5 being at least 50 per cent intramural, type 6 being less than 50 per cent intramural (Figure 6.10)

and type 7 'pedunculated' being attached to the serosa by a stalk (Figure 6.11). In addition to the FIGO types, fibroids may arise within the cervix or very rarely as disseminated nodules within the peritoneum (Leiomyomatosis peritonei).

In many cases fibroids are multiple and include a range of types (Figure 6.12a,b). Long-standing fibroids may calcify.

6.3.1 Leiomyosarcoma

In contrast to fibroids, leiomyosarcoma are very rare (Chapter 15). Pelvic imaging cannot distinguish between sarcoma and fibroids, but typically the peak age of the former is around 60 years and the typical ultrasound appearance is mixed echogenicity with central necrosis and irregular vessels with low impedance and high flow. Whereas the natural history of fibroids is to regress following the menopause, the appearance of a 'fibroid' mass or growth of a fibroid following the menopause – often associated with postmenopausal bleeding – should be regarded as potential malignancy.

6.4 Myometrial Scars

A myometrial scar will appear as a hypoechoic linear defect through the full thickness of the myometrium. Most are in the characteristic position of a lower segment caesarean section (Figure 6.13). Often there is an inverted V shaped defect and just occasionally there is a wide or irregular defect in the myometrium

89

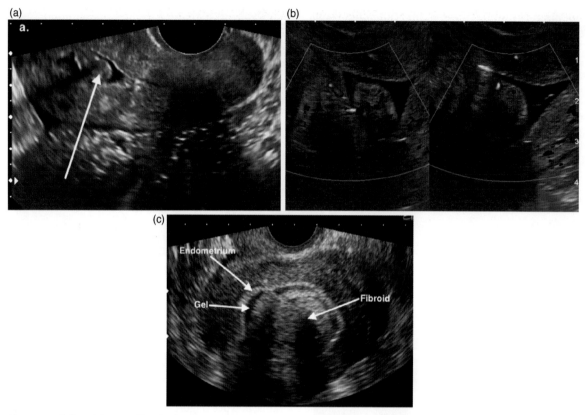

Figure 6.4 (a, b and c) Type 0 fibroids of varying sizes, outlined with gel contrast demonstrating that they lie completely within the endometrial cavity. All three cases had been referred for IUS fitting to manage heavy menstrual bleeding.

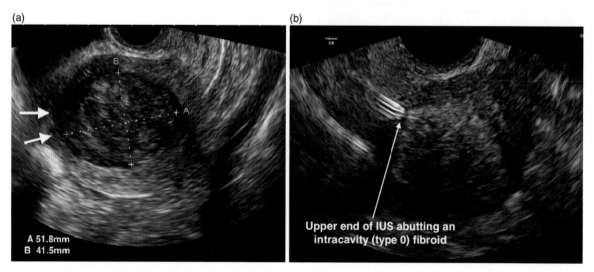

Figure 6.5 (a) Type 1 fibroid – its central location and size are consistent with the fibroid filling the endometrial cavity; however, the thin mantel of myometrium at the uterine fundus (arrows) indicates its depth extends into most of the myometrial thickness. Both the size and myometrial depth of this fibroid make it relatively unsuitable for hysteroscopic resection. (b) A type 0 fibroid is filling the endometrial cavity, resulting in low placement of an IUS.

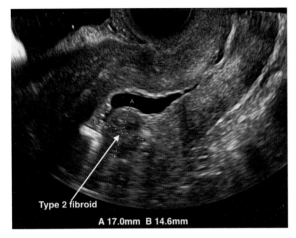

Figure 6.6 A small type 2 fibroid has been outlined by gel contrast in the endometrial cavity. Although more than 50 per cent of this fibroid lies within the myometrium, it is relatively small so there is a 'safe' thickness of myometrium between the fibroid and the uterine serosa such that the resection could be contemplated.

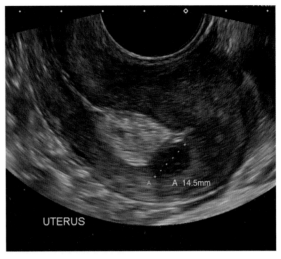

Figure 6.7 A type 3 fibroid measuring 14.5 mm lies 100 per cent within the myometrium just abutting the cavity fundus.

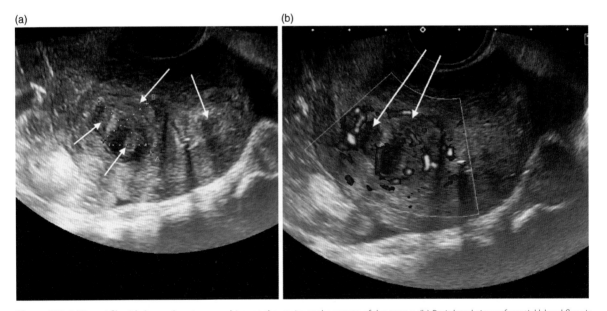

Figure 6.8 (a) Type 4 fibroids (arrows), not encroaching on the cavity or the serosa of the uterus. (b) Peripheral circumferential blood flow is typical of fibroids.

(Figure 6.14a,b). There is currently insufficient data to establish the significance of a myometrial defect in relation to future pregnancy.

6.5 Adenomyosis

Adenomyosis is essentially endometrial tissue invading and forming small cystic spaces in the myometrium and can be considered a variant of endometriosis. It is extremely common in late reproductive years, being found in a high proportion of hysterectomy specimens. Estimates of the frequency range widely from 5 per cent to 70 per cent. Histologically adenomyosis is defined as the presence of ectopic endometrial glands and stroma within the

(a) (b)

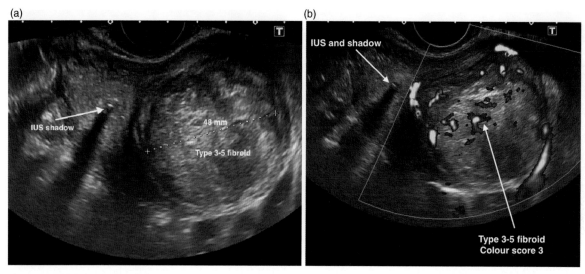

Figure 6.9 (a) Type 3–5 fibroid. This extends from bordering on the cavity to the subserosal surface of the uterus. The position of the endometrial cavity can be judged from the IUS shadow (arrowed). (b) The same image with Doppler demonstrating typical peripheral flow seen with a fibroid.

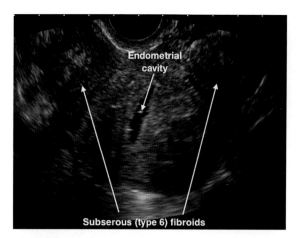

Figure 6.10 Type 6 subserous fibroids (long arrows) with > 50 per cent of the fibroid mass protruding outside the serosal surface. The position of the endometrial cavity is demonstrated by the gel content.

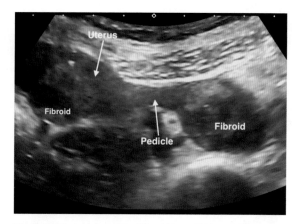

Figure 6.11 A pedunculated fibroid (type 7). The pedicle is arrowed.

myometrium. Most patients with adenomyosis are asymptomatic, but it can be a cause of significant dysmenorrhoea and diffuse uterine enlargement (Figure 6.15a–d). Cysts in the myometrium are a more specific ultrasound feature (Figure 6.15c).[2–4] Adenomyosis is most common on the posterior wall of the uterus adjacent to the recto-uterine space, which results in asymmetric diffuse enlargement of the uterus, although asymmetry is a non-specific finding. Adenomyosis can occur in a localised area, but more often is diffuse through the full thickness of the myometrium giving an ultrasonic appearance of an enlarged globular uterus, particularly with asymmetric thickening of the myometrium and multiple small cystic spaces in the myometrium (Figures 6.15a–c and 11.3). The anechoic spaces are often surrounded by bright tissue that causes radial linear shadows to be cast (sometimes called 'rain in the forest' – Figure 11.3, p. 185). The junctional zone tends to be irregular and interrupted such that the endometrial–myometrial border becomes obscured.

Where the only feature appears to be asymmetric myometrial thickening, it is important to

(a)   (b)

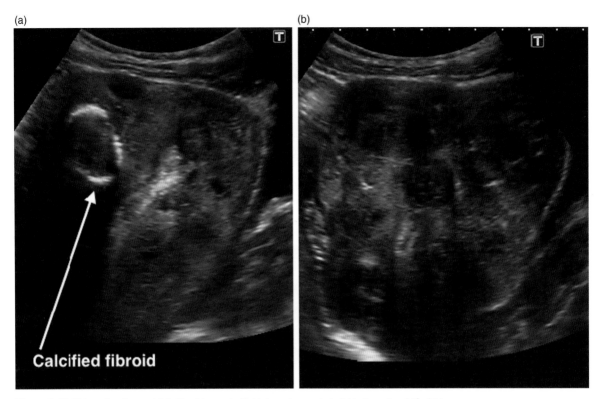

Figure 6.12 This patient has multiple fibroids, most of which are hypoechoic (b) but one is calcified (a).

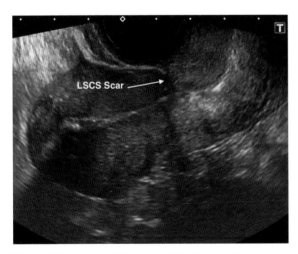

Figure 6.13 A myometrial scar identifying the site of a previous caesarean section.

observe the uterus for consistency of this finding as a uterine contraction may give the same impression but this will not be constant over time (Figure 6.16). The normal uterine vascular pattern with arcuate arteries peripherally giving rise to radial vessels running horizontally through the myometrium is preserved with adenomyosis (Figure 6.15d) but disrupted by fibroids, which typically demonstrate vessels running circumferentially in the periphery of the fibroid.

6.6 Congenital Uterine Anomalies/ Variants

Ultrasound is the most common means of assessing congenital uterine variants, which occur in approximately 1–5 per cent of women and result from incomplete fusion of the Müllerian ducts during early prenatal development (Figure 6.17a–d).

When a variant is identified, it is appropriate to check that both kidneys are present as there is a significantly higher rate of unilateral renal agenesis or pelvic kidney (Figure 6.18) in association with Müllerian tract anomalies.

Uterus didelphys (double uterus) has two cervices with separate endometrial cavities that do not coalesce (Figure 6.19a). There may be an associated longitudinal vaginal septum arising between the cervices, ending superior to the hymen.

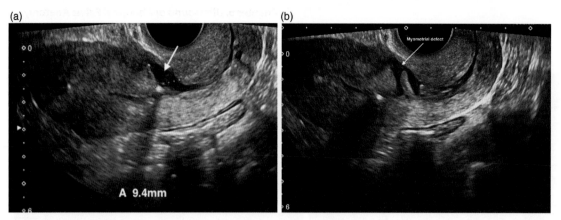

Figure 6.14 (a) A 9.4 mm myometrial defect (arrowed) at the site of a healed caesarean scar is demonstrated following instillation of gel contrast. (b) Irregular tissue within the defect.

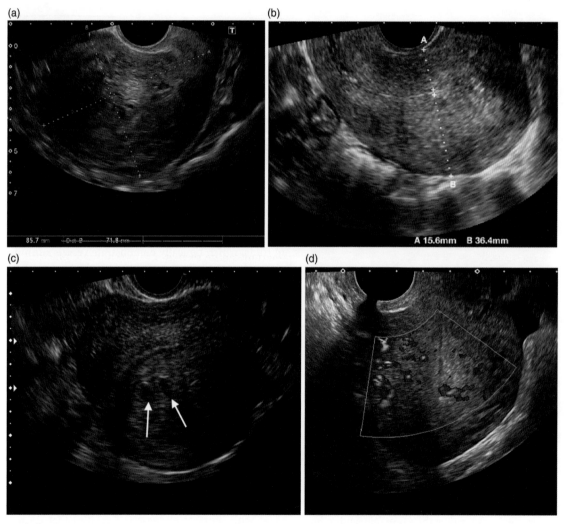

Figure 6.15 (a) Typical features of adenomyosis with diffuse enlargement of the uterine corpus. The endometrial–myometrial border is so indistinct that the endometrium cannot be distinguished, and the thickened myometrium contains multiple small cystic spaces. (b) There is asymmetric thickening differentially greater in the posterior uterine wall and no distinct endometrial–myometrial junction. (c) The uterus is globular but asymmetric with large cystic spaces (arrows) in the thickened posterior wall. (d) This case shows globular enlargement of the uterus which is relatively symmetrical and there is preservation of the radial pattern of blood flow in the inner two-thirds of the myometrium.

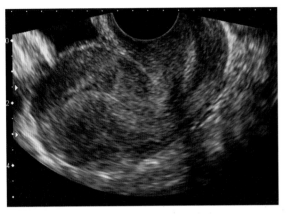

Figure 6.16 A uterine contraction gives the impression of asymmetric myometrial thickness. However, unlike adenomyosis there is no radial shadowing and there are no cystic spaces, and if observed over time it could be confirmed that the contraction and hence the shape is not constant.

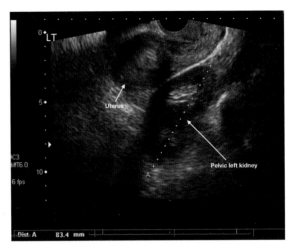

Figure 6.18 A pelvic kidney is demonstrated adjacent to the uterus.

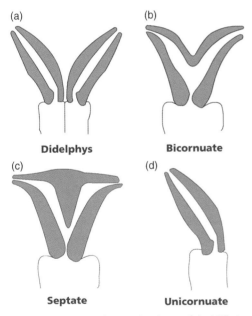

(a) Didelphys   (b) Bicornuate   (c) Septate   (d) Unicornuate

Figure 6.17 Types of incomplete fusion of the Müllerian ducts.

A septate uterus has a midline septum dividing the cavity and has a flat or convex external fundal contour, which is always 10 mm or more above a line drawn between the fundal tips of the endometrial cavities (Figure 6.19c).

On a transverse view moving from the cervix to the fundus the cavity can be seen to divide and the two halves move further apart toward the fundus (Figure 6.20a–d). The cavities show flat medial margins unlike the convex ones seen in a bicornuate uterus. The septum may be complete down to the cervix, or partial (when the uterus is called subseptate – Figure 6.21).

Similarly a bicornuate uterus has a single cervix leading to an endometrial canal that divides into separate right and left cavities each connected to a fallopian tube. The difference from a septate uterus is the convex shape of the fundus or fundal dimple (Figure 6.22a), and the separated endometrial cavities are convex medially and leaf-like in shape. The myometrial margin can be seen as a thin echogenic line dipping between the cavities. Unlike a uterine septum, the tissue separating the two halves of a bicornuate cavity cannot be resected. Pregnancy can arise in either 'horn' (Figures 6.22a,b), and beyond the first trimester the bicornuate shape is not usually obvious.

An arcuate uterus is the most common variant, with no significant clinical associations or implications. The external fundal contour is normal (flat or convex) and the intercornual mid-portion of the endometrial cavity dips down producing a heart-shaped cavity (Figure 6.23). A line drawn from the two cornua to the lower most mid-portion of the endometrium between the cornua has an obtuse angle > 90 degrees.

6.7 The Endometrium

Measuring endometrial thickness is essential in a woman with post-menopausal bleeding and is discussed in more detail in Chapter 4. The accepted convention is that the measurement is made in the

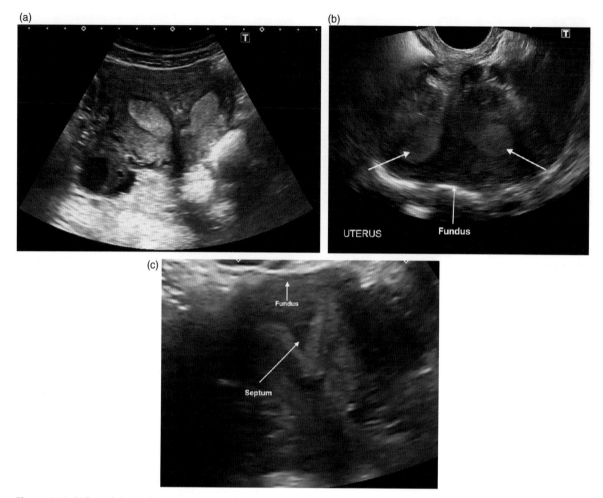

Figure 6.19 (a) Transabdominal view in transverse plane showing a uterus didelphys. The relatively echogenic endometrial outline shows that the two cavities remain separate all the way down to the cervices. (b) Similarly, on the transvaginal image the two endometrial cavities (arrows) do not merge. (NB. It is difficult to image two cervices simultaneously with either TA or TV routes.) (c) A septate uterus with a convex fundus significantly higher than the apices of the bifid cornual regions. The long arrow points to the septum dividing the cavity.

antero-posterior diameter on a long axis image and includes the double thickness. Measurement is made by placing the callipers on the outer edge (or endometrial–myometrial border) on one side to that on the other side where the thickness appears the greatest (Figure 6.24a). In order to obtain a reliable and reproducible endometrial measurement, it is essential to obtain the measurement before endometrial sampling or curettage. Where the endometrial–myometrial border is too indistinct to be seen clearly on ultrasound, the measurement cannot be made and should be reported as such (Figure 6.24b) to avoid misleading clinical evaluation. It is important to visualise the totality of the endometrium from the cervix to the fundus and from cornua to cornua. Where the endometrium cannot be seen clearly due to there being an irregular edge or no distinct difference between the endometrium and myometrium, it cannot be measured accurately and should be regarded as abnormal.[5] It may be possible to enhance the endometrial–myometrial border by filling the cavity with negative contrast (Figure 6.25a,b). Where this clarifies, the endometrial–myometrial border two single thicknesses can be measured and added so the space occupied by contrast is not included in the measurement (Chapter 5).

Endometrial thickening has low specificity for cancer as it can be due to a polyp or clot within the cavity, simple hyperplasia, submucus fibroid(s) or

(a) (b) (c) (d)

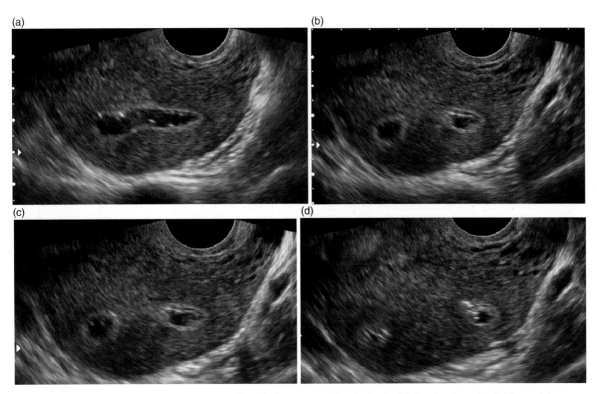

Figure 6.20 A Septate uterus. (a–d) Transverse views from the lower cavity (a) to the fundus (d) showing the cavity dividing and the two halves widely separated at the fundus. Insertion of gel has enhanced the anatomy. There is no dip in the fundal myometrium between the bifid cavity, as would be seen with a bicornuate arrangement.

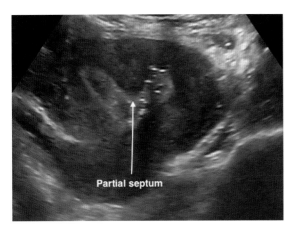

Partial septum

Figure 6.21 A transabdominal view of a subseptate uterus. The fundal myometrium is at least 10 mm above the cornual ends of the cavities and the partial septum divides just the upper cavity into two halves.

artefact, and also may be associated with Tamoxifen therapy (Figure 6.26a,b).

Large polyps typically have a single or two feeding vessels and may be outlined on a stalk by the instillation of negative contrast (Chapter 5). The presence of abundant vascularity in thickened endometrium in a woman of peri- or post-menopausal age is highly suspicious of cancer (Chapter 15), but overall blood flow assessment has low sensitivity and specificity for the diagnosis of endometrial cancer.

6.8 Synechiae

These are fibrotic bands or adhesions that traverse the endometrial cavity (Figure 6.27a,b). They may form due to chronic endometritis or following hysteroscopic surgery to the endometrium, fibroids or a septum, or they may follow morbid placental adherence particularly where manual removal was required. They are unlikely to be diagnosed on conventional ultrasound imaging, but when the cavity is filled with contrast or alternatively when there is a pregnancy in the uterus they are likely to be seen, particularly during the first half of gestation when

(a)　　　　　　　　　　　　　　　　　　　　　(b)

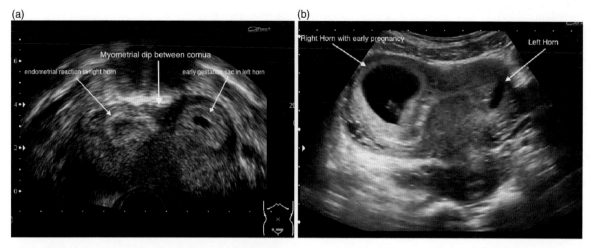

Figure 6.22 (a) An early pregnancy in the left horn of a bicornuate uterus. (b) A pregnancy in the right horn of a bicornuate uterus.

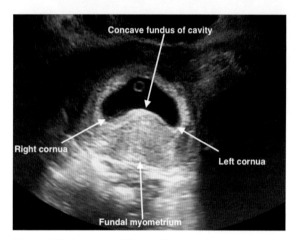

Figure 6.23 A transverse TV view of an arcuate uterus containing an early pregnancy with a yolk sac.

they may incorrectly be diagnosed as 'amniotic bands' (Figure 6.27c).

6.9 Adnexal Masses

6.9.1 Terminology

- An adnexal mass is a structure lying between the uterus and pelvic sidewall that is inconsistent with normal physiology.
- Where it is fluid filled it may contain septae. A septum is defined as a band of tissue connecting one internal wall of a cyst to the opposite internal wall.
- Where a septum does not meet the opposite wall it is termed incomplete (typically seen in diseased fallopian tubes).

- A solid component in an adnexal mass which has relatively high echogenicity is suggestive of tissue (myometrium, ovarian stroma, myomas).
- The 'white ball' in a dermoid is not solid tissue (it is hair, fat and sebaceous material).
- Blood clot tends to have a characteristic heterogenic appearance, but if in doubt should be classified as solid tissue.
- When in doubt, apply gentle pressure with the probe. Pushing on the lesion together with application of Colour Doppler may help, since clot may wobble and will not contain any flow.
- The internal cyst wall is described as smooth or irregular. A solid area less than 3 mm in the cyst wall is an irregular cyst wall (Figure 6.28a). The external wall of the cyst is not taken into account.
- A papillary projection is solid tissue protruding into the cyst cavity measuring at least 3 mm from the cyst wall (Figure 6.28b,c).
- Ascites is free fluid outside the pouch of Douglas (utero-rectal space) (Figure 6.29).

The content of cysts may be

- Anechogenic (clear) (Figure 6.30).
- Low level (Figure 6.31).
- Haemorrhagic (Figures 6.32a–d).
- Mixed (Figure 6.33a,b).
- Ground glass (Figure 6.34a–d).

Many women have what appear to be benign adnexal masses. In most cases removal with surgery

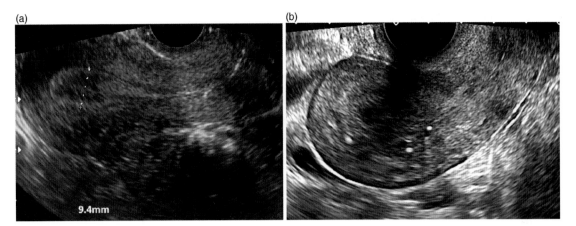

Figure 6.24 (a) A long axis TV view of the uterus demonstrating the endometrial thickness measurement on day 12 of the cycle. (b) The endometrium too indistinct for ultrasound assessment.

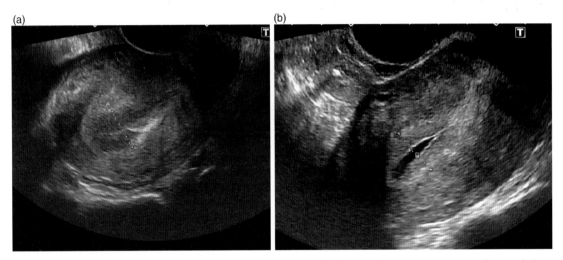

Figure 6.25 (a) The endometrial–myometrial border appears irregular and indistinct so the measurement cannot be regarded as accurate. (b) The endometrium has been enhanced with gel contrast which clarifies a distinct regular endometrial–myometrial junction. The two separate thicknesses can now be measured and added to give the double thickness.

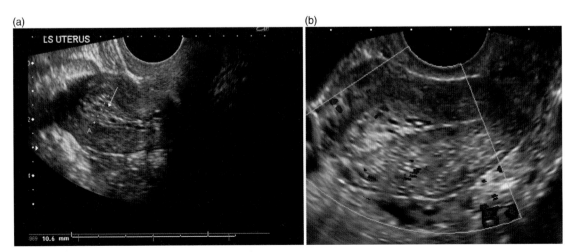

Figure 6.26 (a) Thickened cystic endometrium (arrow) in a post-menopausal woman taking Tamoxifen. (b) Colour Doppler shows small flow in the endometrium (colour score 2).

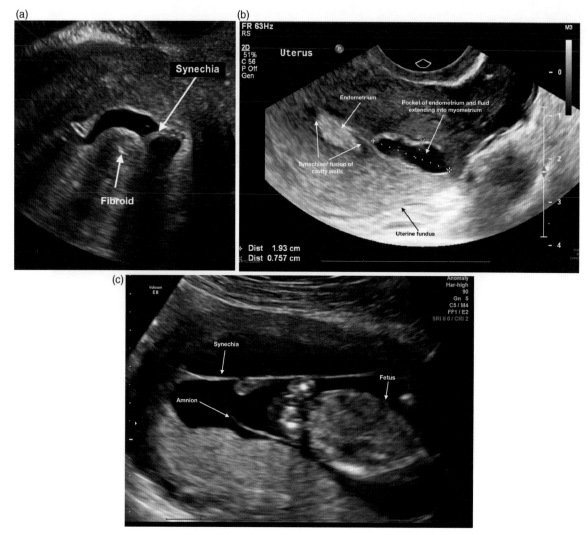

Figure 6.27 (a) This cavity adhesion was revealed when gel contrast was instilled to determine the extent of the submucus fibroid. (b) This scan was performed to investigate return of cyclical bleeding and pain two years following endometrial ablation. It suggests there is fusion of the cavity walls around a pocket of endometrium, and at the fundus there is a fluid-filled pocket within the myometrium. (c) A routine dating scan revealed a cavity adhesion. Although this linear band of tissue appears to run through the gestation sac, it is in reality outside and separate to the sac which fills the space all around the adhesion. With increasing uterine enlargement this type of adhesion will usually disappear.

is not necessary. However, surgery is often performed unnecessarily, for fear that these masses could be malignant. Applying established rules with careful ultrasound assessment should enable differentiation between benign and malignant masses in most cases.

However, there is still a paucity of information available to know how and when to follow up benign masses, or which may have a higher risk of becoming cancer.

The IOTA classification is the best method for distinguishing benign from borderline and malignant adnexal masses.[6] Further detail is included in Chapter 15.

Masses refer to a variety of structures, including but not limited to:

- ovarian cysts: fluid-filled sacs within or attached to an ovary;
- ovarian and metastatic tumours: can be solid tissue or a combination of cysts and solid tissue;

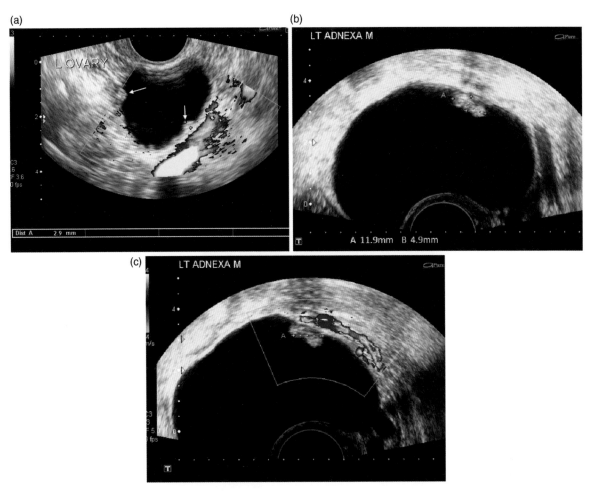

Figure 6.28 (a) An irregular cyst wall with solid projections < 3 mm from the base. (b) To use the IOTA description this is a unlocular-solid cyst with one papilla and a colour score 1 (c). Simple descriptors do not apply. There was no ascites. (c) Doppler shows no flow in the papilla (colour score 1). There are no M and no B features so the nature of this is uncertain and may be borderline.

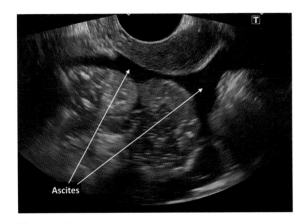

Figure 6.29 Ascites.

- hydro, pyo or haematosalpinges: fluid collections in the fallopian tube;
- fimbrial cysts may be mistaken for ovarian cysts;
- para tubal cysts: fluid-filled collections within the tubal mesentery that may be mistaken for ovarian cysts.

6.9.2 Classification System for Adnexal Masses

Benign Non-ovarian

- paratubal
- hydrosalpinges
- tubo-ovarian abscess
- peritoneal pseudocysts

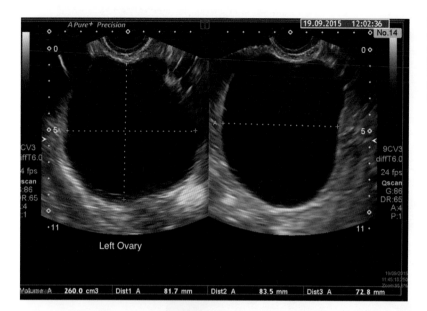

Figure 6.30 A unilocular anechoic mass with regular walls and a maximum diameter < 10 cm is consistent with a simple cyst or cystadenoma. No blood flow was demonstrated. The simple descriptor can be used here to make a diagnosis.

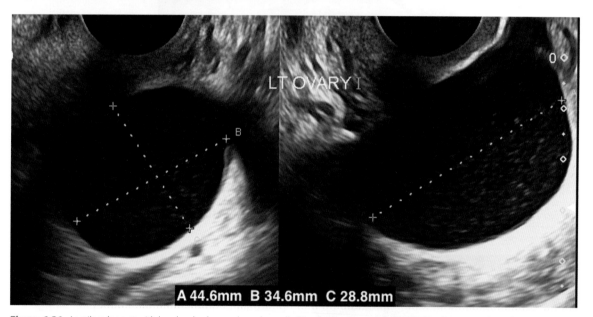

Figure 6.31 A unilocular cyst with low-level echos and regular walls. Simple descriptors can be used to determine this is benign, likely to be a cystadenoma.

- appendiceal abscess
- diverticular abscess
- pelvic kidney

Benign Ovarian:
- polycystic ovaries
- functional cysts
- endometriomas
- serous cystadenoma
- mucinous cystadenoma
- mature teratoma
- fibroma (rare)
- thecoma (very rare, can be hormone secreting).

6.10 Fallopian Tubes

Healthy fallopian tubes are not normally seen on conventional ultrasound imaging. However, when the

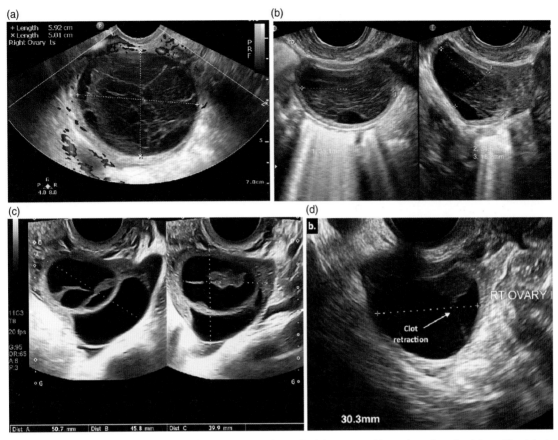

Figure 6.32 (a and b) The reticular or 'cobweb' appearance within each of these cysts with regular walls and no internal flow is instantly recognisable as a haemorrhagic cyst. (c and d) Haemorrhagic cysts will change with resolution over time. Clot retraction can give the appearance of septae. Movement can help to clarify this is clot as it will jiggle.

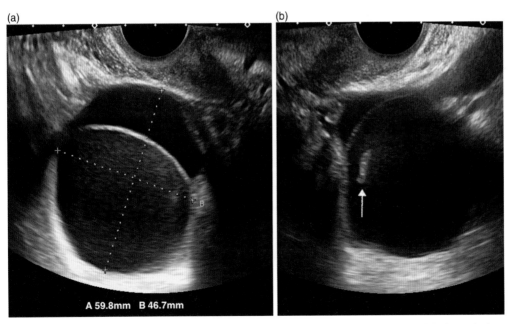

Figure 6.33 (a and b) A mixed cyst showing two locules. The fluid in one locule appears anechoic while that in the bigger locule has low-level echos. The more echogenic area in the bigger locule (arrowed) was not attached to the cyst wall and could be described as 'sludge'.

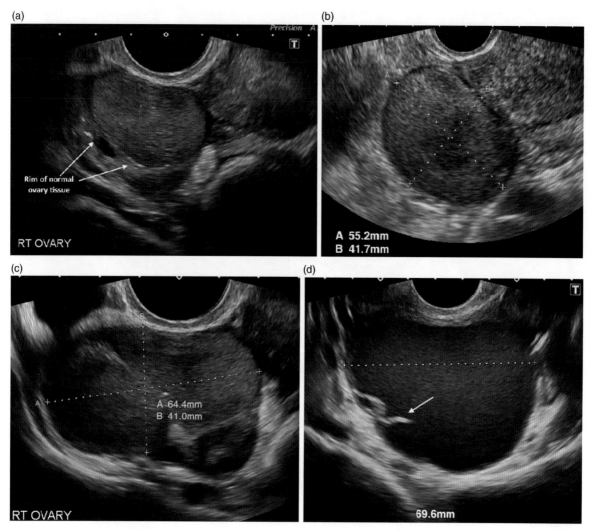

Figure 6.34 The characteristic 'ground glass' appearance within the cyst content and pre-menopausal status of these four different cases make all of these instantly recognisable as endometriomas.

tube is filled with fluid, it can readily be seen. On a longitudinal view it will appear tubular or sausage-shaped with thin walls and incomplete septae (Figures 6.35a–c). On cross-section it may have a cogwheel appearance. The lack of peristalsis helps differentiate it from a fluid-filled segment of bowel. Visualisation of the ovary as a separate structure also helps to clarify whether the fluid-filled structure is tubal in origin. Tubal pathology is typically a complication of chlamydia or gonorrhoea, representing ascending infection involving the tube, or it may be haemorrhage associated with ectopic pregnancy. More rarely it is due to pelvic actinomycosis,

which is typically associated with long-term use of a copper coil which has become colonised.

Upper genital tract Chlamydia is typically asymptomatic, presenting only during investigation of subfertility. Gonorrhoea is more likely to be symptomatic, presenting with fever and pelvic pain, with significant tenderness.

Where the fluid-filled structure is a chronic hydrosalpinx, this will not usually change in appearance on successive scans. Fimbrial cysts can also give rise to a simple cyst within the pelvis. These look very similar to simple ovarian cysts, except that no ovarian

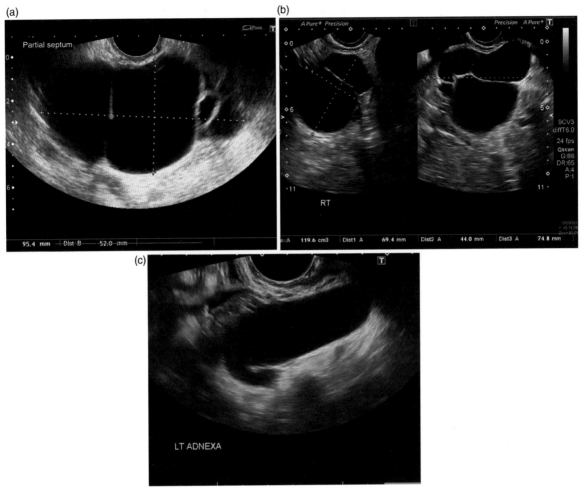

Figure 6.35 (a) A large hydrosalpinx. It is recognisable as tubal due to the incomplete septum. (b) A smaller hydrosalpinx superior to a simple right ovarian cyst. The hydrosalpinx has the typical sausage shape with a clubbed end. (c) A tubular hydrosalpinx with no septae.

tissue will be visible around the cyst capsule and the ovaries may be identified separately.

If there is uncertainty about the nature of a cystic structure, a follow-up scan is useful. Suggested time-scales for follow-up is covered in Section 6.16.

6.11 Tubo-Ovarian Abscess

In severe cases, pelvic infection may also involve the ovary. Ultrasound features can be variable and typic-ally there is mixed echogenicity with abundant blood flow. Sometimes the abnormal tube and adherent ovary can be distinguished (Figure 6.36a) and some-times the appearance may be more bizarre due to differing consistency of the content of the infected

tube (Figure 6.36b). A tubo-ovarian pelvic mass will typically appear as a thick-walled heterogenous com-plex adnexal lesion (Figure 6.36c). Thickened endo-metrium and other signs of hydrosalpinges may be present. Pus-filled fallopian tubes may appear multi-locular and thick walled with incomplete septae, filled with inflammatory echogenic fluid of ground glass or mixed appearance. Pelvic actinomycosis can mimic malignancy (Chapter 10, Case 8).

6.12 Cysts of the Parametrium and Peritoneal Inclusion Cysts

Peritoneal inclusion cysts, also referred to as pseu-docysts, are cystic structures within the pelvis that

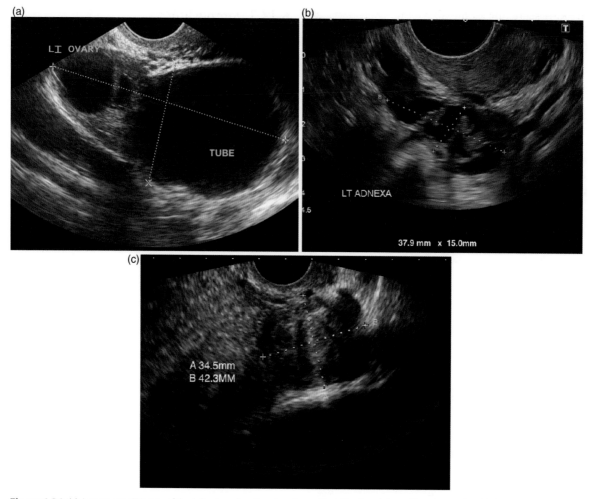

Figure 6.36 (a) A transverse TV view of the left adnexal region showing a dilated hydrosalpinx adjacent to and probably adherent to the left ovary. (b) A TV view of the left adnexal region showing a complex tubular structure with contrasting hyper and hypoechoic areas (measured). There was flow outside but not within the tubular structure. This appearance is consistent with pus within the fallopian tube. (c) A small complex mass in the left adnexal region in a woman with a recent history of pelvic pain and discharge and a long-term IUD. The variable echogenicity, clinical history and pain on applying pressure to the area make an inflammatory tube-ovarian mass most likely. No ovarian structure could be visualised separately in the left adnexa. The differential diagnosis might include a pedunculated fibroid.

entrap peritoneal fluid. These cysts primarily occur following pelvic surgery or infection and result from pelvic adhesions. Ultrasound characteristics include multiple primarily thin but occasionally thick septations that attach to pelvic organs such as the uterus, bowel and ovaries giving unusual shaped fluid collections with angulated rather than ovoid margins (Figure 6.37). The fluid content is typically anechoic, and normal looking ovaries may be seen separately, helping to confirm the diagnosis. Peritoneal inclusion cysts are typically asymptomatic and women are commonly referred with the finding of a septated

pelvic mass diagnosed on CT scan or MRI. Inquiring about the patient's surgical history is important, as pelvic adhesions from prior pelvic surgery is a common aetiological factor for peritoneal inclusion cysts.

6.13 The Ovary: Differentiating Benign Adnexal Pathology from Malignancy

Several models have been developed to characterise adnexal masses on ultrasound in order to improve differentiation between benign and malignant lesions.[7]

The RMI score utilises the ultrasound characteristics (scoring 1 for each of: multilocular cysts, solid areas, metastases, ascites and bilateral lesions and 0 for the absence of these) the Ca 125, and the menopausal status. This algorithm has been widely used as it is simple and reproducible; however, its main disadvantage is that it cannot account for the range of benign pathologies (including endometriosis in pre-menopausal women) which raise the Ca 125 level.[7] The best evaluated alternative strategy is application of the simple rules for evaluating any adnexal mass defined by the IOTA group. B (benign) and M (malignant) descriptors are summarised in Table 6.1.

6.13.1 Simple Descriptors

Certain abnormalities can readily be diagnosed by pattern recognition on ultrasound imaging. These include endometrioma, cystic teratoma (dermoid), simple cyst or cystadenoma, functional cyst (for example, Haemorrhagic), and malignant tumour with ascites.

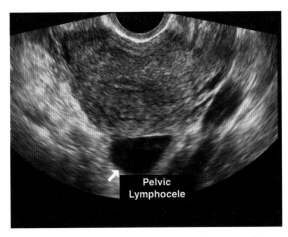

Figure 6.37 Collection of peritoneal fluid within pelvic adhesions (arrowed). The clue that this is not free fluid is that the shape of the collection is not following the contour of the cervix but is angulated where adhesions attach to pelvic structures.

6.13.2 Simple Rules

If the mass is not instantly recognisable, then simple descriptors do not apply and instead simple rules should be applied (Box 6.1).

6.13.3 Adnex Risk Calculator

Adnex estimates the probability that an adnexal tumour is benign, borderline, stage I cancer, stage II–IV cancer or secondary metastatic cancer (that is,

Table 6.1 IOTA Rules

B (Benign) Rules	M (Malignant) Rules
Unilocular	Irregular solid tumour
Presence of solid components where the largest solid component < 7 mm	Ascites (fluid outside the Pouch of Douglas)
Presence of acoustic shadowing	At least four papillary structures
Smooth multilocular tumour with a largest diameter < 100 mm	Irregular multilocular solid tumour with largest diameter ≥100 mm
No blood flow (colour score 1)	Highly vascular (colour score 4)

Table 6.2 Colour Score – Four Categories May Be Applied

Colour Score	Colour distribution	
1	No flow	Simple cyst or follicle (no or min flow)
2	Minimal flow	Endometrioma, benign tumour
3	Moderate flow	Preovulatory follicle, benign tumour (septa and wall)
4	High flow	Corpus luteum tubo-ovarian abscess, ovarian cancer (septa & wall)

Note: The importance of PRF is key to assessment of flow, see Chapter 2 p 24.

Box 6.1 Simple Rules

Rule 1. The mass is classified as malignant if at least one M-feature and no B-features are present.

Rule 2. The mass is classified as benign if at least one B-feature and no M-features are present.

Rule 3. If both M-features and B-features are present, or if no B or M features are present, the result is inconclusive and further investigation is recommended.

metastasis of non-adnexal cancer to the ovary). The model was developed by the IOTA group and is based on clinical and ultrasound data from almost 6,000 women recruited at 24 centres in 10 countries.

It can be accessed at www.iotagroup.org/adnexmodel/

The ultrasound assessment of the mass should answer all of the questions (1–9) that follow.

Box 6.2 Assessment of Adnexal Mass: Menopausal Status and Ultrasound Findings

1. whether the mass is cystic (uni or multilocular), solid and cystic, or predominately solid;
2. the appearance of the internal wall of the cyst:
   - thin smooth capsule
   - thick walled / irregular (projections < 3 mm from base);
3. papillary projections (> 3 mm) measured in number and two perpendicular planes – height and base width, and assessed for flow / colour score;
4. if solid, consider whether:
   - it is echo free or has internal echoes
   - it contains blood clot ('spiders web')
   - there is presence of vascularity within the mass using Colour Doppler
   - there are bright echoes
   - there is any calcification
   - there is acoustic enhancement ('bright up') or shadowing behind the mass
   - there is hair within
   - normal ovary is visible around the mass ('crescent sign')
   - the ovary is seen separate from the mass or not
   - the mass is smooth or irregular in outline
4. the size of the mass
5. if solid, the blood flow (colour score):
   - in the capsule
   - in the solid areas
6. whether the mass is persistent (seen on previous scans)
   - how has it changed?
7. if septa are seen within the mass
   - whether the septa are thin (<3 mm) or thick (>3 mm)
   - whether the septa are complete or incomplete
   - whether there are septal nodules
   - whether there is blood flow in the septa on Colour Doppler
8. if a mass is seen, is there evidence of:
   - free fluid in the recto-uterine space
9. depending on the size and appearance of the mass, whether there is any renal/ureteric dilatation/hydronephrosis

Case Example

A 37-year-old lady was noted to have a right adnexal cystic mass at 20 weeks of pregnancy during a routine anomaly scan. Transabdominal and transvaginal ultrasound assessment showed a multilocular cyst measuring 93.7 × 76.0 × 58.4 mms (Figure 6.38a). There were six locules with no solid areas and septae (some 4 mm thick and some thin). The content of the locules appeared uniformly anechoic on TA imaging but on TV imaging contained low-level echoes. The cyst wall appeared smooth with no irregularity or papillary projections. No colour flow was demonstrated and no free fluid was seen. The left ovary appeared normal. No separate right ovary or normal ovarian tissue was demonstrated around the cyst. Her Ca 125 was 66 U/ml. The IOTA–Adnex model gave a 96.1 per cent chance this was a benign cyst (Figure 6.38b). She was advised it could be managed conservatively and removed at a convenient time after the pregnancy or at delivery in the event she required a caesarean section. A follow-up scan six weeks postnatal showed the cyst appearance was unchanged but the dimensions were smaller (Figure 6.38c).

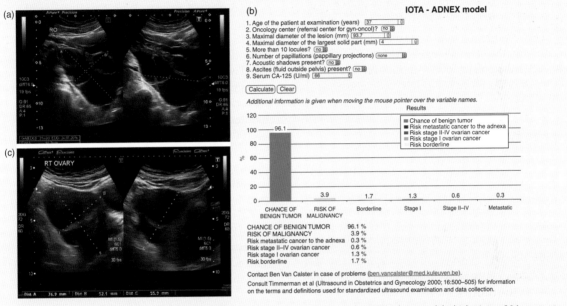

Figure 6.38 (a) A TA view of the multilocular cyst at 20 weeks gestation. (b) Shows the IOTA Adnex model which gives a 96.1 per cent likelihood this cyst will be benign. (c) Shows the appearance of the cyst at six weeks postnatal, which is largely unchanged.

6.14 Benign Ovarian Masses

Terms and Definitions/How to Classify

- Normal Ovary
- Functional Cyst
- Benign Masses
- Borderline Tumour
- Invasive Tumour
- Metastatic Tumour

Normal ovaries and functional cysts have been described in Chapter 4. Tumours are discussed in more depth in Chapter 15. An ovarian lesion is defined as part of an ovary inconsistent with normal physiology. The common benign ovarian lesions are summarised in the sections that follow.

6.14.1 Simple Cysts

These are smooth-walled ulilocular and contain anechoic fluid or fluid with low-level echoes. The majority are functional cysts or cystadenomas (Figures 6.30 and 6.31).

6.14.2 Haemorrhagic Cysts

These result from bleeding inside the ovary, typically in the vascular corpus luteum following ovulation, or other functional cyst. The area of haemorrhage is usually confined by the capsule of the ovary and goes through stages of clot formation, clot lysis, clot retraction and resolution (Figure 6.32a–d). Hence, unlike dermoids and endometriomas, the appearance is dependent on the stage of evolution of the cyst and will resolve spontaneously, usually within eight weeks. The reticular pattern of internal echoes (known as fishnet or cobweb) is due to fibrin strands, which show variable echogenicity. There is no flow within the cyst and circumferential flow in the wall of the cyst. As the clot retracts it may erroneously resemble a papillary projection. However, unlike the papillae in a complex solid/cystic ovarian mass, there will be no blood flow within the solid areas on Doppler imaging. In addition, the clot will 'jiggle' when agitated gently with a transvaginal probe. Alternatively the patient can be asked to move her pelvis to demonstrate this movement.

6.14.3 Endometriosis

Endometriosis, in the absence of endometriomas, is not so readily visible on ultrasound imaging. A structured terminology is being developed to accurately map the location and depth of endometriotic deposits with ultrasound to guide treatment, particularly where surgery is contemplated for complex invasive disease.[8] However this lies beyond the scope of this book. Laparoscopy remains the gold standard for diagnosis. The ovaries are thought to be involved in around 75 per cent of women with endometriosis, and when endometriomas are present in the pelvis, they are easily identified with ultrasound. The most characteristic appearance of an endometrioma is a hypoechoic adnexal cyst filled with homogeneous or 'ground glass' low level echoes (Figure 6.34a–d). These lie within the substance of the ovary, so they are surrounded by a rim of normal looking ovarian tissue (Figure 6.34a). There is good through transmission without acoustic shadowing that would be typical of a dermoid cyst. In other cases, endometriomas appear as cysts with fine septations or with a reticular pattern of septations similar to a haemorrhagic cyst. Endometriomas can be multilocular with areas of anechoic fluid and other areas of complex fluid separated by septations. Septations are typically thin but can be thick. There is no blood flow within an endometriotic cyst, and the presence of blood flow should raise suspicion of an endometriod type tumour. The

main differential however is often from a dermoid. Unlike a dermoid there tends to be excellent sound transmission deep to the lesion with no shadowing. Unlike haemorrhagic cysts, the appearance of endometriomas tends to remain relatively stable over time.

Endometriosis can take on a more sinister appearance in pregnancy, owing to decidualisation of the endometrial tissue (Figure 6.39a,b). Where there is uncertainty about the nature of a cyst, then CT or MRI may give a more definitive diagnosis. Clearly CT cannot be used in pregnancy; however, on MRI, the blood content of endometriomas appears bright on T1-weighted images. With fat saturation the signal remains bright further confirming the content is blood.

Endometriosis infiltrating the peritoneum and bowel wall is difficult to distinguish with conventional ultrasound imaging. The most common site is the rectovaginal septum where small hypoechogenic nodules may be seen on scan when there is deep infiltration. Typically the pelvic structures will not be freely mobile and cannot be demonstrated to slide when applying gentle pressure with the TV probe. The adherence to surrounding tissue may also give fixed angulated cystic structures. When bilateral this may give the classic 'kissing endometriomas' appearance (Figure 6.40). It is appropriate to check the kidneys for evidence of ureteric obstruction when evidence of endometriosis is found or suspected on scan.

6.14.4 Dermoid Cyst (Mature Cystic Teratoma)

Dermoid cysts, or mature cystic teratomas, are a common type of ovarian cyst that occur across the age range and are bilateral in at least 10–15 per cent of cases. They originate from the ovarian germ cells. Dermoids may contain calcifications (about 30 per cent) and can be small and located within an otherwise normal ovary (Figure 6.41), or they may assume different shapes and sizes. They tend to be located superiorly in the pelvis and thus occasionally are out of the range of the TV transducer. The most common ultrasound appearances of a dermoid cyst include the presence of a complex cystic and solid mass, with echogenic internal content that shadows extensively resulting in a characteristic echogenic 'white ball' corresponding to the sebum and hair content (Figure 6.42a). Occasionally there may be a fat–fluid

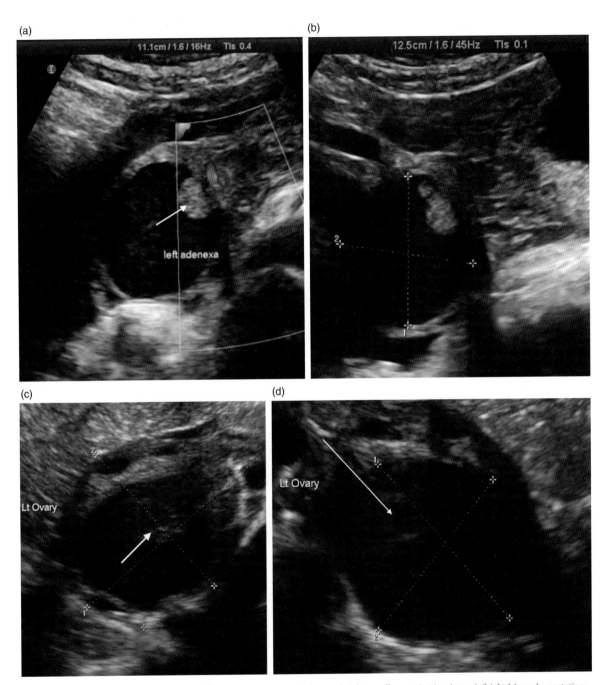

Figure 6.39 (a) An endometriotic cyst in early pregnancy appears to have a bright papillary projection (arrow). (b) At 14 weeks gestation this cyst appears complex with a papillary projection and does not fulfil a simple descriptor. (c and d) At six weeks postnatal the same 'papillary projection' (arrowed) appears comparatively indistinct. Subsequent laparoscopic excision clarified this was an endometrioma. Pregnancy-related hormonal changes leading to decidualisation can result in endometriomas resembling borderline tumours.

level (Figure 6.42b). The appearance of long and short echogenic linear strands correspond to the hair within the fluid content (Figure 6.42c,d). The white echogenic ball is sometimes referred to as the Rokitansky nodule or dermoid plug. The presence of excessive papillary projections within a dermoid cyst, in addition to the presence of vascularity on Colour Doppler evaluation, should raise the suspicion for the presence

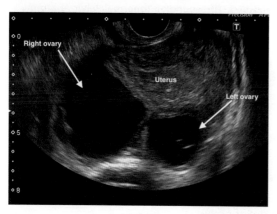

Figure 6.40 Bilateral ovarian cysts that are relatively anechoic with abnormal shape fixed to the back of the uterus and obliterating the pouch of Douglas, sometimes referred to as 'kissing endometriomas'.

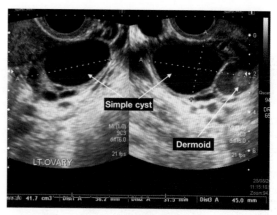

Figure 6.41 A small dermoid (long arrow) located in an otherwise normal ovary.

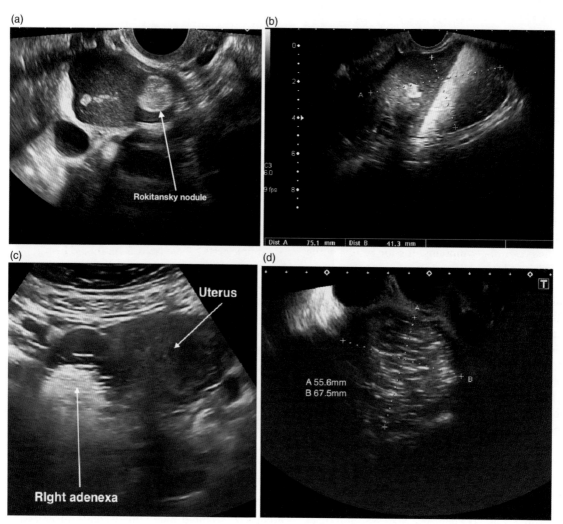

Figure 6.42 (a) A complex cystic solid ovarian mass with white ball (arrow), also called a 'Rokitansky nodule'. (b) This unilocular mass with mixed echogenicity, a fat fluid level and shadows can instantly be categorised as a dermoid. (c) TA view shows a right adnexal mass with bright and dark areas. (d) TV view clarifies this is a unilocular mass with mixed echogenicity, including linear bright strands (representing hair) and acoustic shadows. This can instantly be categorised as a dermoid.

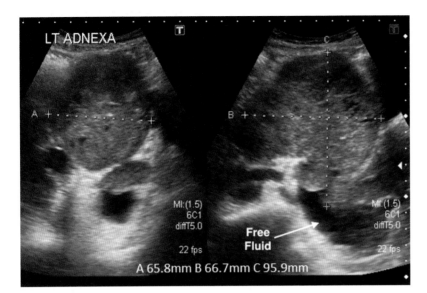

Figure 6.43 Presentation with pain. The left adnexal mass does not have normal-looking ovarian structures but has the typical appearance of ovarian oedema and has some surrounding free fluid. This enlarged oedematous appearance is typical of ovarian torsion. Colour flow imaging is less reliable for diagnosis of torsion as variable flow may be seen.

of immature or neuronal elements and the need for further evaluation.

6.15 Adnexal Torsion

Patients presenting with an adnexal torsion are typically symptomatic with acute pelvic pain and tenderness. Although there are sonographic signs suggestive of adnexal torsion, ultrasound is not always diagnostic and there should be a high index of suspicion based upon the presenting symptoms. Torsion results in the obstruction of lymphatic and venous drainage of the ovary and tube, and thus the ovary becomes enlarged, globular and oedematous (Figure 6.43). Comparison with the contralateral ovary may be helpful. Sometimes a torted ovary is found in an unusual location such as anterior to the uterus, and/or an ovarian mass such as a cyst, which has predisposed the ovary to torsion, may be seen. Doppler imaging may show absent or diminished flow, but this must be interpreted with caution as variable degrees of torsion result in differing findings. Haemorrhagic infarction may occur and result in the presence of fluid with varying degrees of echogenicity. Colour flow and pulsed wave Doppler ultrasound cannot confirm or rule out the diagnosis as the degree of vascular occlusion may vary. Intraperitoneal fluid may be present and is thought to result from transudate from the capsule of the ovary with lymphatic and venous obstruction. The most consistent feature is an oedematous enlarged ovary in association with acute onset of severe pain.

6.16 Follow-Up

This is a grey area and resources to enable follow-up are limited. Recommendations have been published in the United States in a consensus statement by the Society of Radiologists in Ultrasound.[9] No similar recommendations exist in UK but the following would generally be agreed.

Simple cysts (reproductive age)

- follicles/simple cysts < 3 cm diameter are considered normal;
- simple cysts ≥ 3 cm but < 5 cm should be reported but do not require follow-up;
- simple cysts 5–7 cm should be described with a statement that this is almost certainly benign and a follow-up scan in 12 months considered;
- simple cysts > 7 cm are difficult to evaluate completely with ultrasound so further imaging, for example, MRI or surgical removal, considered;

Simple cysts (post-menopausal)

- simple cysts < 1 cm are not important and do not need follow-up;
- simple cysts of > 1 cm and < 7cm can be described as almost certainly benign. A follow-up should be considered in 12 months;

Simple cysts > 7 cm: at any age require further evaluation and surgical removal should be considered;

Thin walled cysts with a single thin septation or focal calcification (almost always benign)

- follow-up as for simple cysts;

113

Haemorrhagic cysts (reproductive age) typically resolve within 8 weeks.

- > 5 cm 8–12 weeks. If smaller, follow-up is not required;

Dermoid cysts where not removed

- 12 months is suggested to ensure stability;

Endometrioma where not surgically removed

- 12 months suggested to ensure stability;

Cysts with indeterminate but probably benign characteristics

- Reproductive age: 6–12 weeks;
- Post-menopausal: consider removal.

For cysts with a higher possibility of malignancy, conservative management with ultrasound follow-up is not appropriate.

6.17 Summary

Ultrasound is the imaging of choice for any woman with a suspected pelvic pathology. Taking a careful history and doing a systematic scan is key to making a diagnosis. Ultrasound has good sensitivity and specificity for distinguishing benign and malignant ovarian pathology. The most common pelvic masses are fibroids. Adenomyosis is also a common cause of uterine enlargement that has characteristic features on ultrasound.

The FIGO classification can be used to describe fibroids, but in practice evaluation of submucous fibroids is most important since the extent to which these distort the endometrial cavity determines suitability for treatment options.

Where an adnexal mass is present, the IOTA classification should be used to describe the lesion. Applying simple descriptors (pattern recognition) enables a high proportion of masses to be diagnosed. Where the mass is not instantly recognisable, applying simple rules enables the mass to be categorised as benign, uncertain or malignant.

References

1. Munro MG, Critchley H, Fraser IS. (for the FIGO menstrual disorders working group). The FIGO classification of causes of abnormal uterine bleeding in the reproductive years. *Fertil Steril.* 2011;95:2204–2208.

2. Dueholm M. Transvaginal ultrasound for diagnosis of adenomyosis: a review. *Best Pract Res Clin Obstet Gynaecol.* 2006;20(4):569–582.

3. Van den Bosch T, Dueholm M, Leone FPG et al. Terms, definitions and measurements to describe sonographic features of myometrium and uterine masses: a consensus opinion from the Morphological Uterus Sonographic Assessment (MUSA) group. *Ultrasound Obstet Gynecol.* 2015;46:284–298.

4. Gordts S, Brosens JJ, Fusi L, Benagiano G, Brosens I. Uterine adenomyosis: a need for uniform terminology and consensus classification. *Reprod Biomed Online.* 2008;17(2):244–248.

5. Leone FPG, Timmerman D, Bourne T et al. Terms, definitions and measurements to describe the sonographic features of the endometrium and intrauterine lesions: a consensus opinion for the International Endometrial Tumor Analysis (IETA) group. *Ultrasound Obstet Gynecol.* 2010;35:103–112.

6. Kaijser J, Bourne T, Valentin L, Sayasneh S, Van Holsbeke C, Vergote I, Testa AC, Franchi D, Van Calster B, Timmerman D. Improving strategies for diagnosing ovarian cancer: a summary of the International Ovarian Tumor Analysis (IOTA) studies. *Ultrasound Obstet Gynecol.* 2013;41:9–20.

7. Management of suspected ovarian masses in premenopausal women. Green-top Guideline No. 62 RCOG/BSGE Joint Guideline 1 November 2011.

8. Guerriero S, Condous G, van den Bosch T et al. Systematic approach to sonographic evaluation of the pelvis in women with suspected endometriosis, including terms, definitions and measurements: a consensus opinion from the International Deep Endometriosis Analysis (IDEA) group. *Ultrasound Obstet Gynecol.* 2016;48:318–332.

9. Levine D, Brown DL, Andreotti RF et al. Management of asymptomatic ovarian and other adnexal cysts imaged at US: society of radiologists in ultrasound consensus conference statement. *Radiology.* 2010;256:943–954.

Resources

IOTA apps (risk calculator). www.iotagroup.org.

Pregnancy Ultrasound for SRH Work

Mary Pillai

7.1 Introduction   115
7.2 Service Operational Issues   115
7.3 Interpretation of hCG   116
7.4 The Ultrasound Examination   116
7.5 Dating   118
7.6 Dating in the Second Trimester   120
7.7 Multiple Pregnancy   124

7.8 Abnormal Findings in Early Pregnancy   125
7.9 Criteria to Define Miscarriage   127
7.10 Management Following Diagnosis of Failed
     Pregnancy   129
7.11 Ultrasound during Surgical Abortion   130
7.12 Ultrasound in the Management of
     Complications   131

7.1 Introduction

This chapter focuses on the level of knowledge essential for practitioners providing ultrasound to pregnant women presenting for care within SRH services.

Currently within the UK, the NHS commissions around two-thirds of abortions within the independent sector. Where provision remains within NHS services, this is predominantly within SRH services. These services are a very important resource for specialist training in abortion care, which at the present time is not included as a core competency within obstetrics and gynaecology training.

Services are more correctly called 'pregnancy advisory' since women attending may be ambivalent and seeking to clarify their options regarding the pregnancy. No assumption should be made that any woman attending will proceed with abortion. There is considerable overlap with early pregnancy clinics, since a proportion of women presenting will have early pregnancy complications such as PUL (pregnancy of unknown location), PUV (pregnancy of uncertain viability) or ectopic pregnancy.

Abortion care can be, and in resource-poor settings often is, provided without ultrasound.[1] However, scanning considerably improves the overall quality of care through clarification of the following:

1. Confirmation of the pregnancy location.
2. Assessment of gestational age (dating).
3. Detection of signs of a failing or failed pregnancy.
4. Detection of multiple pregnancy.
5. Detection of uterine anomaly or pathology that may increase the risks of abortion procedures.
6. Detection of adnexal pathology.

The ability to clarify these findings is key to maximising safety and efficacy, and so ultrasound provision is routine normative practice in services providing abortion care within the UK.

7.2 Service Operational Issues

There is a general consensus that ultrasound in the first trimester should be performed transvaginally, due to closer positioning of the transducer and the greater resolution possible. However, in a busy clinical setting this needs to be balanced against the greater convenience and acceptability of transabdominal ultrasound. The most important objectives in a pregnancy advisory service are locating and dating an early pregnancy, and these objectives can be achieved in most cases using the transabdominal route. It is entirely reasonable to adopt a pragmatic approach and perform a routine transabdominal scan, and then selectively ask women to proceed to the transvaginal approach only where the findings are uncertain, or to better clarify unexpected pathology. It is helpful to ask women not to empty their bladder for two hours prior to their appointment. In the author's experience it is unnecessary and even counter-productive to ask women to drink a specified amount, as this tends to result in the bladder being over distended and uncomfortable during the scan, particularly if they are kept waiting.

Within the UK, it is recommended that women should be seen for assessment within five days of requesting a pregnancy advisory appointment.[2] The high-sensitivity pregnancy tests currently available over the counter can result in women who are concerned about an episode of contraceptive failure or non-use, doing serial tests and having a positive result earlier than a pregnancy can be detected with ultrasound. A biochemical pregnancy may be detected up to one week before a period is missed and around 2–3 weeks before the first evidence of the pregnancy on ultrasound. When a pregnancy is confirmed biochemically but cannot be visualised on ultrasound, it is called PUL. In this circumstance management should include checking a pregnancy test definitely is positive and then taking a careful menstrual history, clarifying whether the woman knows when conception most likely occurred and when any pregnancy test first became positive. If this information fits with the pregnancy being less than five weeks, then explaining that it is too early to see on scan and arranging a rescan in one week is the most appropriate course of action. Conversely, if she should be more than five weeks, then the possibility of ectopic location becomes higher. A history of any pain should be noted and a more thorough ultrasound examination of the adnexal regions performed, noting any free fluid or inhomogenous mass. An initial quantitative hCG level is also key to safe management. Where the woman is symptom free and there are no abnormal adnexal findings, then a review in 48–72 hours will be appropriate. It will depend on local arrangements whether this may be more appropriate within an early pregnancy assessment service and this will result in transfer to a service managing women with wanted pregnancy. It is very unfortunate if at that stage an intrauterine pregnancy has appeared and a referral is then required for a further appointment at the pregnancy advisory service. So where possible the patient pathway should support a second appointment 48–72 hours later within the pregnancy advisory service. As a rule if the pregnancy cannot be located at a second appointment then appropriate management is a serial hCG level with referral to the early pregnancy service.

7.3 Interpretation of hCG

The concept of there being a discriminatory zone above which ultrasound should visualise the pregnancy and below which a pregnancy will not be seen has outlived its usefulness. In the case of a viable intrauterine pregnancy, this hCG threshold could be anywhere from 1,000 to 3,000 mIU/ml or more. However, the rise and fall of hCG levels in both ectopic pregnancy and incomplete miscarriage is very different from normal pregnancy, and ultrasound signs may be present to assist the diagnosis if the uterus and adnexal regions are carefully evaluated regardless of the hCG level.

7.4 The Ultrasound Examination

The beginning of any pelvic ultrasound examination should be an overview of the pelvis without magnification (initial survey) performed in two anatomical planes. The uterus, its relative position and content, adjacent structures and any free fluid should be noted. Following this overview, the area of interest, usually the pregnancy, should be magnified to optimise the image and any measurements. A structure being measured should ideally fill two-thirds of the screen, and this can most appropriately be achieved using both the depth and the zoom options.

The first sonographic sign of pregnancy is an eccentrically placed, spherical sac, usually with an echogenic rim, measuring 2–4 mm diameter situated within one layer of the decidua (Figure 7.1). This is sometimes called the *interdecidual sac sign*. Assuming a 28-day cycle with ovulation around mid-cycle, the earliest this will be seen is 4–5 weeks from the LMP date. It could easily be confused with an endometrial cyst (Chapter 4/Figure 4.25 of endometrial cyst/s), which is typically the same size and position but does not typically have a spherical echogenic double layer border. However, this distinction is not always clear in practice.

Once the implantation sac is around 3–4 mm, its trophoblastic borders typically appear echo bright. This echogenic ring is a very important sign that also helps distinguish a very early pregnancy from a fluid collection between the decidual layers, known as a 'pseudo sac' (Figure 7.2).

A viable gestation sac will usually double in size every 2–3 days, but failure to do so is not a reliable sign that the pregnancy is failing.[3] An MSD can be calculated as the mean of the sagittal, transverse and

(a) (b)

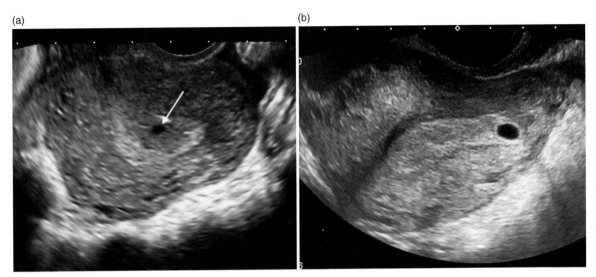

Figure 7.1 Week 4–5. (a) An eccentrically placed 2–3 mm sac (arrow) implanting within one layer of the endometrium. By dates she was 4 weeks 3 days. (b) The same pregnancy at 4 weeks 5 days showing a more evident echogenic rim and a doubling in the sac size.

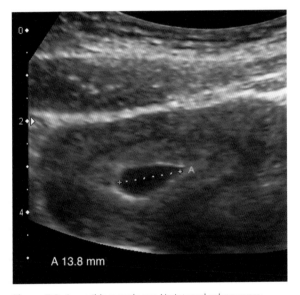

A 13.8 mm

Figure 7.2 A possible pseudo sac. No internal echoes were present. The fluid lies between rather than within the decidual layers, and assumes the shape of the endometrial cavity, resulting in a pointed edge.

coronal diameters of the sac (measured from the inner border to the inner border of the surrounding trophoblast), but the MSD is not recommended for dating. A yolk sac appears as a small highly echogenic ring within the gestation sac and is generally seen by the time the sac reaches 8 mm (Figure 7.3), but may be visible with a smaller sac size, or may appear later (see Table 7.1). This equates to five weeks' gestation. The

yolk sac has a diameter of around 2 mm at 5 weeks increasing to around 6 mm at 12 weeks. When the yolk sac appears abnormally small or large, this is usually a sign of an abnormal or failing pregnancy (Figure 7.4).

The first detection of the embryo is around six weeks with the appearance of a thickened area in the free wall of the yolk sac. This earliest appearance of the embryo adjacent to the yolk sac has been likened to a 'diamond or signet ring' (Figure 7.5).

The embryo is attached to the yolk sac by the vitelline duct, but this structure is not visible.

The amniotic sac appears as a thin reflective membrane inside the gestation sac just after the appearance of the yolk sac. It can be seen as a separate membrane within the gestation sac up to the time the chorion and amnion fuse at around 13–14 weeks.

The embryo develops within the amniotic sac while the yolk sac lies outside the amnion (Figure 7.6). The gestation sac varies in size, but the amniotic sac size is closely related to the size of the embryo between 6 and 10 weeks.

The size of the embryo increases rapidly at around 1 mm per day. Cardiac activity is usually visible as soon as the embryo can be seen, and in most cases by six weeks or an embryo size of 5 mm (Figure 7.7). However, considerable controversy has surrounded the diagnosis of non-viable early pregnancy. In most pregnancies, a yolk sac will be visible when the gestation sac measures 8 mm, a fetal node or embryo will be visible by the time the sac is around 16–20 mm

(a) (b)

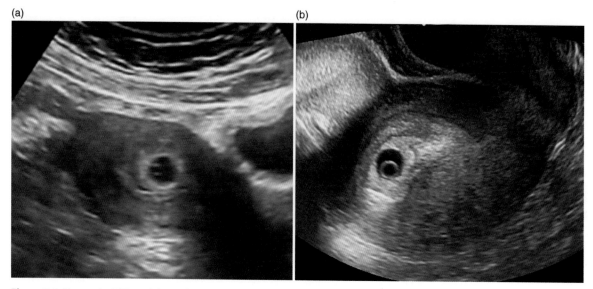

Figure 7.3 Five weeks. (a) Transabdominal view of a yolk sac within a normally situated early gestation sac, surrounded by fluid, trophoblast, decidua and myometrium. (b) The same pregnancy viewed transvaginally. The embryo and amnion are not yet visible.

and cardiac pulsations will be visible by the time the embryo measures 5 mm. In a minority of 'viable' pregnancies the appearance of the yolk sac, the embryo or cardiac pulsations has been shown to fall beyond these limits. In October 2011, two papers provided evidence that guidelines for the diagnosis of failed pregnancy were unsafe.[3,4] A systematic review concluded that existing guidelines were based on inadequate information.[5] Following these publications, the RCOG changed its guidance to a diagnostic threshold of an empty gestation sac with MSD > 25 mm or no cardiac activity present in an embryo of 7 mm or more.[6] In December 2012, the UK National Institute for Health and Care Excellence adopted the recommendations of the RCOG.[7]

The recommendations of the current guidance is appropriate where continuation of the pregnancy is desired, but may be inappropriate in a pregnancy advisory setting where a high proportion of women are seeking to end their pregnancy. In this circumstance, once the possible scan interpretations are explained, the woman's preference for either proceeding with termination without delay, or a follow-up appointment to clarify viability in 1–2 weeks is more appropriate to determine the management.

7.5 Dating

Menstrual dates are notoriously unreliable in a high proportion of pregnancies, and dating can much more

reliably be estimated by performing biometric measurements and using recommended charts.[8] In the first trimester, the CRL of the embryo is the recommended method for dating from 6 to 14 weeks and is the most accurate way to date pregnancy. An important consideration that may need explanation to women attending a pregnancy advisory service is the fact that the age of the fetus or embryo is expressed in 'weeks of gestation' calculated from the first day of LMP. This corresponds to approximately 14 days more than the date of conception. When women either know a particular date that conception occurred or they are hoping to pinpoint the conception date based on ultrasound dating, understanding that the weeks of gestation is different from the timing of conception becomes very important. Most ultrasound equipment has gestational age (dating) charts already input and will automatically give the average gestation for any particular measurement. It is essential that the operator ensures that the correct chart is programmed into the ultrasound system consistent with that nationally recommended.

7.5.1 CRL

CRL measurements can be carried out transvaginally or transabdominally. At very early gestations, care must be taken to avoid inclusion of the yolk sac. During the embryonic phase (6–10 weeks), this is the measurement of the longest distance in any scan plane

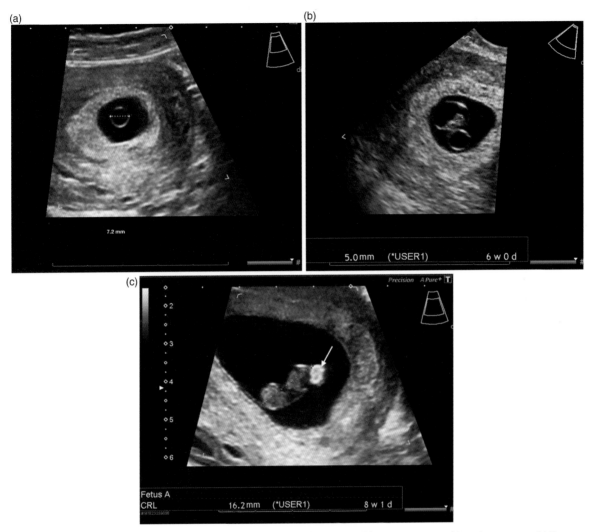

Figure 7.4 Abnormal yoke sac. (a) The yolk sac appears unusually large for the size of the gestation sac in this early pregnancy. (b) One week later the amniotic sac and embryo have appeared. No cardiac activity was detectable; however, as the embryo was less than 7 mm, a further scan was performed one week later, when the findings were unchanged. (c) An abnormally shaped yolk sac (arrow). No cardiac activity was detected in the embryo and a diagnosis of non-viable pregnancy confidently made at this single scan, as the embryo was bigger than 7 mm.

from the cranial to the caudal ends of the embryo. At 6–7 weeks, the embryo has the appearance of a grain of rice and the cranial and caudal ends cannot be defined (Figures 7.6–7.8).

Provided one technically acceptable section and measurement is obtained, then that is the best one to use and there is no need to repeat it several times.[8] Otherwise the best of three discrete measurements – or the mean of three if they are all similar – is recommended.

The CRL grows rapidly at a rate of 1.1 mm per day. At 8–9 weeks some body curvature gives a 'kidney bean' appearance (Figure 7.9). At this stage limb buds and spontaneous movement of the embryo may just be discernible.

At 9–11 weeks midgut herniation is a normal feature (Figure 7.10) and should not be misdiagnosed as a fetal anomaly (abdominal wall defect).

At 11–14 weeks, detail of the fetal anatomy is much clearer and the fetal position has a significant effect on the CRL measurement. Although very exacting measurement of the CRL is required for antenatal combined screening for Downs syndrome, a difference of one or two days within the context of SRH work makes very

119

(a)

(b)

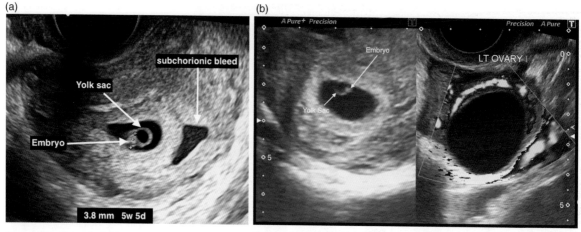

Figure 7.5 Six weeks. (a) Six weeks showing the early embryo developing adjacent to the yolk sac. Coincidentally a subchorionic bleed is visible outside the gestation sac. (b) A six-week gestation sac with early embryo and a corpus luteum cyst in the left ovary.

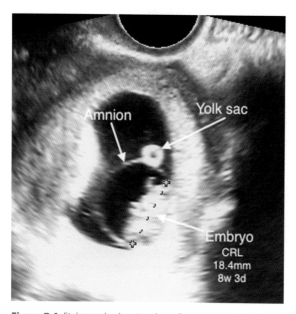

Figure 7.6 Eight weeks showing the yolk sac now outside the amniotic sac. The embryo is growing inside the amniotic sac, so is now separate from the yolk sac.

little difference to the management options. A midline sagittal section of the whole embryo or fetus should be obtained, with a line between the crown and the rump horizontal (perpendicular) to the ultrasound beam and not more than 30 degrees from the horizontal (Figure 7.11). The fetus should be in neutral position, not too flexed or hyperextended. In neutral position, fluid should be visible between the fetal chin and the chest. It is important that the measurement does not include the vitelline duct in early pregnancy

as this will overestimate the CRL and gestational age. It is also important that the CRL should not include limbs/yolk sac for same reason.

An accurately performed CRL in the first trimester has a range (from 5th to 95th Centile) of plus or minus six days. Where measurements are inexpertly performed such that the correct measurement plane or correct placement of calipers is not achieved, the error will further widen the range.

7.6 Dating in the Second Trimester

Although a majority of women presenting with an unwanted pregnancy will do so in the first trimester, some will present later. It is therefore necessary that pregnancy advisory services are able to date these pregnancies with an appropriate degree of accuracy in order to be able to advise the women about their options. In the second trimester, measurements of the head and femur have traditionally been used for dating. These structures can be measured from around 13 weeks, but a well-measured CRL is likely to be most accurate up to 14 weeks (Figure 7.11). Biometric charts are available for a range of structures including the cerebellum, the abdomen and all the long bones. The later a pregnancy is dated after the first trimester, the less accurate is the estimation of gestational age since fetal size shows more natural variation. By mid-gestation, there is considerable fetal size variation, so where dating occurs as late as 20–23 weeks the estimated gestational age range is close to plus or minus two weeks. How this variation should be managed in regard to the 24-week threshold set by the UK

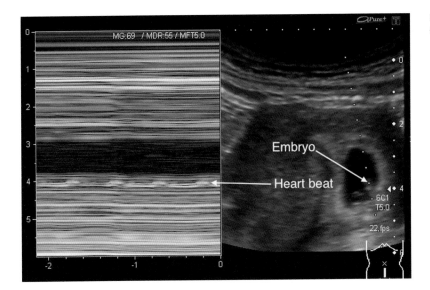

Figure 7.7 M-mode demonstrating cardiac activity in an early embryo.

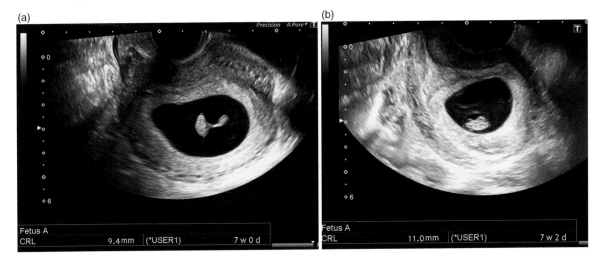

Figure 7.8 At seven weeks the embryo appears straight like a grain of rice.

Abortion Act is unclear and so far is lacking any professional guidance. Therefore, it is largely left to the discretion of individual services.

Owing to the increasing range of possible gestation with later dating, more accuracy will be obtained by composite measurement (at least three and preferably four different fetal structures). These could be the HC, the cerebellum, the AC and the FL. If the correct anatomical section of the fetal head cannot be obtained due to fetal position, then it is very important to include measurements of other structures for which the best images are possible. The cineloop option (usually activated by moving the trackball once the image is frozen) is very helpful when doing fetal measurements, as fetal movement frequently prevents freezing at the point the image is optimal. The ability to rewind 3–5 seconds of captured imaging enables a return to the optimal image for doing the measurement.

7.6.1 Head Measurement

The recommended charts are those of Altman and Chitty,[8] where HC is derived from the BPD and OFD using the equation HC = π(BPD+OFD)/2.

The BPD, OFD and HC measurements should be measured in a transverse section of the fetal head at the level of the fetal ventricles. The placement of the

(a)   (b)

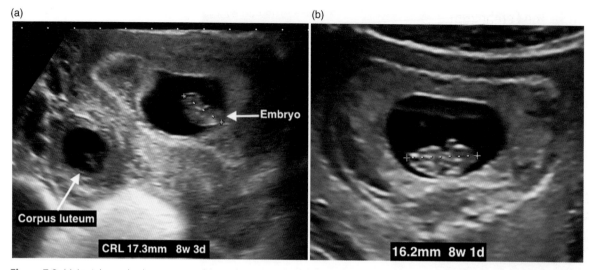

Figure 7.9 (a) At eight weeks, the curvature of the embryo changes the appearance to a kidney bean, and (b) limb buds begin to appear.

(a)   (b)

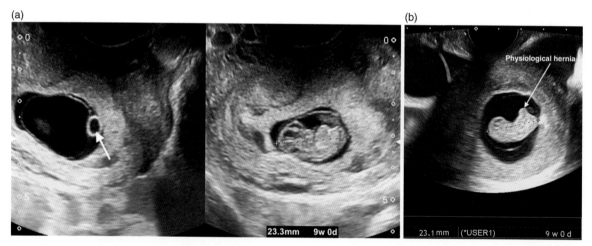

Figure 7.10 A nine-week pregnancy. (a) Showing the yolk sac outside the amnion (arrow) and the embryo inside the amniotic sac. (b) Physiological small bowel herniation at nine weeks (arrow).

callipers should be on the outer to outer borders of the skull. The sonographic landmarks confirming the correct measurement plane include:

- The head shape should resemble a rugby football.
- The midline echo (falx) should be horizontal.
- The midline echo should be broken one-third of the way from the front by the septum cavum pellucidum, which appears as a small box.
- The hemispheres should appear symmetrical either side of the midline.
- The ventricles appear either side of the midline (although typically only the anatomy in the distal hemisphere is clear owing to the deflection of the beam by the skull).

- The choroid plexus should be visible within the posterior horn of the ventricle in the distal hemisphere.
- The cerebellum should not be visible.

Where the ellipse facility is available for the HC, the ellipse should trace the outer border of the skull (Figure 7.12a, b).

The BPD measurement will depend on the head shape. Where the head is long and narrow (dolicocephalic), it will substantially underestimate the gestational age, so it should not be used in isolation without other measurements, but may be used together with the OFD to calculate the head circumference.[8]

7.6.2 The Cerebellum

Measuring a single structure will be less reliable than several structures. The fetal cerebellum is relatively less affected by growth problems than other measurements, particularly the femur, and is a relatively easy landmark to recognise and obtain the correct views for measurement from 18 weeks onwards. The transcerebellar plane is an axial (slightly oblique) view at the level of the posterior fossa. The plane is easily

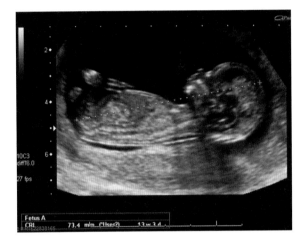

Figure 7.11 First trimester dating. Thirteen weeks demonstrating the criteria for CRL measurement. The crown and the rump of the fetus are clearly shown in a sagittal view with the tip of the nose visible. The fetal attitude is correct with fluid visible between the chin and the chest and the plane of measurement is less than 30 degrees from the horizontal.

obtained by angling the transducer posteriorly about 45 degrees from the BPD plane. The cerebellum is easily recognisable and should be measured from the outer to outer border at its widest point (Figure 7.13).

7.6.3 FL

The recommended charts are those of Altman and Chitty.[5] The femur should be imaged as close as possible to the horizontal plane to avoid underestimating the length. Care should be taken to include the whole femur diaphysis in the image and to place the callipers accurately on the diaphyseal ends, but it is important to avoid measuring spur artefacts that can falsely extend the femur length giving an overestimated gestational age (Figure 7.14).

7.6.4 AC

The AC is measured on a transverse section of the upper fetal abdomen that is as close as possible to circular in shape to avoid errors in the measurement. A transverse section should include the spine and aorta posteriorly, the umbilical vein in the anterior third of the abdomen and the fetal stomach (Figure 7.15). A section of the fetal rib may be seen laterally on either side. The calipers should be placed on the outer skin edge to measure the transverse diameter and the anterior–posterior diameter at 90 degrees to each other. Where the ellipse option is available, place one calliper on the skin over the spinous process and

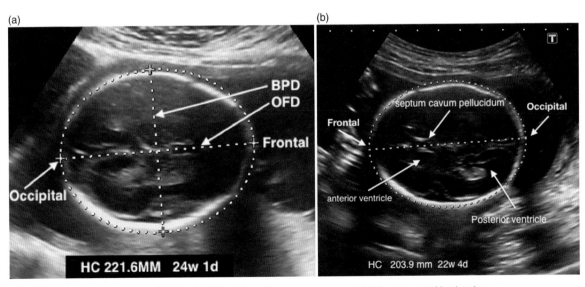

Figure 7.12 The second trimester fetal head. (a) Head circumference measurement. (b) The intracranial landmarks.

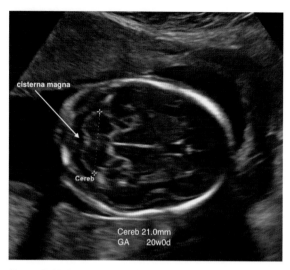

Figure 7.13 A transverse cerebellar view.

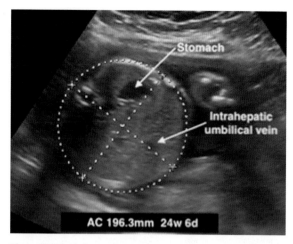

Figure 7.15 Abdominal circumference showing the stomach and intrahepatic vein. These landmarks determine the correct level for measurement.

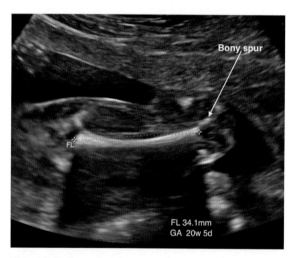

Figure 7.14 Femur length.

7.7 Multiple Pregnancy

Twinning occurs in around 1 in 80 spontaneous conceptions, and so will be encountered in the pregnancy advisory setting. No assumption should be made that this information is of no importance to women in the pregnancy advisory setting. Although most women are very surprised at the finding of a twin pregnancy, sometimes this factor may be influential in a woman's decision to continue or end the pregnancy. The type of chorionicity determines the relative risk of complications, and therefore the level of surveillance required and the risk of perinatal morbidity and mortality in the event the woman decides to continue the pregnancy. All dizygous twins (from two fertilised ova) have separate placentas and are dichorionic–diamniotic. Around 25 per cent of monozygous twins (from one fertilised ovum) are also DCDA having developed the dichorionic placental type following embryo division at a very early stage. Overall around 80 per cent of twins are DCDA. Chorionicity is much more easily diagnosed on ultrasound in the first trimester, compared with later pregnancy. Dichorionic placentae have no shared placental vascular connections and do not need surveillance for twin–twin transfusion syndrome. The development of this complication in a proportion of MCDA accounts for a much higher rate of perinatal morbidity and mortality.

Dichorionic twins have two gestation sacs and a thick membrane between their amniotic cavities. Chorionic tissue can be seen between the layers of

the other on the skin edge of the opposite side of the section keeping the abdomen symmetrical either side of the callipers. The ellipse should then be opened out by rolling the trackball sideways until the ellipse is perfectly overlaid on the skin contour. When the ellipse is not well-aligned with the skin contour, it is usually possible to swing the whole ellipse by calliper movement.

The main limitations of the AC are that it is not always symmetrical and its size will vary with fetal respiration and body flexion/extension. It has greater variability than other structures so it should never be used in isolation to date pregnancy.

membrane, giving rise to the characteristic 'lambda' sign (also called the 'delta' or 'twin-peak' sign) (Figure 7.16).

It is important not to mistake an area of subchorionic fluid (bleed) for a twin gestation sac (Figure 7.5a). If one apparent sac does not contain an embryo or yolk sac while the other does then it is not appropriate to diagnose twins.

Approximately 75 per cent of monozygous twins will be monochorionic. Monochorionic twins have one gestation sac but each twin has its own amniotic sac. The dividing membrane between each sac is thin

and inserts in a characteristic 'T' configuration onto the shared placenta (Figure 7.17).

Much more rarely monochorionic twins are in a single amniotic sac, and exceptionally they can be conjoined, but such consideration is beyond the scope of this book, as is discussion of higher order multiple pregnancies.

7.8 Abnormal Findings in Early Pregnancy

The shape of the sac is variable so the mean sac diameter is calculated from the mean of its greatest sagittal, transverse and coronal planes. A mean sac diameter of 25 mm or more with no embryo is considered diagnostic of failed pregnancy (Figure 7.18).[3–6,9,10]

A finding of subchorionic haematoma is relatively common in the first trimester. It appears as a crescent-shaped hypoechoic fluid collection between the decidua and the gestation sac (Figures 7.5a and 7.19). When large, it may considerably distend the endometrial cavity and exceed the size of the pregnancy (Figure 7.20). Although most patients will have bled overtly, it is 'silent' in around 30 per cent who have not experienced any vaginal bleeding. This finding is associated with an increased risk of pregnancy loss in women continuing the pregnancy. However, in many cases it resolves and is not usually detectable after 25 weeks.

A range of fetal anomalies may be recognisable in the first trimester, but this is not within the remit of a

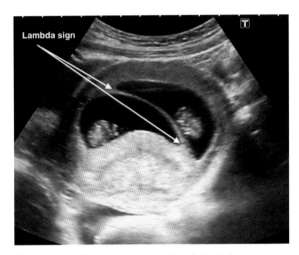

Figure 7.16 DCDA twins demonstrating the lambda sign.

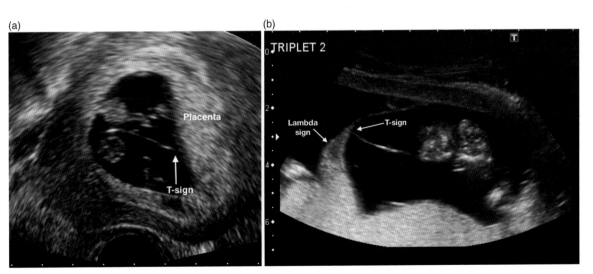

Figure 7.17 (a) MCDA twins demonstrating the T-sign. (b) A triplet pregnancy arising following two embryo replacement IVF, showing both the lambda sign and the T-sign identifying the MCDA fetuses separate to the DCDA fetus.

pregnancy advisory service and therefore beyond the scope of this chapter. The only exception to this would be recognition of acrania (Figure 7.21). This is part of the spectrum of neural tube disorders, and the recurrence risks for a neural tube defect in future pregnancy are increased compared with the background rate. The recurrence risk can be reduced by up to 75 per cent (from 4 per cent to 1 per cent) with high dose preconception folic acid (5 mg daily) and for this reason it is good practice to share the information where acrania is obvious on a dating scan performed in a pregnancy advisory service.

7.8.1 Gestational Trophoblastic Disease

Partial hydatidiform mole (coexisting with a fetus – Figure 7.22) and complete hydatidiform mole (no fetus present – Figure 7.23) are the commonest types of gestational trophoblastic disease and have an incidence of 1 in 700 and 1 in 1,500–2,000 pregnancies respectively. Although they will rarely be encountered in pregnancy advisory work, their recognition is important due to their potential for bleeding and the importance of performing surgical evacuation and

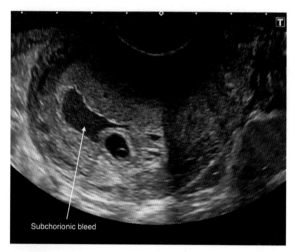

Subchorionic bleed

Figure 7.19 A subchorionic haematoma. The gestation sac is normally situated but a hypoechoic area of fluid between the decidua and the trophoblastic ring represents a subchorionic bleed.

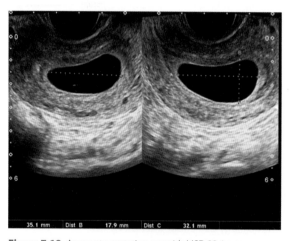

Figure 7.18 An empty gestation sac with MSD 28.4 mm.

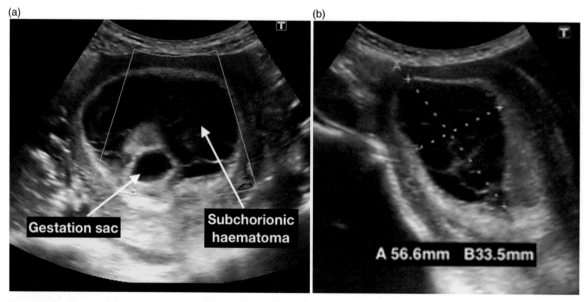

(a) | (b)

Gestation sac

Subchorionic haematoma

A 56.6mm   B33.5mm

Figure 7.20 A large subchorionic haematoma.

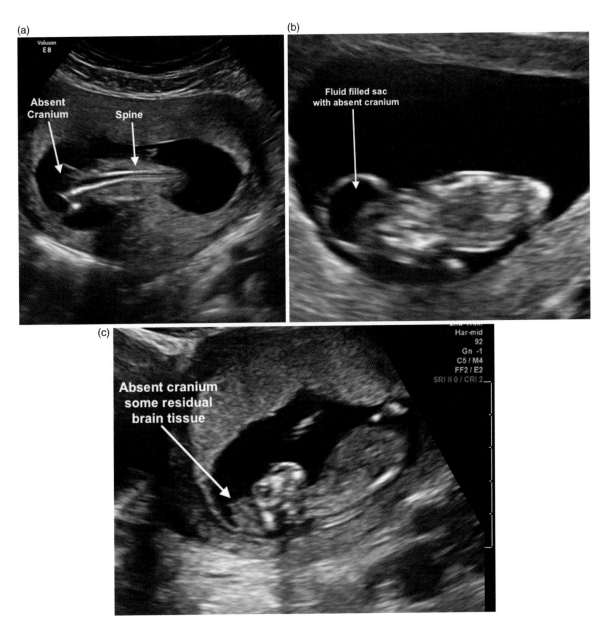

Figure 7.21 (a–c) Fetal acrania cases at 11–13 weeks.

sending all tissue obtained for histology. Ultrasound in early pregnancy is not as striking as in the mid-trimester pregnancy, but the presence of large abnormal-looking placental tissue with multiple small cystic spaces should raise a suspicion of the diagnosis. This should be managed with careful surgical evacuation of the uterus by an experienced operator, and submission of all the tissue removed for histological examination, which remains the gold standard for diagnosis.

7.9 Criteria to Define Miscarriage

Large prospective studies have shown that the criteria established in the 1990s for defining a failed pregnancy are unacceptable.[3–5] A CRL of 5 mm with no visible cardiac activity was associated with a false positive rate as high as 8.3 per cent when used to diagnose early pregnancy failure, and an empty gestation sac measuring 16 mm had a false positive rate of 4.4 per cent. A further study demonstrated significant

(a)   (b)

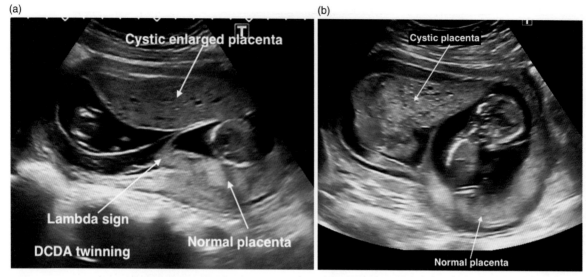

Figure 7.22 (a) Partial molar pregnancy in one of a DCDA twin pair. (b) The placenta is large and bright with multiple small cysts and a very different appearance to the placenta of the co-twin.

inter- and intra-observer variability in MSD and CRL measurement, whereby an MSD measurement of 20 mm by one examiner could translate to a measurement of anywhere between 16.8 mm and 24.5 mm for a second examiner. A study following women with an empty sac concluded that growth rates for the gestation sac and embryo could not predict viability accurately.[3] However, when a sac was empty on initial scan, the absence of a visible yolk sac or embryo on a second scan performed seven days or more later was always associated with a failed pregnancy.[10] Guidelines have changed, both in the UK and more widely. Currently a diagnosis of failed pregnancy requires that an embryo with no demonstrable cardiac activity must measure 7 mm or more. Where there is no visible embryo an empty sac must have an MSD of 25 mm or more (Tables 7.1 and 7.2).[6,7,9]

A transvaginal scan should be done in all cases where a failed early pregnancy is suspected. If there is doubt, particularly where the above diagnostic criteria are not fulfilled, then the pregnancy should be considered as a PUV. In that circumstance, there should be a re-scan at an interval of at least one week, unless the woman has come to a clear decision for termination and does not wish to wait. Where the 'empty' MSD is below 12 mm then a more appropriate re-scan interval is two weeks.[10]

Although recommending a re-scan is appropriate for a wanted pregnancy, the existing revised guidelines are not aimed at women attending a pregnancy advisory service and need to be put in context. In the setting of a pregnancy advisory service, the woman's preference should always be explored. No assumption should be made that the information about uncertain viability will not be important to her. Some women will choose to wait and see if the pregnancy fails, while others will want to proceed as a termination to end the pregnancy without delay.

Additional data on pregnancy outcome has been used to evaluate the performance of cut off values of CRL and MSD in diagnosing failed pregnancy. This has helped clarify the best interval for a repeat scan.[10]

With gestation beyond 70 days (for example, pregnancy test was positive at least 49 days earlier):

- an MSD ≥ 18 mm with no embryo was 100 per cent specific for miscarriage;
- an embryo with CRL ≥ 3 mm with no heart activity was 100 per cent specific for miscarriage.

For repeat scans:

- a pregnancy with an embryo with no heart activity on initial scan and a repeat scan ≥ 7 days later was 100 per cent specific for miscarriage;
- a pregnancy with no embryo and an MSD < 12 mm in which the sac size had not doubled after ≥ 14 days was 100 per cent specific for miscarriage;

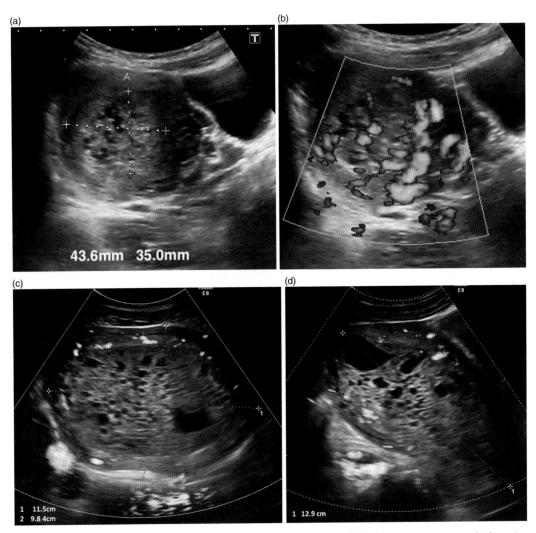

Figure 7.23 Complete molar pregnancy. (a and b) At seven weeks the uterus is filled with tissue containing multiple cystic spaces, high blood flow and no embryo. (c and d) At 12 weeks the uterus is significantly large for dates and filled with echogenic tissue with multiple cystic spaces and no fetus.

Table 7.1 False Positive Rates for Diagnosis of Miscarriage Based on MSD and CRL[4]

Empty Gestation Sac		
Mean sac diameter	False positive (%)	Viable at F/U
MSD 16 mm	FPR 3.3	1 in 30
MSD 20 mm	FPR 0.5	1 in 200
MSD ≥ 25 mm	FPR < 0.1	< 1 in 1,000
Embryo with no cardiac activity		
CRL 5 mm	FPR 3.6	1 in 30
CRL 6 mm	FPR 0.9	1 in 110
CRL 7 mm	FPR 0	0

- a pregnancy with no embryo and MSD ≥ 12 mm with no embryo heart activity after ≥ 7 days was 100 per cent specific for miscarriage.

7.10 Management Following Diagnosis of Failed Pregnancy

Where failed pregnancy is diagnosed, the management options are the same as for women seeking termination but with three important differences:

1. Women can be offered expectant management. This may not be appropriate where the pregnancy/fetal size is more than 12 weeks, and is most appropriate where the size is under 10 weeks.

129

Table 7.2 Society of Radiologists

Findings Diagnostic of Early Pregnancy Loss	Findings Suggestive but Not Diagnostic of Early Pregnancy Loss
CRL of 7 mm or more with no heartbeat	CRL less than 7 mm and no heartbeat
MSD of 25 mm or more with no embryo	MSD of 16–24 mm and no embryo
Absence of embryo with heartbeat 2 weeks or more after a scan showing a sac with no yolk sac	Absence of embryo with heartbeat 7–13 days after a scan showed a gestation sac with no yolk sac
Absence of embryo with heartbeat 11 days or more after a scan showing a gestation sac with a yolk sac	Absence of embryo with heartbeat 7–10 days after a scan showed a gestation sac with a yolk sac
	Absence of embryo for 6 weeks or longer from the LMP
	Enlarged yolk sac (> 7 mm)
	Small gestation sac in relation to the embryo size (< 5 mm difference between MSD and CRL)

Source: *Ultrasound Guidelines for Ultrasound Diagnosis of Early Pregnancy Loss.*

Where expectant management is chosen, it is appropriate to offer a follow-up appointment in 2–3 weeks and re-offer the option of surgical evacuation if there is no change in this time.

2. Women can be offered medical management, which is also most appropriate with pregnancy size less than 10 weeks. This can be as a single stage procedure with misoprostol 400–800 mcg, which a woman can take away to self-administer at home at a time of her choosing. There is no indication to give mifepristone with a failed pregnancy.

3. The abortion forms (HSA 1 & 4) are not required.

Contraindications to expectant management include suspected infection, suspected molar pregnancy, a bleeding tendency or when conservative management is not wanted by the woman. Knowledge of the figures for success with various management options is important to help the woman make a fully informed choice (Table 7.3).

7.11 Ultrasound during Surgical Abortion

There is a lack of randomised trials of care provision with and without ultrasound. Within the author's service, introduction of ultrasound availability during procedures and training of doctors has resulted in a significant reduction in failed procedures and an increase in confidence around difficult procedures. All the doctors who perform surgical procedures have become competent at using ultrasound to guide difficult dilatation, to complete difficult procedures and routinely at D & E procedures. Increasingly the doctors are choosing to do a routine check at the end of all surgical

Table 7.3 Management of Miscarriage by Outcome

Method of Management	Miscarriage Classification	Success Rate (%)
Expectant	Intact sac	28–76
	Incomplete	80–94
Medical	Intact sac	52–92
	Incomplete	70–96
Surgical	Intact sac	95–100
	Incomplete	95–100

Source: MIST BMJ 2006.

procedures. This also means that a surgical procedure can be offered to women who are five and six weeks, owing to the increased confidence with which the operator can confirm the pregnancy has been removed.

The ability to guide the procedure when any uterine anomaly has been identified (Figure 7.24), when there is extreme ante or retro flexion, or when any difficulty is encountered at dilatation has significant potential to avoid complications. The transabdominal probe is placed showing a sagittal plane of the uterus and the transducer angled towards the pelvis to include the upper cervix within the image. The sterile towel on the abdomen can be used by the operator to assist finding the best image, which is then held in place by an assistant. The passage of the dilator can then be followed. Where resistance has been encountered at the level of the internal os, use of guidance most often demonstrates this is due to the attempted insertion having been applied in the wrong direction. Visualisation enables easy correction of this and in most cases the dilator then readily passes into the

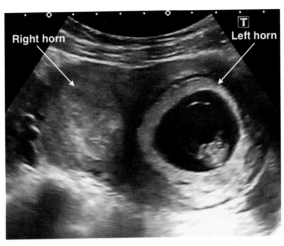

Figure 7.24 A bicornuate uterus with a pregnancy in the left horn.

cavity. It has also been our impression that the application of suprapubic pressure from the transducer during imaging seems to stimulate 'opening' of the internal os, such that no resistance is sometimes felt where previous attempts had met with significant resistance.

Ultrasound can also be extremely useful to ensure correct placement where an intrauterine device is inserted at the end of the procedure. Sometimes a strong myometrial contraction on completion of the termination may close the cavity such that it feels as if the fundus has been reached but the operator is aware that it feels too low. Simultaneous ultrasound enables placement correctly at the fundus while minimising any risk of perforation or false passage.

7.11.1 Dilatation Evacuation

Using ultrasound to guide retrieval of parts that are too large to pass down the suction catheter confers significant benefits:

- It reduces the number of times forceps need to be passed into the cavity and therefore the duration of the procedures. Intuitively this should enhance safety.
- It enables the operator to be confident that the procedure is complete.
- It removes the need for the very distasteful practice of checking the fetal parts at the end of the procedure.
- It greatly enhances the ability to safely supervise trainees learning the procedure.

7.12 Ultrasound in the Management of Complications

The commonest complication following termination is prolonged bleeding. Within our service, around 5 in 100 women require a follow-up due to physical symptoms following an MTOP and around 1 in 100 following a surgical termination. The most common reason by far is prolonged bleeding. A proportion of MTOP cases require follow up due to persistence of a positive pregnancy test at or beyond four weeks after their procedure. This is much less common where a low sensitivity pregnancy test is used.

Women with prolonged bleeding or a prolonged positive pregnancy test are offered a scan. The commonest finding with prolonged bleeding and/or a persistent positive test is a small amount of RPC (Figure 7.25a), often with high myometrial flow extending into the RPC (Figure 7.28c).

In women presenting with acute miscarriage or during medical abortion, clots and the gestation sac may be found within the cervix or lower uterus (Figure 7.26).

Where the presentation is with protracted bleeding following a pregnancy, the demonstration of blood flow helps to distinguishing between RPC and blood clot within the endometrial cavity (Figure 7.27). In a proportion with protracted bleeding and/or a persistently positive PT, myometrial hypervascularity is demonstrated (Figure 7.28c), but it is unclear how or when this should influence the management. The range of the duration of bleeding is very wide. Where no retained products can be visualised, bleeding may reflect infection (endometritis). Management should be determined by the clinical presentation. In most cases the appearance of some 'RPC' is not significant and watchful management is most appropriate. Where the woman has significant bleeding and or pain, management with antibiotics and a further dose of misoprostol should be considered (Table 7.3). Where a significant volume of retained products remain with persistent symptoms, then surgical evacuation is likely to be the fastest and most convenient means to resolution, but if the woman declines then further misoprostol and antibiotics may shorten the time interval to return to normal. Any re-instrumentation of the uterus (that is, prior surgical termination) or where prolonged retention products of conception is identified increases the risk of associated infection, and antibiotics should be administered prior to surgical

(a)   (b)

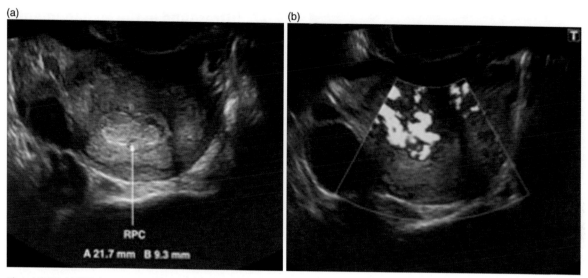

Figure 7.25 (a) RPC shows as irregular bright tissue surrounded by more hypoechoic myometrium. (b) Colour Doppler shows flow in the tissue and through an area of the surrounding myometrium.

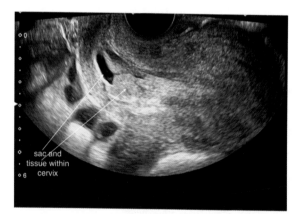

Figure 7.26 Twenty-four hours after mifepristone this lady returned for misoprostol, reporting she had quite heavy bleeding and wondered if she had passed the pregnancy. Tissue is visible in the lower endometrial and upper endocervical canal. Applying gentle pressure with the probe or asking the woman to cough will often demonstrate relative movement of the tissue called the 'sliding sign'.

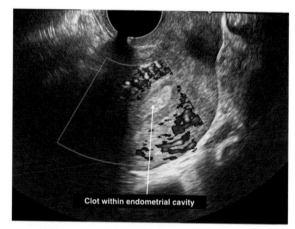

Figure 7.27 Clot within the endometrial cavity. No colour flow will be demonstrated within clot.

evacuation. The woman should be advised that with conservative management the time to resolution can take several weeks.

Case History: A nulliparous 20-year-old requested medical termination at 5 weeks and 4 days (Figure 7.28a,b). She bled as expected following mifepristone and misoprostol. The bleeding settled after ten days, but two weeks later she started bleeding again. Almost four weeks later the bleeding had not settled and was intermittently heavy. She presented back to the service seven weeks after the medical termination with continuing bleeding and an ultrasound scan which showed some fluid (blood) in the endometrial cavity, which otherwise appeared empty. An area of myometrial hypervascularity extending through the full thickness of myometrium was noted (Figure 7.28c).

Presentations like these following early medical abortion are not uncommon. This is much less common following surgical abortion procedures.

The patient described had an implant inserted at the time of her initial medical procedure. She was managed with a course of antibiotics and progestogen

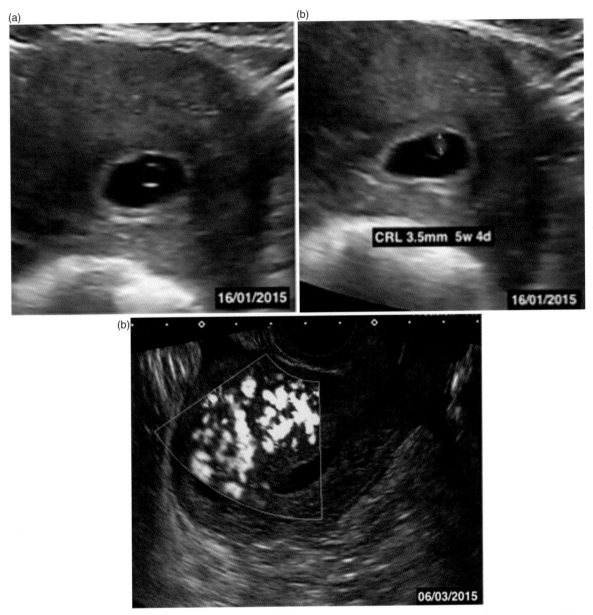

Figure 7.28 (a and b) Case history: Early pregnancy appearance on the day mifepristone was taken. (c) Ultrasound appearance more than seven weeks later showing high flow through the myometrium and fluid in the endometrial cavity.

to induce a medical curettage, and reviewed two weeks later. The bleeding settled whilst taking the tablets, and on withdrawal of the progestogen she had a moderate bleed. When reviewed there was a much smaller area with high flow and her bleeding was noted to be much improved.

Currently there is a lack of clarity on how to manage cases with protracted bleeding following medical termination and persistence of elevated hCG levels. Where there is significant tissue this should be surgically evacuated and submitted for histology to rule out gestational trophoblastic disease, although this would be extremely rare where the preceding pregnancy appearance was normal. Experience has shown that protracted bleeding following MTOP settles eventually but this can take weeks or even months.

References

1. *Safe abortion: technical and policy guidance for health systems.* 2nd edition. WHO 2012. ISBN 978 92 4 154843 4.

2. Care if women requesting induced abortion. Evidence based guideline number 7. *RCOG* November 2011 www.rcog.org.uk/globalassets/documents/guidelines/abortion-guideline_web_1.pdf

3. Abdallah Y, Daemen A, Guha S, Syed S, Naji O, Pexsters A et al. Gestational sac and embryonic growth are not useful as criteria to define miscarriage: a multi-center observational study. *Ultrasound Obstet Gynecol.* 2011;38:503–509. (Level II-3)

4. Abdallah Y, Daemen A, Kirk E, Pexsters A, Naji O, Stalder C et al. Limitations of current definitions of miscarriage using mean gestational sac diameter and crown-rump length measurements: a multicenter obser-vational study. *Ultrasound Obstet Gynecol.* 2011;38: 497–502. (Level II-3).

5. Jeve Y, Rhana R, Bhide A, Thangaratinam S. Accuracy of first-trimester ultrasound in the diagnosis of early embryonic demise: a systematic review. *Ultrasound Obstet Gynecol.* 2011;38:489–496.

6. Royal College of Obstetricians and Gynaecologists. Addendum to GTG No 25 (Oct). The management of early pregnancy loss. RCOG Press; 2011.

7. Ectopic pregnancy and miscarriage: diagnosis and initial management. *NICE guidelines* (CG 154) December 2012.

8. Loughna O, Chitty L, Evans T, Chudleigh T. Fetal size and dating: charts recommended for clinical obstetric practice. *Ultrasound.* 2009; 17:161–167.

9. Doubilet PM, Benson CB, Bourne T, Blaivas M, Barnhart KT, Benacerraf BR et al. Diagnostic criteria for nonviable pregnancy early in the first trimester. Society of Radiologists in Ultrasound Multispecialty Panel on Early First Trimester Diagnosis of Miscarriage and Exclusion of a Viable Intrauterine Pregnancy. *N Engl J Med.* 2013;569:1443–1451.

10. Preisler J, Kopeika J, Ismail L, Vathanan V, Farren J, Abdallah Y et al. Defining safe criteria to diagnose miscarriage: prospective observational multicentre study. *BMJ.* 2015; 351:h4579.

Ultrasound Assessment of a Potential Ectopic Pregnancy

Karen Easton

8.1   Introduction   135

8.2   Attributing Factors   135

8.3   Confounding Diagnostic Factors – Clinical Presentation   135

8.4   Signs and Symptoms   136

8.5   Diagnosis of an Ectopic Pregnancy   138

8.6   Where to Find an Ectopic Pregnancy   138

8.7   Ultrasound in the Diagnosis of Ectopic Pregnancy   138

8.8   Masses in the Fallopian Tube   143

8.9   Ovarian Findings   145

8.10 Less Common Findings   145

8.11 Colour Doppler Assessment   148

8.12 β-hCG   148

8.13 Ultrasound Assessment during the Treatment of Ectopic Pregnancy   149

8.14 Summary   149

8.1 Introduction

Ectopic pregnancy is defined as a pregnancy outside the endometrial cavity of the uterus. Figure 8.1 is a diagrammatic view of ectopic sites. The prevalence is 1–2 per cent in all pregnancies.[1] There is an increased incidence associated with IVF pregnancies (4.5 per cent).[2] Between 2006 and 2008, more than 35,000 women (in England and Wales) were diagnosed with an ectopic pregnancy and 6 of them died. Four of these deaths may have been associated with inadequate care.[2] Most ectopic pregnancies (98 per cent) are found in the fallopian tube, but they can occur anywhere outside the uterus or even within the uterine wall (caesarean scar ectopic) or cervical ectopic pregnancy within the inner and outer cervical os (Figure 8.2). The combination of loss of a wanted pregnancy with potential loss of fertility can cause considerable distress and adversely effect the quality of life.[3]

The condition is still one of the causes of maternal death but with the increased use of ultrasound scanning in experienced hands, most cases are diagnosed and managed without the woman coming to major harm. The condition still confounds even the most experienced healthcare providers and should not be taken lightly. Transvaginal ultrasound combined with serum β-hCG assessment is the best way to diagnose ectopic pregnancy.[1,3,4]

8.2 Attributing Factors

Causes of ectopic pregnancy include damage to the body of the fallopian tube, or to the cilia. Recognised predisposing factors include:

- History of infertility
- IVF
- STI
  – Past chlamydia infection, including a raised chlamydia antibody titre in women who have never knowingly had chlamydia
  – Past gonorrhoea infection
- Past tubal ligation sterilisation or tubal reconstruction
- Intrauterine contraceptive device (overall IUCs reduce the risk of ectopic compared with no contraception use)
- Endometriosis.

The infections described are often sub-clinical with the woman being unaware she has suffered one or more.

8.3 Confounding Diagnostic Factors – Clinical Presentation

The bowel, urinary and reproductive organs are all intimately positioned within the pelvis. All of these structures can give rise to similar symptoms in early pregnancy. This causes half of all ectopic pregnancies

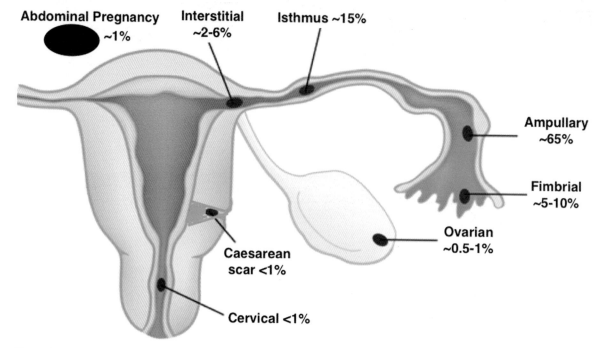

Figure 8.1 Locations of Ectopic pregnancy.

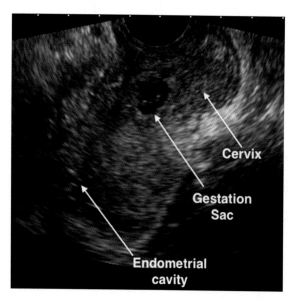

Figure 8.2 Cervical Ectopic. These are rare, accounting for <1 per cent of ectopics. Risk factors include previous curettage, previous caesarean section and IVF.

to be missed at first consultation. For this reason, a high index of suspicion is needed and a low threshold for doing a pregnancy test. Pregnancy testing should be routine in girls and women of reproductive potential who present with pain or a change in their bleeding pattern. Despite the advances in technology and competence with this over the past 10–15 years, a good history remains the key to diagnosis in most cases of ectopic pregnancy. In order to view the pelvis with the best chance of visualising an ectopic, its history should be looked into which will give vital clues as to where to look and what may be found.

8.4 Signs and Symptoms

The classic clinical signs of ectopic pregnancy are as follows: a positive pregnancy test – no matter how faint the test line is on any pregnancy test, it should be read as pregnant.

Ectopic pregnancy can be relatively asymptomatic, or it can cause severe pain, haemodynamic instability and maternal death. However, usually, the woman will complain of unilateral, lower abdominal pain, which is persistently in the same place, becoming worse over time. She will often have an orangey-brown vaginal loss as the fallopian tube begins to distend and ooze, progressing to red loss as the tube ruptures. There may be no revealed bleeding but only fluid visible in the pelvis, usually in the recto- uterine pouch (Pouch of Douglas), and an empty uterus (Figure 8.3). Where the content of fluid is blood, there may be evidence of clot/fibrin within the fluid (Figure 8.3d).

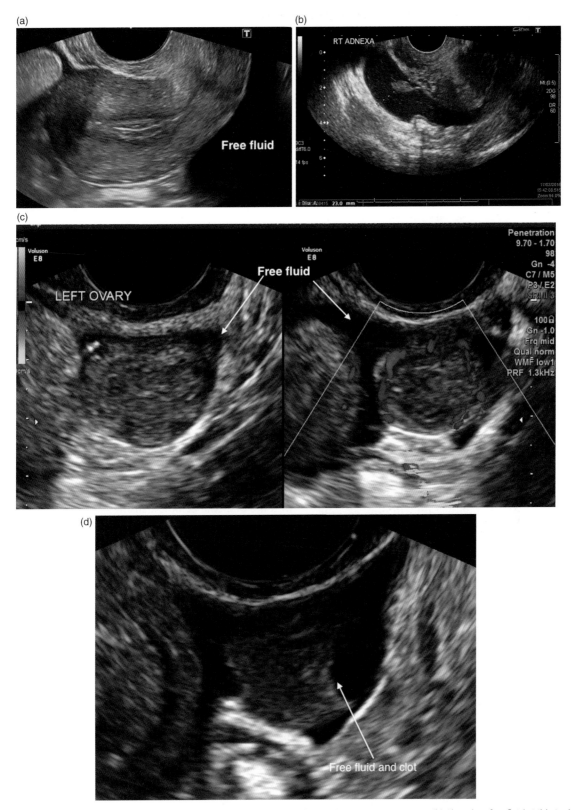

Figure 8.3 (a) Transvaginal scan showing an empty uterus with free fluid in the recto-uterine space. (b) Abundant free fluid visible in the recto-uterine space with no evidence of an intrauterine pregnancy. Possible clot or fibrin is visible within the fluid consistent with blood. (c) Free fluid is also seen around the ovaries. (d) Free fluid containing clot. This will wobble when gently probed with the transducer or if the woman moves her pelvis.

Classically:

- Bleeding – is evident in most cases, but is not always present.
- Pain – often unilateral in the iliac fossa. Most cases of lower abdominal pain, even unilateral iliac fossa pain, are not due to ectopic pregnancy.

  However, many women, especially those in some of the high-risk groups such as those with endometriosis, PID or a history of these conditions, or those with painful periods, have pain at times during their cycle and some have pain up to 100 per cent of the time. So, differentiating between normal and a new pathology can be fraught with difficulty.

> **Important** – *At the point of rupture, a woman who has been agitated, in significant pain and restless, may become more settled. This is the time to insert large bore cannulae, take blood for group and save, full blood count and serum β-hCG, monitor vital signs constantly and alert the theatre team.*

8.5 Diagnosis of an Ectopic Pregnancy

Women of reproductive age with lower abdominal pain and/or bleeding per vaginum (PV) should have a pregnancy test taken on seeking medical help from general practitioners, emergency departments or early pregnancy units. If positive, ectopic pregnancy should be assumed until excluded, due to the risk of morbidity and mortality associated with the condition. Historically, a diagnosis of ectopic pregnancy was most often made at laparoscopy, and the threshold for laparoscopy was a symptomatic woman with a positive pregnancy test and absence of a pregnancy within the uterus on scan. However, with the advent of high-resolution transvaginal ultrasound, positive visualisation of the ectopic pregnancy is achieved in 70–90 per cent of cases. The remaining 10–30 per cent are PUL. In 2016, The Royal College of Obstetricians and Gynaecologist Green Top Guidance stated that transvaginal ultrasound is the diagnostic tool of choice for ectopic pregnancy.[5]

Most healthcare facilities now have access to serum β-hCG tests which are useful in assessing women for the progress of a pregnancy of unknown location or progressing pregnancy. It is important to familiarise oneself with the assay and levels at which one's unit assay is likely to show a gestation sac within the uterus on transvaginal ultrasound. Progesterone is not a useful indicator of ectopic pregnancy.[5]

The presence of an intrauterine pregnancy in natural conception greatly reduces the risk of ectopic pregnancy, although it does not completely exclude the condition (see heterotopic pregnancy).

8.6 Where to Find an Ectopic Pregnancy

Most ectopic pregnancies are found within the fallopian tube (see Figure 8.1). Tubal ectopic pregnancies should be positively identified, if possible, by visualising an adnexal mass that moves separate to the ovary.[5]

- Tubal Ectopic – 93–97 per cent (Figure 8.4a–c):
  - ampullary: most common ~80 per cent of tubal ectopics and ~65 per cent of all ectopics
  - isthmal ectopic: ~15 per cent of tubal ectopics (Figure 8.5)
  - fimbrial ectopic ~5 per cent of tubal ectopics and ~ 5–10 per cent of all ectopics
- Interstitial or cornual ectopic 2–6 per cent; also essentially a type of tubal ectopic (Figure 8.6a, b)
- Ovarian ectopic – ovarian pregnancy; 0.5–1 per cent (Figure 8.7)
- Cervical ectopic – cervical pregnancy; rare < 1 per cent (Figure 8.2)
- Caesarian scar ectopic – site of previous Caesarian section scar; rare (Figure 8.8b)
- Abdominal ectopic: rare; ~1.4 per cent (Figure 8.9a, b)
- Heterotopic pregnancies – particular risk of IVF pregnancies 1 per cent[3] (Figure 8.10a)

Approximately 7 per cent of ectopic pregnancies are outside the fallopian tube, but they account for disproportionate morbidity.

8.7 Ultrasound in the Diagnosis of Ectopic Pregnancy

No specific ultrasound appearances are diagnostic of an ectopic pregnancy unless a viable embryo/fetus is identified outside the endometrial cavity. All women with a positive pregnancy test should be treated as an ectopic pregnancy until a pregnancy is seen in the uterus, as many ectopic pregnancies are not visible outside the uterus at first examination. Half of all ectopic pregnancies are misdiagnosed, or not seen at first presentation.[1]

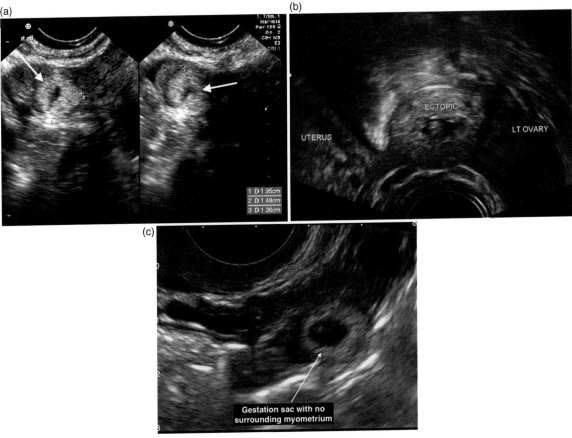

Figure 8.4 (a) A transvaginal image of the right adnexal region. There is a gestation sac (arrowed) that is not surrounded by myometrium so the appearance resembles a 'doughnut' or 'bagel'. (b) A left tubal ectopic lying between the uterus and the left ovary. (c) It is unclear from the image what structures are adjacent to this gestation sac, except it is clearly not within the uterus. The ectopic shows the typical 'bagel' or 'doughnut' appearance.

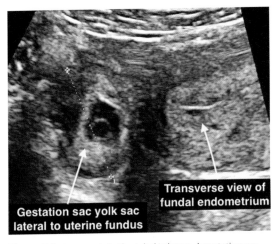

Figure 8.5 An ectopic in the tubal isthmus. A gestation sac containing a yolk sac is visible immediately adjacent to the right lateral margin of the uterus. It lies outside the myometrial margin so is likely to be in the tubal isthmus.

8.7.1 The Endometrium

There is no particular endometrial appearance that is characteristic of ectopic pregnancy. It can appear thick or thin, layered or uniform.

The first ultrasound finding of an intrauterine pregnancy at around four and a half weeks is the intra-decidual sac sign (Figures 8.11a), where a small sac is seen implanting in thickened decidua on one side of the endometrial cavity, so appearing eccentrically placed. This sign is not universally reliable.[5,6] Decidual cysts can be mistaken for an intradecidual sac, and decidual cysts are common in normal and ectopic pregnancies. These are located within the endometrial–myometrial junction, often multiple and usually without an echogenic rim (Figure 8.12b). There is the risk that a decidual cyst may be mistaken for the intradecidual sign. Follow-up of these women is

139

(a)
(b)

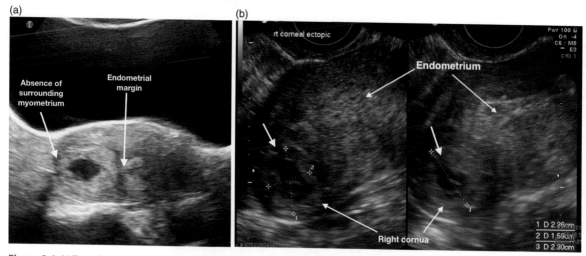

Figure 8.6 (a) Transabdominal transverse view at the level of the uterine fundus showing a gestation sac in the interstial myometrium outside the endometrial cavity and with an incomplete myometrial layer surrounding the sac. (b) Transvaginal transverse view also shows the gestation sac is adjacent to but not within the cornual part of the endometrial cavity.

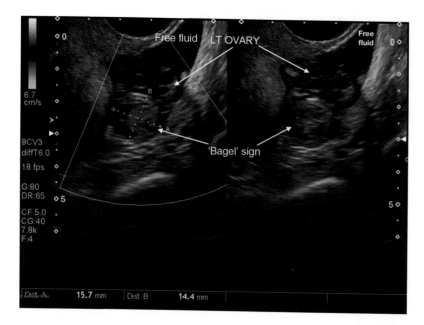

Figure 8.7 This well-defined spherical structure in a woman with a positive PT and empty uterus appears attached to the left ovary. It is not possible on scan to definitively determine whether an ectopic is ovarian or adjacent to the ovary. Ovarian ectopics account for 0.5–1 per cent of ectopics and predisposing factors include intrauterine contraceptive use, IVF and PID.

important, both with ultrasound and serum β-hCG levels, which will be discussed in the next section. Within a week of the intradecidual sign appearing, a yolk sac should be visible within the sac of a viable intrauterine pregnancy, reasonably excluding ectopic pregnancy in most cases.

At around five weeks' gestation, a 'double decidual sign' is caused by the chorionic villi surrounded by a crescent-shaped fluid-filled area and in turn surrounded by the decidua vera. This sign is highly indicative of an intrauterine sac, especially if seen in conjunction with a yolk sac (Figure 8.11b, c). It is too early to clarify whether a pregnancy is viable so where this is of concern, women with a double decidual sign should still be followed up, usually by re-scanning them in 10–14 days, to confirm viability.[4] If a clinician is in any doubt, the β-hCG level can be repeated.

At 5–6 weeks, in many pregnancies a fetal pole will be visible on ultrasound or cardiac pulsations

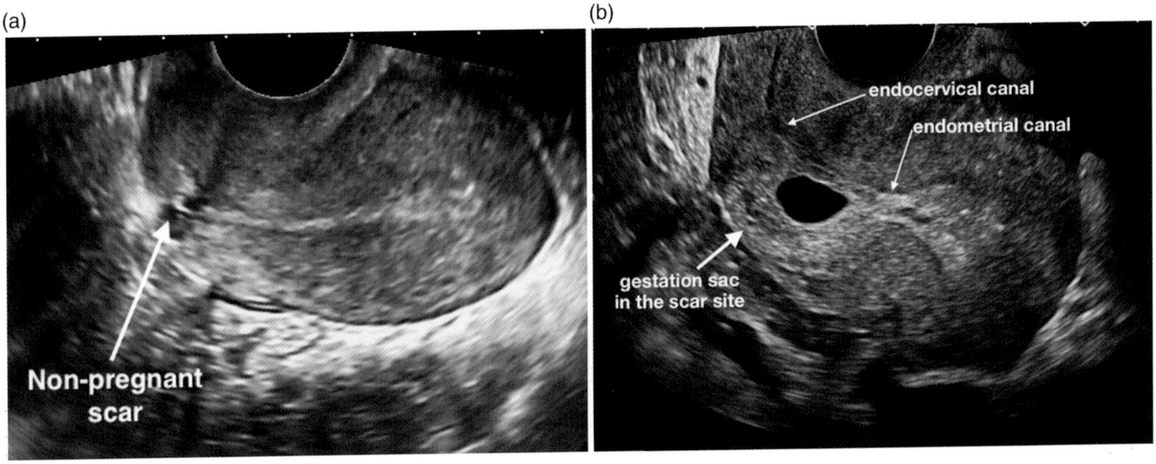

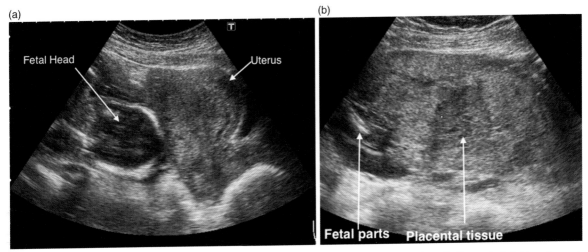

Figure 8.8 (a) There is a myometrial defect at the site of a caesarean scar in this retroflexed non-pregnant uterus. (b) A subsequent pregnancy shows features of a scar ectopic. The higher the number of previous caesareans the greater the risk of scar ectopic. The gestation sac in (b) lies within the scar close to the empty endometrial cavity. There is no visible myometrium between the sac/placenta and the serosal surface of the uterus. The placentation may grow towards the bladder or towards the endometrial cavity. If the pregnancy continues there is a high risk of placenta accreta.

Figure 8.9 (a) An advanced abdominal pregnancy. The uterus lies to the left and the fetal head to the right. No amniotic fluid can be seen surrounding the fetus, although the fetal kidneys and bladder were visible on review of the fetal anatomy. (b) The mass of placental tissue lies within the peritoneal cavity not surrounded by myometrium and with little or no evidence of amniotic fluid. Some fetal long bones can be seen adjacent to the placenta.

can be seen within the sac (Chapter 7). It is prudent to see both a fetal pole and cardiac pulsations before a definitive diagnosis of viable intrauterine pregnancy is made.

Interdecidual fluid or a 'pseudosac' may also be misdiagnosed as an early pregnancy. A pseudosac may be present in 10–20 per cent of ectopic pregnancies. This is a fluid collection within the endometrial canal surrounded by a single echogenic rim (Figure 8.13) as opposed to the double echogenic rim seen with the 'double decidual sac' sign (Figure 8.11a–c).

It is agreed that transvaginal ultrasound is the diagnostic tool of choice for the diagnosis of ectopic pregnancy and that abdominal ultrasound can augment this with an assessment of ovaries and surrounding areas, the kidneys and liver (specifically the hepato-renal fossa, also called Morisson's Pouch) to assess for large volume haemoperitoneum

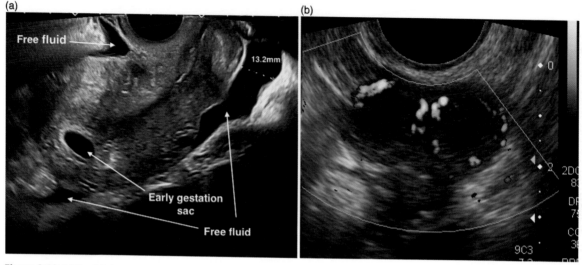

Figure 8.10 (a) Possible heterotopic pregnancy – there is an intrauterine gestation sac but also an abnormal amount of fluid surrounding the uterus. Free fluid above the level of the fundus is a significant amount, especially when fluid is present under the diaphragm and around the liver. (b) Two corpora lutea demonstrated with a single intrauterine pregnancy necessitates consideration of the possibility of heterotopic pregnancy where symptoms or other ultrasound findings could reflect this rare diagnosis.

(Figure 8.14) which collects in the fossa as it is the most dependent part of the body with the patient lying supine.[7] This is particularly important in women who have had IVF, or in whom an intrauterine pregnancy is not seen with confidence; this examination is imperative to diagnosis.[3] Free fluid may also be seen on transabdominal imaging of the pericolic gutters, perihepatic and perispinal regions. If large volumes of free fluid are seen, urgent management in the form of surgery is indicated and should be expedited.

On ultrasound, the pelvis should be imaged in at least two planes (normally sagittal/long axis and transverse/short axis) ensuring that the examination is not just focused on the uterus, tubal regions and the ovaries. Visualising out to the pelvic wall and down to the cervix and vagina is essential for a thorough assessment. In addition, high-resolution assessment of the endometrial cavity is required to visualise small intrauterine gestation sacs (Figures 8.11 and 8.12). Thereafter, detailed assessment of both adnexal regions is required, not only the side of the reported pain, but the opposing side too. The ovaries are assessed followed by concentration on the areas between the uterus and the ovaries to assess the fallopian tubes for masses, as this is the area where most ectopic pregnancies occur. When a pregnancy test is positive and there is no evidence of an IUP on ultrasound, any

adnexal finding other than a corpus luteum should be considered suspicious of an ectopic pregnancy until proven otherwise (Figure 8.15a, b).

8.7.2 Typical Adnexal Features

A 'doughnut' or 'bagel' sign is the most characteristic feature of an ectopic pregnancy in the adnexa (Figures 8.4, 8.5, 8.15a–c).

An 'inhomogenous mass' is the description given to a mass of differing echo texture that is sometimes seen at the ectopic site (Figure 8.16a–c). These can be found above, below or adjacent to the ovary, so a careful assessment of these areas is of great importance, as is recording of any masses or abnormalities. Occasionally, an ectopic pregnancy may appear as a solid mass in the adnexa surrounded by a ring of vascularity shown on Colour Doppler imaging (Figure 8.15a). This should be differentiated from the corpus luteum (Figure 8.17). The site of the corpus luteum may lead the operator to believe that the mass will be on the same side, but in one-third of cases the ectopic pregnancy is on the contralateral side.

8.7.3 Interactive Imaging

Gentle palpation of the area between the operator's free hand and the probe can show the mobility of masses found. This helps to differentiate between

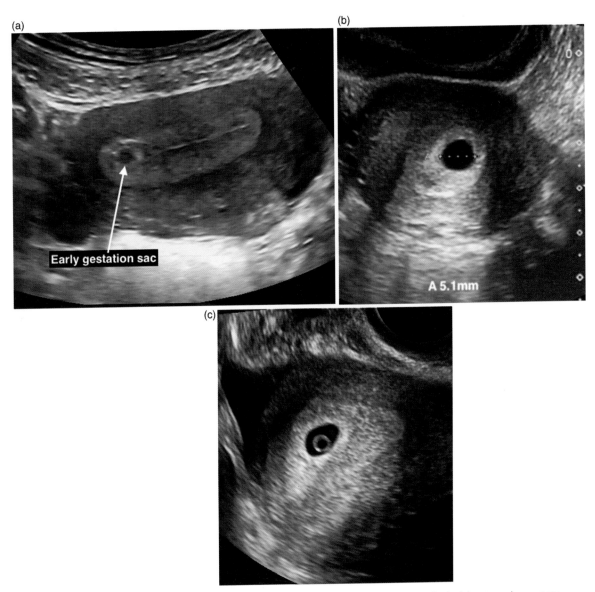

Figure 8.11 Double decidual or intradecidual sac sign. Transabdominal (a) and transvaginal images (b, c) of the uterus demonstrate gestational sac surrounded by two hyperechoic curvilinear lines. The inner line represents *deciduas capsularis*, the outer line represents *deciduas vera* (parietalis). Also note the yolk sac in (c).

ovarian masses that move with the ovary and the separate mobility of an ectopic pregnancy within the fallopian tube.

A defined or suspected ectopic pregnancy should be measured in three dimensions to help inform the treatment options most appropriate (Figures 8.4, 8.6, 8.16). Following this, it is important to assess the recto-uterine pouch for any evidence of free fluid (Figures 8.3, 8.10a, 8.16c), as this allows any treatment

plans to be assessed for risk of rupture with more confidence.

8.8 Masses in the Fallopian Tube

As this is the most common site of ectopic pregnancy, following on from an assessment of the endometrium, the area between both sides of the ovary and uterine wall must be carefully assessed (Figures 8.3c–8.7 and

(a)

(b)

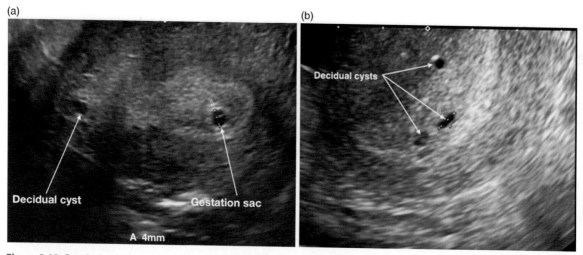

Figure 8.12 Decidual cysts do not typically have a bright edge but more importantly do not have the double decidual sac sign.

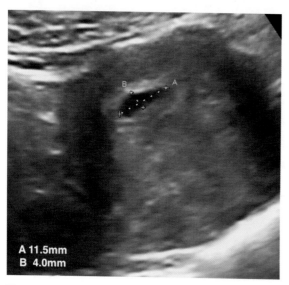

Figure 8.13 A pseudosac – fluid between the decidual layers. There is no specific appearance of the endometrium with tubal ectopic. In about 20 per cent there may be fluid in the cavity.

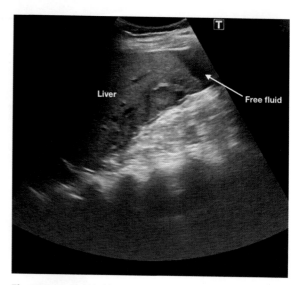

Figure 8.14 Fluid in Morrison's Pouch indicating a significantly abnormal amount of free fluid.

8.15–8.17). Normal fallopian tubes are rarely seen, but a swelling or mass, a fluid-filled sac (ring) with or without yolk sac may be seen or a live (embryo) ectopic pregnancy seen outside the uterine cavity. This is diagnostic for ectopic pregnancy (Table 8.1).

Most ectopic pregnancies arise in the ampullary portion of the fallopian tube. Typically, the enlargement of the fallopian tube will be due to bleeding into the wall and lumen of the tube rather than the conceptus. This is usually demonstrated as an amorphous mass.

A careful assessment of myometrium is required to assess the amount of myometrial tissue surrounding a gestation sac. This should be approximately 5 mm when measured in all planes around a sac which is located high in the cornua or interstitial part of the uterus; this is important to rule out interstitial or cornual pregnancy (Figure 8.6). The operator may wish to confirm findings with a second operator, as the diagnosis of a cornual pregnancy is more difficult to manage clinically. An undiagnosed cornual pregnancy may reach a more advanced stage of development compared with tubal pregnancy, and bleeding can then be torrential if rupture occurs.

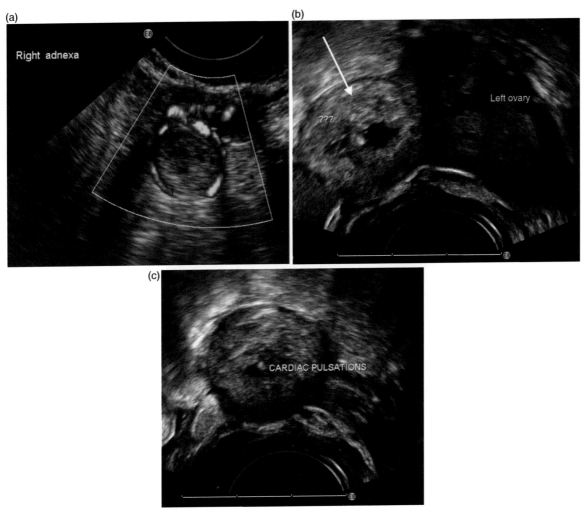

Figure 8.15 (a) A solid mass in the right adnexa surrounded by a peripheral ring of vascularity is suspicious for an ectopic. It should not be mistaken for the corpus luteum as it is not obviously within the ovary. (b) A mass lying adjacent to the left ovary (arrowed) has the more characteristic appearance of the bagel or doughnut sign. Both of these cases had a positive pregnancy test with an empty uterus. Right and left ampullary tubal ectopic pregnancies respectively were subsequently confirmed. (c) Within the classic 'bagel' sign in this case an embryonic heart beat was visible demonstrating a 'live ectopic'.

8.9 Ovarian Findings

The most common finding in the ovary is the corpus luteum (yellow body), a normal pregnancy-related structure that can vary in appearance and size (Figures 8.17–8.18 and Chapter 4). It is situated within or exophytic to the ovary, whereas most ectopic pregnancies are within the fallopian tube. Even a cyst that appears complex (mixed echo texture) is more likely to be a corpus luteum than an ectopic pregnancy (Figure 8.18). The wall of a corpus luteum is usually much more hyopechoic than that of an ovarian ectopic pregnancy. Gentle manipulation between the vaginal probe and the operator's free hand will show whether the mass moves with or is separate from the ovary. A haemorrhagic ovarian cyst will evolve as the blood within it changes (Figure 8.19).

Ovarian ectopic pregnancy is extremely rare. It can appear as a ring-like structure intimately related to the ovary (Figure 8.7), a ring with yolk sac, or a live embryo, as with tubal ectopic pregnancy.

8.10 Less Common Findings

Cervical ectopic pregnancies account for less than 1 per cent of ectopic pregnancies. They are centred in

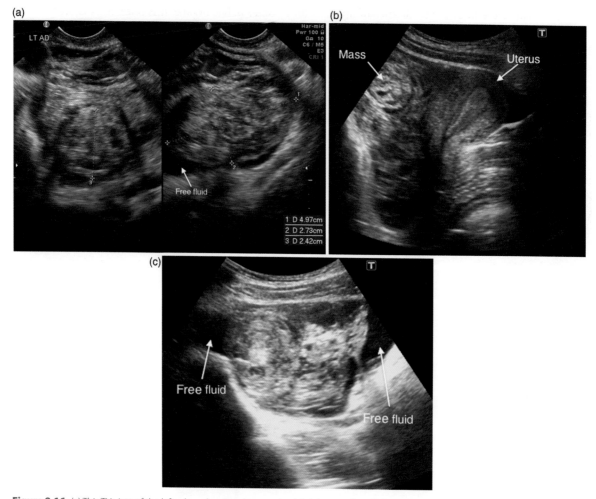

Figure 8.16 (a) This TV view of the left adnexal region shows a sizeable inhomogenous mass with surrounding free fluid. (b) Viewed transabdominally in longitudinal section, the uterus appears pushed forwards by the sizeable mass behind. A normal endometrial echo is demonstrated with no sign of a pregnancy. (c) Significant free fluid around the mass (arrows).

the cervix (Figure 8.2) and enlarge the cervical canal. It is important to routinely locate the cervical canal and follow this upwards to the endometrial canal to ensure that any ectopic pregnancy located outside the endometrial cavity is not misinterpreted as a normal implantation. Cervical ectopics show an empty uterus, a barrel-shaped cervix, a gestational sac present below the level of the internal cervical os, the absence of the 'sliding sign' and blood flow around the gestational sac using Colour Doppler.[5]

Where a pregnancy is located in the upper cervix, it may grow into the lower segment of the uterus and the pregnancy may continue.

Most pregnancies that implant in the cervix will miscarry, and sometimes it is unclear whether a sac

seen in the cervix is a normally located pregnancy in the process of miscarriage. An on-going cervical pregnancy can be differentiated from a miscarriage in progress by cardiac pulsations at or after about six weeks' gestation. Profuse bleeding at the time of surgical management of a cervical pregnancy often occurs due to the amount of fibrous tissue in the cervix. Because of this risk, referral to a senior clinician should occur without delay where cervical pregnancy is suspected.

8.10.1 Scar Ectopic Pregnancy

These are on the increase, probably due to the rise in caesarean section rates. An empty uterus, empty cervical canal but a developmental sac in the anterior lower segment of the uterus with absence of myometrium between the bladder wall and the sac is indicative of scar ectopic pregnancy (Figure 8.8b).

8.10.2 Abdominal Pregnancy

This is a very rare condition that usually develops in the ovarian ligaments, but can develop elsewhere in the pelvis where it takes blood supply from omentum or other pelvic organs. It is often not diagnosed until relatively late, when the risk of life-threatening emergency to the mother and child is high. Live birth has occasionally resulted from abdominal pregnancy, but major blood loss should be anticipated at delivery and procedures and expertise in place to manage this. (Figure 8.9a, b)

8.10.3 Ultrasound Appearances in Heterotopic Pregnancy

Experience and improved techniques in infertility units are making the practice of returning several embryos during IVF less prevalent. However, this is not the case for all units or individual women and many women undergoing such treatment may have sub-fertility due to tubal damage, which renders

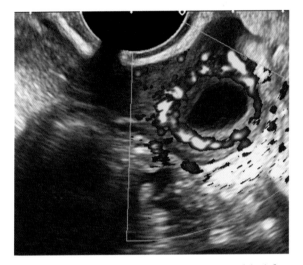

Figure 8.17 A typical corpus luteum of pregnancy with high flow resembling a 'ring of fire'. Colour Doppler cannot differentiate a corpus luteum from an ectopic; however, a corpus luteum will have surrounding ovarian tissue; it will move with the manipulation of the ovary and it will not have the thick echogenic ring seen with decidua.

Table 8.1 PPV for Adnexal Ultrasound Findings

Ultrasound Sign	PPV for Ectopic (%)
Live embryo in extrauterine sac	100
Adnexal mass with a yolk sac or non-viable embryo	Close to 100
Complex or solid adnexal mass Example – tubal ring	95
Echogenic tubal ring/doughnut separate from the ovary	90–95

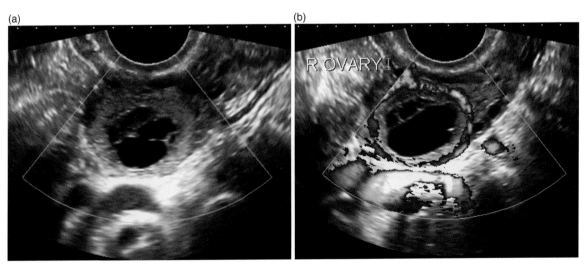

(a) (b)

Figure 8.18 (a) A corpus luteum with haemorrhage within. The apparent echogenic ring is accentuated by haemorrhage within the luteal cyst, but is not a decidual ring. (b) Colour Doppler gives the characteristic high circumferential flow seen in a corpus luteum.

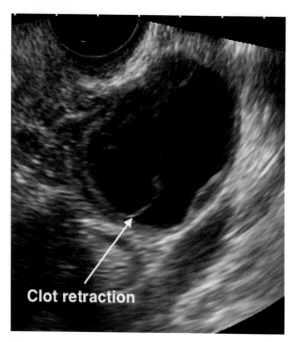

Clot retraction

Figure 8.19 Clot retraction within a resolving ovarian haemorrhagic cyst. A thin rim of normal ovarian tissue can be seen around the cystic area.

them at greater risk of ectopic pregnancy. It is important to know that, if a pregnancy is achieved by IVF, the risk of ectopic pregnancy is two to four times more likely than with spontaneous conception, and heterotopic pregnancy should not be discounted in the event of a live intrauterine pregnancy being seen. It is also more prevalent in women undergoing ovulation induction. Careful assessment of both adnexae should still be performed and recorded, even where an intrauterine pregnancy is seen, as the risk of heterotopic pregnancy rises from around 1 in 30,000 with natural conception to 1 in 100 with multiple embryo transfer at IVF, and is thought to be rising.[5] Where more than one embryo has been replaced at IVF, or where more than one corpora lutea is identified in a natural conception (Figure 8.10b), visualising an early intrauterine pregnancy does not reliably rule out a co-existing heterotopic pregnancy. Where there are symptoms, particularly in the context of more than a normal amount of free fluid (Figure 8.10a) the possibility of an ectopic co-existing with a normal intrauterine pregnancy needs to be considered and very careful evaluation of the possible sites performed.

8.11 Colour Doppler Assessment

Some ectopic pregnancies will demonstrate high circumferential blood flow (Figures 8.3c and 8.15a) reflecting low impedance and high diastolic flow that often surrounds a tubal ectopic pregnancy, particularly where the pregnancy is still 'viable'. This can be mistaken for a corpus luteum (Figures 8.17 and 8.18b), so this hypervascular appearance is only a differential of ectopic pregnancy when it can be demonstrated as being separate from the ovary. It is a useful image to capture when an ectopic pregnancy is suspected, as it will differentiate it from bowel loops.

8.12 β-hCG

This hormone is secreted from the pregnancy and works in conjunction with progesterone secreted by the corpus luteum to support the development of the embryo and fetus until 11–16 weeks when the placenta is established. β-hCG is detected in maternal blood samples by radioimmunoassay as early as 7–8 days after ovulation, although in most units, pregnancy tests will be positive (>2 mIU/ml) by 10 or 11 days post-luteinising-hormone surge (or hCG injection in IVF pregnancies). Generally, the rise in β-hCG levels is 63–100 per cent in 48 hours, although in very early pregnancies, this rise can be slower.[8] Levels peak at about 8–10 weeks and then begin to fall, remaining at lower levels throughout the remaining pregnancy (Table 8.2).

8.12.1 The Discriminatory Zone (An 'Outdated' Concept)

This is the level at which an intrauterine pregnancy is expected to be seen, but is now generally regarded as a flawed concept owing to this range of β-hCG showing considerable variation. Ultrasound features of ectopic pregnancy may be present at relatively low levels of β-hCG so the indication for ultrasound and its interpretation should be based on the clinical history and not the β-hCG level. Calculations and models incorporating β-hCG used in the diagnosis of pregnancy location contain imperfections.

8.12.2 Progesterone

A single assessment of maternal progesterone blood levels can give an indication whether a pregnancy is likely to be on-going or failed. Low levels usually

Table 8.2 Reference Ranges for Beta hCG (using the Roche Cobas® analyser) during the First Half of Pregnancy

Weeks of Gestation	β--hCG (mIU/ml)
3	6–71
4	10–750
5	217–7138
6	158–31795
7	3697–163563
8	32065–149571
9	63803–151410
10	46509–186977
12	27832–210612
14	13950–62530
15	12039–70971
16	9040–56451
17	8157–55868
18	8099–58176

indicate non-viability but, like the β-hCG level, it does not tell the clinician where the pregnancy is situated in the pelvis.

8.13 Ultrasound Assessment during the Treatment of Ectopic Pregnancy

Traditionally, active treatment options for ectopic pregnancy have largely fallen into two categories:

Surgery – Laparotomy and more recently laparoscopic salpingectomy for ectopic pregnancies within a fallopian tube or partial oophorectomy in the case of an ovarian ectopic pregnancy were, until relatively recently, seen as the treatment of choice for many ectopic pregnancies due to the perception that it is a serious gynaecological condition with high levels of morbidity and a risk of mortality. This is still the treatment of choice in a haemodynamically unstable woman. However, as the maternal age is rising and risks of pelvic damage becoming more prevalent, other modes of treatment are being considered.

Methotrexate – Although not currently licenced for use for the treatment of ectopic pregnancy, a single dose treatment is used in many units (50 mg/m^2). This can cause side effects and the current advice following treatment is to wait three months before conceiving again to allow folic acid pathways to normalise before the next pregnancy. Folic acid supplementation is important to minimise the risk of neural tube defect in the next pregnancy.[9]

An emerging alternative – Conservative – This alternative option is emerging for carefully selected women.[10] The management is based on natural demise of small ectopic pregnancies or PUL. It is essential that the woman understands the need to seek medical intervention quickly should symptoms of abdominal pain, bleeding or shoulder tip pain (a sign of diaphragmatic irritation from haemorrhage within the abdomen) occur. She must be willing to undergo follow-up for reasonably long periods of time (up to 147 days has been recorded), to allow natural resolution of ectopic pregnancy.[9,11] The decision to manage an ectopic pregnancy in this way relies on accurate ultrasound assessment of the size and position of the 'ectopic' (if seen) as well as β-hCG levels below 1500 mIU/ml where the ectopic pregnancy is seen within the fallopian tube or 2000 mIU/ml in the case of a PUL.

Fertility outcomes are similar for the methods described.

During treatment, whether with methotrexate or conservative management, ultrasound surveillance of the woman may be repeated in the presence of worsening or new symptoms, or in order to assess the efficacy of treatments and review management as required. This should be carried out in the normal way as others.

8.14 Summary

The term PUL is appropriate where ultrasound fails to clarify the pregnancy location in a woman with a positive pregnancy test. A systematic approach is required to avoid misdiagnosis and to ensure timely diagnosis and management where the pregnancy is ectopic.

There are numerous locations for ectopic pregnancy and characteristic ultrasound findings in a high proportion of cases, which have been reviewed in this chapter. Expectant management is appropriate in certain cases where the woman is stable as spontaneous resolution will often occur.

References

1. Jurkovic D, Wilkinson H. 2011 Diagnosis and management of ectopic pregnancy. *BMJ* 2011;342:d3397.

2. *Saving Mothers' Lives: Reviewing Maternal Deaths to Make Motherhood Safer 2006–2008: The Eighth Report of the Confidential Enquiries into Maternal Deaths in*

the United Kingdom; Centre for Maternal and Child Enquiries (CMACE); March 2011 www.hqip.org.uk/assets/NCAPOP-Library/CMACE-Reports/6.-March-2011-Saving-Mothers-Lives-reviewing-maternal-deaths-to-make-motherhood-safer-2006-2008.pdf

3. The Ectopic Pregnancy Trust 2016 – What is an ectopic pregnancy. www.ectopic.org.uk/patients/what-is-an-ectopic-pregnancy/ accessed 11.3.2016

4. *NICE 2012.* Ectopic pregnancy and miscarriage: diagnosis and initial management. *NICE guidelines* [CG154], December 2012.

5. Elson CJ, Salim R, Potdar N, Chetty M, Ross JA, Kirk EJ. 2016 on behalf of the Royal College of Obstetricians and Gynaecologists. Diagnosis and management of ectopic pregnancy. Green-top Guideline No.21, November 2016.

6. Laing FC, Brown DL, Price JF, Teeger S, Wong ML. Intradecidual sign: is it effective in diagnosis of an early intrauterine pregnancy? *Radiology.* 1997;204:655–660.

7. Chiang G, Levine D, Swire M, McNamara A, Mehta T. The intradecidual sign: is it reliable for diagnosis of early intrauterine pregnancy? *AJR Am J Roentgenol.* 2004;183:725–731.

8. Steinkampf MP, Guzick DS, Hammond KR, Blackwell RE. Identification of early pregnancy landmarks

by transvaginal sonography: analysis by logistic regression. *Fertil Steril.* 1997;1:168–170.

9. Sowter MC, Farquhar CM, Petrie KJ, Gudex G. A randomised trial comparing single dose systemic methotrexate with laparoscopy for the treatment of unruptured tubal pregnancy. *BJOG: Int J Obstet Gynaecol.* 2001;2:192–203.

10. Mavrelos D, Nicks H, Jamil A, Hoo W, Jauniaux E, Jurkovic D. Efficacy and safety of a clinical protocol for expectant management of selected women diagnosed with a tubal ectopic pregnancy. *Ultrasound Obstet Gynecol.* 2013;42:102–107.

11. Turan V. Fertility outcomes subsequent to treatment of tubal ectopic pregnancy in younger Turkish women. *J Pediatr Adolesc Gynecol.* 2011;5:251–255.

Further Reading

Shapiro BS, Cullen M, Taylor KJ, DeCherney AH. Transvaginal ultrasonography for the diagnosis of ectopic pregnancy. *Fertil Steril.* 1988;3:425–429.

Schurz B, Wenzl R, Eppel W, Reinold E. Early detection of ectopic pregnancy by transvaginal ultrasound. *Arch Gynecol Obstet.* 1990; 1:25–29.

Ultrasound Imaging of Progestogen-Only Subdermal Contraceptive Implants*

Paul O'Brien

9.1 Introduction 151
9.2 Locating the Implant 152
9.3 Ultrasound Requirements for Implant Imaging 153
9.4 Visualising the Implant 153
9.5 Ultrasound Appearances of the Structures within the Arm 155
9.6 Adipose Tissue 157
9.7 Fascia 157

9.8 Muscle 157
9.9 Blood Vessels 157
9.10 Nerves 158
9.11 Removal of Deeply Sited and Non-palpable Implants 159
9.12 Use of Ultrasound in the Management of Implant Complications 161
9.13 Tips on How to Avoid Deep Insertion 161
9.14 Summary 161

9.1 Introduction

Sophia, age 17, presents to a community sexual health service with a request for her sub-dermal contraceptive implant to be removed. This was fitted at the time of a surgical termination of pregnancy, whilst Sophia was anaesthetised. The pregnancy was unplanned, but she was ambivalent about her decision, as she had always been of the opinion that abortion was 'wrong'. She felt 'persuaded' to have the implant fitted by both the doctor and her mum.

The nurse seeing her in the sexual health service is very enthusiastic about the fact that Sophia has no bleeding with the implant, but somehow this just didn't feel 'right' to Sophia and she no longer needs contraception. After a long discussion, the nurse agrees to remove the implant and give Sophia some time to consider which method of contraception she would like to use in the future. Unfortunately, the implant is not palpable. Fortunately, the nurse has been on a recent training event, highlighting appropriate investigations under the circumstances.

She explains that Sophia will be referred for an ultrasound scan to a colleague in a neighbouring service with experience of removing impalpable implants and that the implant will likely be removed at that appointment.

Fully impalpable implants are uncommon. Prior to any attempted removal of a fully impalpable implant, ultrasound location is mandatory. There is no good data to estimate the rate of deep implants, but a figure of 1 in 1,000 insertions suggested by the manufacturer has been cited.[1] The rate probably varies with country and training.

Sophia's nurse did one of the most important things in managing a deep implant – recognising the extent of one's skills and referring to an expert with experience in ultrasound location and removal of deeply sited implants.

Although this chapter deals with ultrasound imaging of impalpable contraceptive implants, much of the chapter relates, of necessity, to the applied anatomy of the upper arm. Important vulnerable neural and vascular structures need to be identified using ultrasound and avoided to ensure safe removal of the implant. The manufacturer of Nexplanon® advises that 'exploratory surgery without knowledge of the exact location of the implant' is strongly discouraged. Removal of deeply inserted implants should be conducted with caution in order to prevent damage to deeper neural or vascular structures in the arm and should be performed by clinicians familiar with the anatomy of the arm. Before we remove impalpable implants, we must know precisely where in the arm they lie.

* Figures in the chapter were provided by Mary Pillai.

There are two contraceptive implants in wide use. Nexplanon® is a single radiopaque, non-biodegradable, progestogen-only, flexible white rod containing 68 mg of etonogestrel. It replaced the similar, but non-radiopaque Implanon® in 2011. The rod is 40 mm long and 2 mm wide. Nexplanon® has an ethylene vinyl acetate copolymer hormone impregnated core (also containing barium sulfate, which does not alter its appearance on ultrasound, but makes it radiopaque). It is encased in an ethylene vinyl acetate skin. Jadelle® (Norplant-2) is a two-rod non-biodegradable, progestogen-only, flexible silicone implant, with each rod containing 75 mg of levonorgestrel in a polymer matrix. Jadelle is slightly bigger than Nexplanon® (43 mm long and 2.5 mm wide). The Jadelle rods are also a little softer and more flexible. Both devices have a similar appearance on ultrasound.

When the device is palpable, the most common method of removal is the 'pop out' technique where a small incision is made over one end of the implant that is elevated by applying pressure to the other end. However, sometimes devices are deceptively palpable, yet are still difficult to remove. A device that cannot be 'popped up' for a simple removal because the ends are embedded in subcutaneous tissue and cannot be removed by simple dissection of encapsulating fibrous tissue can usually be removed using the 'U technique'. With this technique the implant is grabbed at the centre of the device using either a mosquito or a modified vasectomy/ring forceps (Figure 9.1) without the use of ultrasound. Most failed removals occur because the ends of the device cannot be freed. More widespread training in the U technique will reduce the number of referrals to specialists for ultrasound-assisted removal.

9.2 Locating the Implant

Ultrasound will always be required when a device is impalpable.

This may be assisted by finding the insertion scar. Unless the device has been inserted into muscle, it will usually be located immediately proximal to the scar. Devices not felt by inexperienced clinicians will frequently be felt at the specialist centre and may not require ultrasound guidance for removal. Sometimes a device not easily palpable and missed on first examination will be located, or at least just felt, with the right hand of the operator (for a device in the left arm) whilst the left hand supports the patient's hand, allowing the upper arm musculature to relax. The suspected location can then be confirmed with ultrasound.

An implant inserted into a muscle does not develop a fibrous thickening around it, as occurs subdermally. Consequently an implant within muscle is not fixed and may be found up to 10 centimetres from its original position (Figure 9.2). An implant inserted in the middle third of the upper arm, but deep in the biceps muscle may be found in the axilla. If the implant cannot be located, the search with ultrasound must be directed upwards towards the axilla and down to the elbow. Likewise, a device inserted into the triceps can

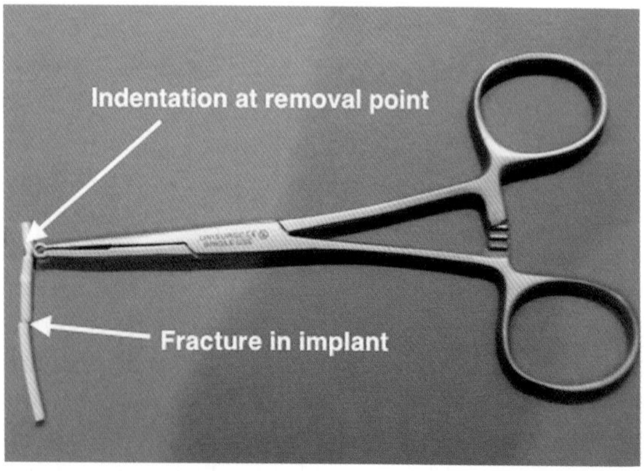

Figure 9.1 Ring forceps for U technique of implant removal. In this case the implant was palpable but there was a palpable fracture midshaft (arrow). The pop out technique will not be effective where the implant is fractured so the U technique was used.

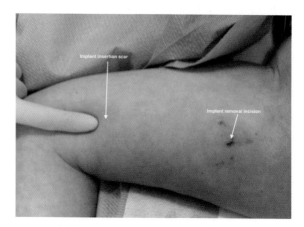

Figure 9.2 This implant removed in this case had never been palpable. It was located with ultrasound and was positioned deeply within the axillary end of biceps muscle. This was her first implant and the insertion scar was more than 10 cm distal to the implant. The punctures either side of the removal incision are from a green needle that was passed under the implant to enable safe removal through a small puncture.

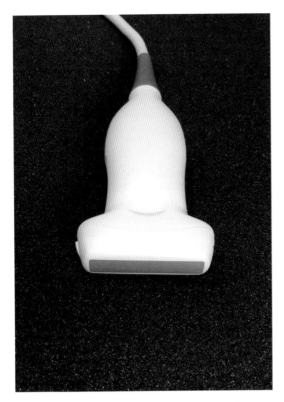

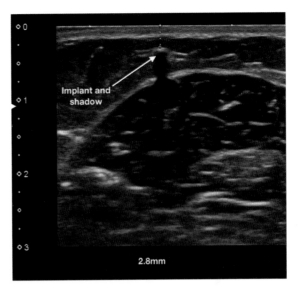

Figure 9.4 Transverse image of the upper arm showing the white (hyperechoeic) edge of the implant nearest the transducer. The acoustic shadow can be seen behind the implant. This implant is normally positioned and easy to palpate.

Figure 9.3 Example of a high frequency linear transducer.

move to either end of the muscle and therefore this area needs to be examined in its entirety before the presence of a device can be excluded.

If the implant is not found in the arm presented, it is appropriate to check the other arm with ultrasound even when the woman feels sure which arm it was fitted into.

9.3 Ultrasound Requirements for Implant Imaging

A high-frequency linear array transducer (10 MHz or greater frequency) is most appropriate to locate deeply sited contraceptive implants (Figure 9.3). The appropriate system preset is selected (typically musculoskeletal) and then the settings are adjusted to optimise the image (Chapters 2 and 17). The benefit associated with turning off compound imaging (multibeam) is discussed in this section.

The most prominent and helpful sonographic feature in detecting implants is the posterior acoustic shadow, sometimes called the 'eclipse sign' (Figure 9.4). In many medical ultrasound examinations of superficial structures, compound image setting is switched on. Compound imaging uses multiple beams to image the same tissue multiple times, but from different angles. With beams angled and oriented along different directions, the echoes from multiple acquisitions are averaged together into a single composite image. The resulting image has reduced levels of speckle, noise, clutter and refractive shadows with improved margin definition. Enhancement and shadowing artefacts are decreased, but this may be a disadvantage in the case of locating a foreign body where the acoustic shadow helps differentiate it from normal anatomical structures.[2] Once the implant is located, compound imaging is turned on.

9.4 Visualising the Implant

The transducer is generally held such that the ulnar aspect or the finger of the operator rests against the patient's arm to stabilise the transducer. This allows fine controlled movements of the probe on the patient's arm (Figure 9.5).

Almost all use of ultrasound to locate and remove deep implants is done with the linear transducer placed across the upper arm, perpendicular to the long axis of the arm so the beam is perpendicular to the lie of the implant. The implant is less well seen when viewed along its length or long axis because there is

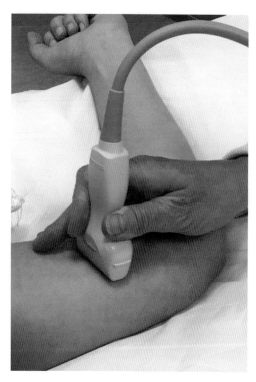

Figure 9.5 Transducer applied transversely to the inner aspect of the arm to locate a non-palpable implant.

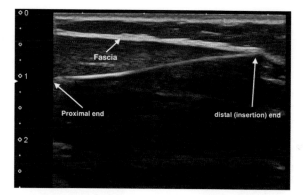

Figure 9.6 This longitudinal view along the length of the implant demonstrates the implant and the acoustic shadow are much less obvious compared with in the transverse view. In this case the implant has been inserted under the fascial sheath and at a downward angle, so the proximal end lies deeper than the distal end. There is minimal subcutaneous tissue. It is under the muscle fascia throughout its length and was never palpable.

less chance of insonating the device at 90 degrees and hence a weaker reflective echo (Figure 9.6). The ultrasound beam is reflected off the edge of the implant closest to the probe, which is seen as a short hyperechoeic (bright) line or dot. The proximal edge of the implant is therefore visible on ultrasound, but the implant itself occupies a 2 mm hypoechoeic area behind it.

Generally, however, it is often the acoustic shadow cast by the implant rather than the implant itself that is seen first. When imaging perpendicular to the implant the acoustic shadow appears as a narrow hypoechoeic (dark) band running deep from the implant (Figure 9.4). No other structure in the upper arm gives a similar appearance, and looking for the shadow behind the implant is the easiest way to find it. With the transducer applied transversely across the gelled inner arm (Figure 9.5), slide the probe up and down to find the acoustic shadow. By sliding the probe up and down the arm, the shadow can be seen as a narrow uninterrupted outline for 4 cms representing the length of the implant. If the implant is not obvious then moving the probe left and right across the medial

aspect of the arm may locate it. Most devices will be discovered on the inner aspect of the upper arm.

Despite clear instructions from the manufacturer of Nexplanon to insert the device 8–10 cms above the medial epicondyle of the humerus, sometimes the device is inserted in the upper or lower third of the arm. Alternatively, the device may be found to have migrated above or below the insertion scar, particularly if it is within muscle (Figure 9.2). If the device is not located in the recommended position in the middle third of the upper arm, the search is extended to include a thorough examination of the upper arm from the midline anteriorly to the midline posteriorly, a full 180 degrees and from the axilla proximally to the elbow distally. Occasionally the device is not inserted in the recommended reclining position, but instead with the user sitting upright with the arm elevated. Insertion in this position can result in the device being inserted anywhere on the posterior upper arm and the examination needs to be extended over the whole area of triceps muscle, guided by the insertion scar.

Once one is familiar with the appearance of implants on ultrasound, they are generally easy to identify. Without that experience, however, devices can be difficult to locate and this is the reason that specialist referral centres with experience of both accurately locating impalpable implants and removing them is recommended for women with implants that are either difficult to feel or impalpable.[3]

On occasion patients and clinicians will report being able to feel an implant immediately after

(a)   (b)

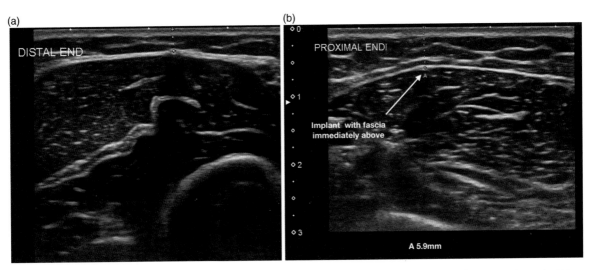

Figure 9.7 Transverse images of the arm 4 cm apart showing (a) the distal end and (b) proximal end. The implant appears located within the fascia throughout its length. It had never been palpable.

insertion, but when it comes to removal it cannot be palpated. Where a device is inserted in adipose tissue deep to the subdermal plane, weight gain will make it more difficult to palpate. However, it will only be completely impalpable where insertion has inadvertently punctured the deep fascia of the upper arm. Non-palpable implants are usually within or below the fascia (Figures 9.6, 9.7 and 9.8), and devices within muscle can migrate (Figure 9.2).

Nexplanon and Jadelle (Norplant 2) are radiopaque and can be easily visualised on X-ray. When they are not palpable, their position can be identified on X-ray relative to a paper clip fixed as a marker on the overlying skin. However, X-ray provides no information on the depth of the device or any adjacent structure that needs to be avoided. Attempted removal based on location by soft tissue X-ray is therefore not recommended. MRI can be used to demonstrate the device and surrounding soft tissue, but as the device might relate differently to surrounding structures at removal with the arm in another position it is less useful than real-time location with ultrasound. Ultrasound has the advantage of being a bedside tool and with appropriate aseptic technique can be used to guide removal.

9.5 Ultrasound Appearances of the Structures within the Arm

Figure 9.9 shows the essential anatomy of the arm relevant to managing deeply sited or non-palpable

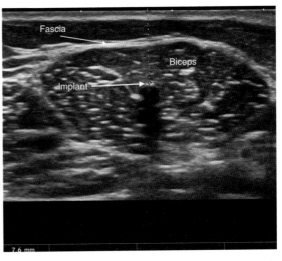

Figure 9.8 Transverse image of arm at the level of the middle of the shaft of the humerus, showing a single rod implant lying within biceps muscle deep to the fascia. This implant had never been palpable.

implants. Initially the manufacturer instructions were to insert at the site of the groove between biceps and triceps (Figure 9.9). However, as shown in the figure, this is in close proximity to main neurovascular structures. Injury to these structures has occurred during attempted removal of deeply sited implants and this led to a revised recommendation that insertion should avoid the sulcus between biceps and triceps. The Clinical Effectiveness Unit of the UK Faculty of Sexual

155

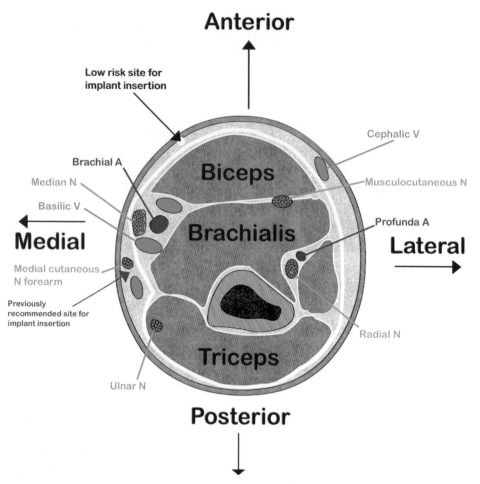

Figure 9.9 Diagram showing the anatomy of the upper arm as seen in transverse section approximately 10cm above the elbow. Artwork courtesy of Mark Pountney, University of Liverpool.

Table 9.1 The Ultrasound Characteristics of Anatomical Structures

	Echogenicity	Transverse	Longitudinal	Compressibility	Doppler
Nerve	Mixed -hyperechoic perineurium	Honeycomb	Fascicular	–	No
Muscle	Mixed	'Starry night' / speckled	Feather like	–	No
Vessel	Anechoic	Round anechoic	Long anechoic	(A) + (V) ++	Yes
Ligament	Hyperechoic	Broom end	Fibrillar	–	No

and Reproductive Healthcare supports the manufacturer's advice that Nexplanon insertion should avoid the sulcus between biceps and triceps and further recommends insertion over biceps muscle, to avoid the potential for injury to the ulnar nerve.[4]

Once the implant and the tissue in which it lies have been identified, it is important to determine what structures lie in close proximity. Ultrasound defines the boundaries between tissues of differing echogenicity. When the ultrasound beam encounters tissue with different acoustic impedance such as the transition from fat to fascia and fascia to muscle, a part of the beam is reflected and is seen as hyperechoic or white. Different anatomical structures may be identified by their individual ultrasound characteristics, as detailed in Table 9.1.

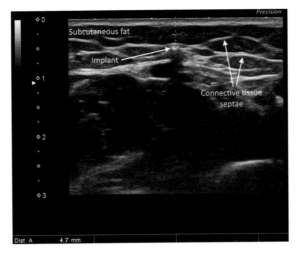

Figure 9.10 Implant 4.7 mm deep in subcutaneous fat and connective tissue. The referring clinician thought it was not palpable, but once its position was clarified with ultrasound, it could be palpated.

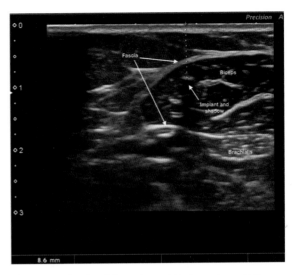

Figure 9.11 Implant 8.6 mm deep within biceps beneath the fascia. The implant was not palpable and the patient had never been able to palpate it.

9.6 Adipose Tissue

Subcutaneous adipose tissue has low echo intensity and appears as dark fat interspersed with hyperechoic (white) linear echoes running mostly parallel to the skin. These represent connective tissue septae (Figure 9.10).

9.7 Fascia

The brachial deep fascia of the arm is a sheet of fibrous connective tissue binding the structures of the upper arm (Figure 9.11). It lies deep to subcutaneous fat, and appears hyperechoeic on ultrasound.

9.8 Muscle

Immediately deep to the fascia of the upper arm are the biceps muscle anteriorly, the anterior brachialis behind biceps becoming superficial towards the elbow and the triceps posteriorly. The sonographic appearance of muscle is distinct and can be discriminated from important surrounding structures such as nerves and blood vessels. The boundaries of the muscle are clearly visible as white hyperechoeic lines. In the transverse plane, perpendicular to the long axis of the muscle, the muscle has a speckled appearance ('Starry night' Figures 9.4, 9.8, 9.11).

9.9 Blood Vessels

The brachial artery is easy to identify. It descends into the upper arm at the axilla, passes down the medial aspect of the arm into the antecubital fossa in front

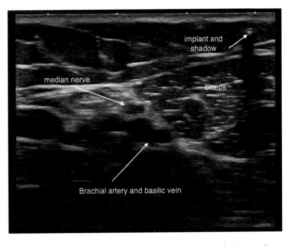

Figure 9.12 Medial aspect of the arm approximately 10 cm above the elbow. Vessels show as round anechoic structures.

of the elbow joint. The basilic vein, often multiple, is found in close proximity (Figures 9.9, 9.12, 9.13). Blood vessels are readily compressible by applying pressure to the transducer, and the artery can be seen pulsating. Pressure of the transducer on the arm can be used to distinguish arteries from veins. The thin-walled veins will readily collapse with minimal pressure. Thicker walled arteries at higher pressure will not so readily compress; however, with modest pressure of the transducer on the arm, both will collapse. No other structures are compressible in this way. By turning on Colour Doppler any area with movement

157

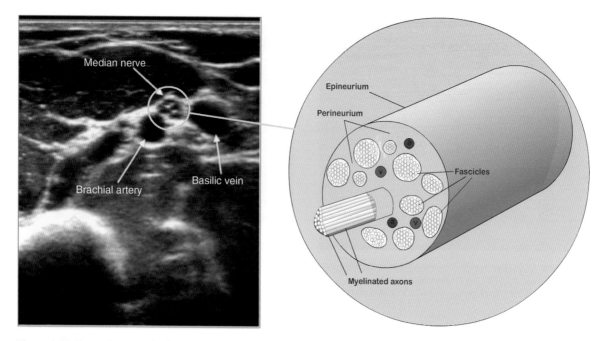

Figure 9.13 The median nerve lies between the brachial artery and basilic vein. The adjacent diagram shows an enlarged transverse section through the nerve showing fascicles.

will light up. This will distinguish blood flow from still structures. Movement toward the transducer is usually coded red and away from the transducer coded blue.

9.10 Nerves

The nerves of the upper arm are recognised by their characteristic appearance. Nerves are described as having a fascicular appearance on ultrasound (like a bunch of bound reeds or straws seen end on) running down the arm (Figures 9.13–9.15). Groups of nerve fibres are bound in fibrous tissue (perineurium) and several of these run within the nerve trunk bound together by epineurium. It is the outer perineurium of the fascicles that appears on ultrasound as hyperechoeic tubes surrounding a hypoechoic core of nerve cells or axons (Figure 9.13). The nerve tissue itself is the hypoechoic inner core of the 'fascicles'. Nerves can be difficult to identify on a simple cross-section from adjacent fibrous tissue. However, with the linear transducer lying transverse to the long axis of the arm, nerves maintain their character as the transducer is moved up and down the entire arm as they run from the axilla to hand, whereas tendons and ligaments insert around the elbow (Figure 9.15).

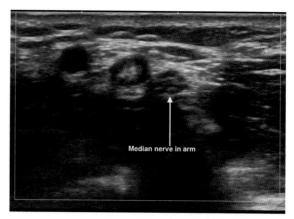

Figure 9.14 Proximity of the median nerve to blood vessels.

Knowledge of the nerve distribution in the arm is necessary for safe removal of deeply sited implants. The important nerves for deep implant removal are the median, ulnar and medial cutaneous nerves of the forearm.

The *median* nerve originates from the brachial plexus hugging the brachial artery, usually lying first lateral to the artery, then crossing anteriorly to the artery in the middle third of the arm, before running medial to the artery in the distal arm and into the antecubital fossa. With the ultrasound transducer held against the medial aspect of the arm (Figure 9.5),

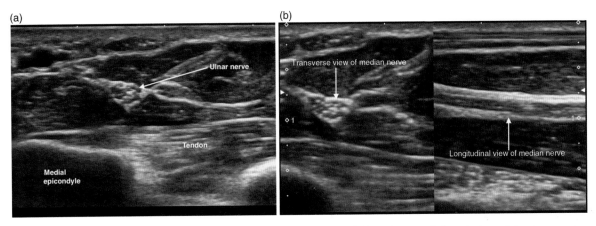

Figure 9.15 (a) Ulnar nerve just above the elbow much more superficially located. (b) Median nerve in forearm shown in transverse and longitudinal section.

the median nerve will be found in close proximity to the brachial artery (Figures 9.12 and 9.13). In 6 per cent of the population the median nerve is bifid and may lie either side of the artery.

The *ulnar* nerve enters the arm medially, close to the brachial artery, and continues down the medial side of the brachial artery as far as the middle of the upper arm. Here it pierces the medial intramuscular septum to lie in the fascia over the medial edge of the triceps and descends to the medial aspect of the elbow joint before leaving the upper arm behind the medial epicondyle of the humerus. The ulnar nerve can be seen on ultrasound at the elbow, immediately behind the medial epicondyle, irrespective of the morphology of the woman, immediately beneath the skin close to the bone (Figure 9.15a). Following a tubular structure to the elbow and seeing it course behind the medial epicondyle can be the easiest way to confirm the structure is the ulnar nerve.

The *medial cutaneous nerve of the forearm,* another branch of the brachial plexus, runs close to the medial side of the brachial artery and basilic vein to the middle of the upper arm where it pierces the deep fascia to run superficial to supply the skin of the medial side of the forearm. Of the nerves of interest in the upper arm only the medial cutaneous nerve of the forearm lies above the fascia in part of its course. The diameter of the nerve is small and it can be difficult to locate on ultrasound.

The radial nerve is of little concern in implant removal as it is tucked away in the posterior compartment of the upper arm and runs behind the humerus and then to the forearm in the lateral aspect of the antecubital fossa.

9.11 Removal of Deeply Sited and Non-palpable Implants

Three techniques are used to remove deep contraceptive implants.

9.11.1 U Technique

With the arm in a stable position, the implant is visualised with ultrasound and the exact position marked on the overlying skin (Figure 9.16a), usually over the most superficial part of the implant. A small 2–4 mm incision is made and with blind dissection, using either a small artery forceps or a ring forceps, the implant is felt and grasped. It is then delivered through the incision and any residual fibrous tissue released.

9.11.2 Open Technique

This is used for deeper sited implants and those below the brachial deep fascia. Similar to the U Technique, ultrasound is used to locate the implant and the skin over implant is marked. A larger 15 mm incision is made over the long axis of the implant. With the aid of retractors and dissection, the implant is located by touch. A ring or small mosquito forceps is then inserted and the implant grasped, any fibrous sheath released and the implant removed.

9.11.3 Needle-Lift Technique

As with the other techniques, the implant is first located with ultrasound and adjacent structures carefully noted. Appropriate aseptic techniques are used including placing the transducer in a sterile cover

(a)   (b)   (c)

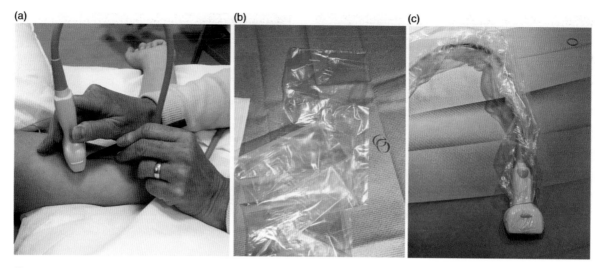

Figure 9.16 (a) Marking the position of a non-palpable implant. (b) A sterile transducer cover. (c) The probe inside the cover.

(a)   (b)   (c)

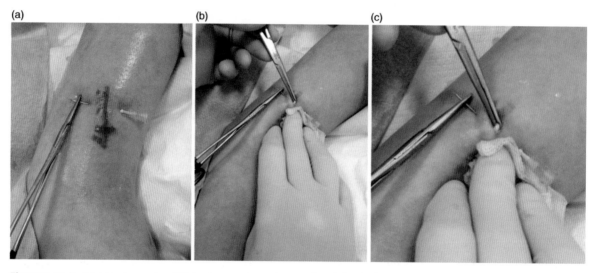

Figure 9.17 (a–c) Removal procedure. This implant was 3 mm above and medial to the brachial artery and 2.5 mm above and lateral to the median nerve and lay parallel to these structures. Guided insertion of the needle lifted it up away from these structures.

(Figure 9.16b) with sterile gel applied inside and outside (Figure 9.16c), and cleansing the skin with alcohol wipes or surgical skin prep. Although shown here (Figure 9.17a), with this technique marking of the skin is unnecessary as real-time ultrasound is used to guide a needle under the implant. The transducer is applied transversely and to the posterior side of the deep implant so that a transverse view of the midpart of the implant is visible in the periphery of the field of view. Using the 'heel in' technique, pressure is applied to the lower edge of the transducer while raising the upper end off the skin and a little sterile acoustic gel applied in the gap. A 21 gauge needle on a 2 or 5 ml syringe filled with lidocaine is aligned to the plane of the ultrasound beam. As the tip of the needle is placed on the skin, the ultrasound image shows it traversing the gel before it pierces the skin to the side of the implant. The tip of the needle, which is kept in view all the time, is advanced under the implant while lidocaine/adrenaline is injected. The needle is then angled

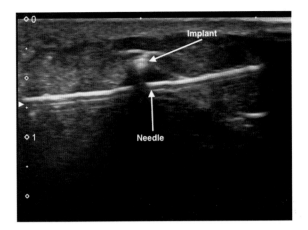

Figure 9.18 Needle placed under a subfascial implant.

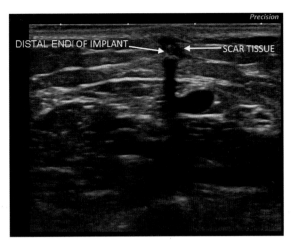

Figure 9.19 Implant surrounded by scar tissue

upwards using counter pressure on the skin of the arm to pierce the skin beyond the implant (Figure 9.17a). Application of a small artery forceps to the exposed tip of the needle will protect both the patient and the operator (ideally it should be closer to the sharp tip than in Figure 9.17a). The implant is now fixed to the skin (Figure 9.18) and can be removed through a small 3 mm incision (Figure 9.17b, c). Blunt dissecting frees the area over the implant and the implant is grasped with ring forceps through the deep fascia. The forceps are raised and angled and the deep fascia incised along the plane of the implant. The implant is exposed, grasped and removed.

Experience with ultrasound needle imaging can be learned with in-vitro training using a phantom with an implant inserted around 1 cm depth in the jelly.[5]

On occasion an impalpable device located on ultrasound will be left in situ. This might be because the device is still within the product license or because the woman does not wish to conceive again and prefers to leave it. However, in other circumstances ultrasound location of a deeply sited implant will often be followed by removal.

9.12 Use of Ultrasound in the Management of Implant Complications

Where there is a complaint of neurological symptoms, ultrasound can readily determine the proximity of the implant to the ulnar or median nerves. Where there have been failed removal attempts with a palpable implant, there may be evidence of scar tissue surrounding the implant (Figure 9.19). Where there is suspicion of infection, this can be confirmed with ultrasound showing fluid around the implant (Figure 9.20a, b). In this circumstance, removal of the implant is the only course likely to resolve the infection. Failure to remove despite continued symptoms can result in severe infection (Figure 9.21). A new implant can be fitted at the same time, but should always be placed in the other arm using completely new disposable items and good aseptic technique to avoid any possibility of contamination.

9.13 Tips on How to Avoid Deep Insertion

Recent published correspondence has clarified an important technique for avoiding deep insertion. After the needle bearing the implant has penetrated the dermis, it should be withdrawn until the bevel is seen and then insertion continued after the angle of the needle has been adjusted parallel to the skin surface.[6,7]

9.14 Summary

The vast majority of subdermal implants are correctly inserted and easily palpable. The key to safe removal of a non-palpable implant is accurate localisation with ultrasound by an appropriately skilled clinician who can identify the implant and its relationship to anatomical structures in the upper arm.

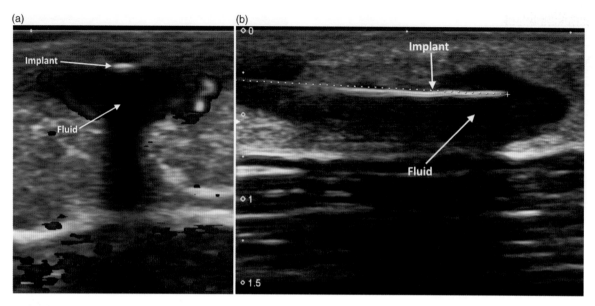

Figure 9.20 (a) Transverse and (b) longitudinal views of implant surrounded by fluid. The fluid is confirmation there is infection within the implant track.

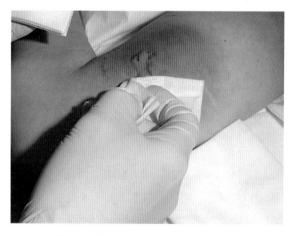

Figure 9.21 Arm with a severely infected implant.

Ultrasound is the method of choice. MRI has less reliability at locating a non-palpable implant, and also does not assist the actual removal procedure. Knowledge of the anatomy of the upper arm and the appearance of structures on ultrasound is essential to ensure successful removal using a minimally invasive technique and avoidance of injury to vulnerable structures.

References

1. Walling M. How to remove impalpable Implanon® implants. *J Fam Plann Reprod Health Care* 2005;31:320–321.

2. Gabriel H, Shulman L, Marko J, Nikolaidis P. Compound versus fundamental imaging in the detection of subdermal contraceptive implants. *J Ultrasound Med* 2007;26:355–359.

3. Mansour D, Walling M, Glenn D, Egarter C, Graesslin O, Herbst J, et al. Removal of non-palpable etonogestrel implants. *J Famm Plann Reprod Health Care* 2008;34:89–91.

4. Statement from Clinical Effectiveness Unit. Intravascular insertion of Nexplanon®. June 2016.

5. Nicholson RA, Crofton M. Training phantom for ultrasound guided biopsy. *Br J Radiol* 1997;70; 192–194.

6. Walling M. Inserting the etonogestrel contraceptive implant. *J Fam Plann Reprod Health Care* 2016;42:75.

7. Searle S, O'Brien P, Rowlands S. Comment on inserting the etonogestrel contraceptive implant. *J Fam Plann Reprod Health Care* 2016;42:158.

Chapter 10

Ultrasound Imaging in Relation to Intrauterine Contraception[*]

Zara Haider

10.1	Introduction 163		10.5	Size of the Frame 170	
10.2	Types of IUC 163		10.6	Frameless IUCs 171	
10.3	Performing a Scan to Check IUC Position 164		10.7	Difficult IUC Fittings 172	
10.4	Complications of IUC Fitting 167		10.8	Conclusions 173	
			10.9	IUC Case Studies 174	

10.1 Introduction

IUC are rapidly reversible, highly effective contraceptive methods. There are 168 million IUC users worldwide,[1] 83 per cent of these users being in Asia.[2] Data from community contraceptive services shows that only around 9 per cent of women in the UK use intrauterine contraception.[3] Use is significantly higher in the Nordic countries.

Ultrasound is the first line imaging modality for evaluating IUC position and assessing for complications, for example, in cases of pelvic pain, abnormal bleeding, threads which are not visible or after a difficult insertion. Problems associated with IUC include malposition, expulsion and perforation (partial or complete). Most IUC is inserted without the need for ultrasound guidance.

Sonography is the most commonly used modality to evaluate IUC because:

1. It provides the additional benefit of demonstrating the morphology of the uterus enabling assessment of IUC placement (Figure 10.1a, b, c, d). This is particularly useful when there is a defect within the uterine cavity. Historically, plain film X-ray was used, but this could not clarify the position within the uterus; it could only confirm whether a device was present.
2. Ultrasound is considered cost-effective and safe when conducted by a trained operator.
3. There is no risk of radiation exposure.

Ultrasound is a useful adjunct to history taking and examination when a patient presents with pain or bleeding and an IUC in situ. Sonography is ideally recommended prior to the removal of an IUC where the threads are not visible, to verify, before any attempt is made to locate the threads or the device, that the device is indeed in situ. After a difficult insertion, the use of ultrasound to verify correct IUC location is reassuring to both clinician and patient. Clinics that provide a specialist service for complex cases may use transabdominal ultrasound simultaneously to guide difficult intrauterine procedures (Video clip).

10.2 Types of IUC

Currently, IUCs fitted in the developed world are broadly of two different types:

1. Copper containing IUCs (copper wire on a plastic T-shaped frame licenced for use for 5–10 years or copper beads on a polypropylene thread licenced for use for 5 years, called GyneFix®). Copper is spermicidal and promotes a local foreign body inflammatory reaction in the endometrium, creating an inhospitable environment for implantation of the embryo (Figure 10.1a, c).
2. Hormonal IUCs (also known as the IUS – Figure 10.1b, d). Available devices currently contain two different amounts of synthetic progestogen (52 mg or 13.5 mg Levonorgestrel) within a reservoir surrounded by a rate-limiting membrane,

---

[*] Figures and the cases described in this chapter were provided by Mary Pillai.

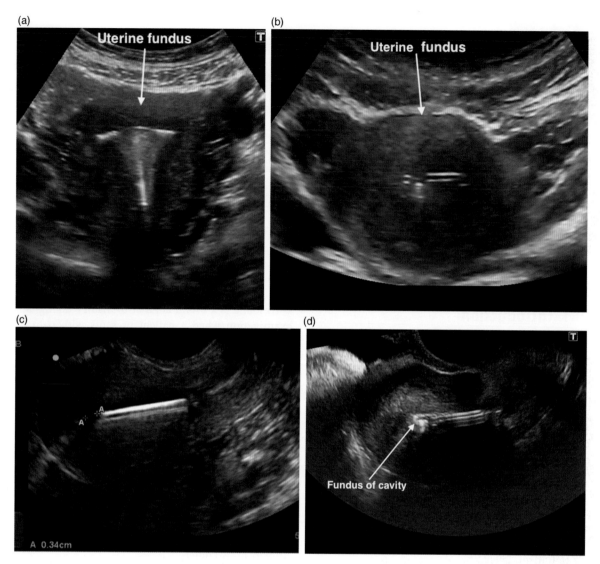

Figure 10.1 (a) A banded IUD correctly sited – easily seen on transverse TA view owing to the uterus being anteverted and the echogenic copper content. (b) IUS showing the arms of frame correctly sited – easily seen on TA transverse view owing to uterine anteversion. (c) IUD frame correctly sited on TV sagittal view showing the copper stem. (d) IUS frame correctly sited on TV sagittal view; the reservoir over the stem of the frame shows as four parallel lines.

currently licenced for five and three years respectively. Progestogen thickens the cervical mucus making it less penetrable to sperm and suppresses the growth of the endometrium, leading to an endometrial environment unfavourable for embryo implantation.

Worldwide there are many different IUC designs. Women may still present with inert devices in situ, for example Lippes loop and the stainless steel Chinese ring. (Figure 10.2a, b).

10.3 Performing a Scan to Check IUC Position

The transvaginal route provides higher resolution, although it does not always allow better assessment of the position of the intrauterine device, as illustrated in Figure 10.1.

The operator should record the normality and position of the uterus (anteverted, retroverted, axial), and any pathology identified. The location of the IUC should be determined and its position in relation to

(a) (b)

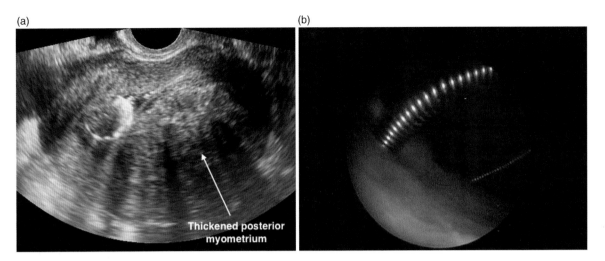

Figure 10.2 (a) Ultrasound image of Chinese IUD at cavity fundus. (b) Picture of the same case taken at hysteroscopy. Attempted outpatient removal failed owing to the distance to the device – a 6 cm posterior wall fibroid (not shown in this image). At hysteroscopy no thread was found on the device, and no suitable instrument for grasping the IUD could pass down a hysteroscope channel. Ultrasound-guided retrieval with Hartman forceps was successful.

(a) (b)

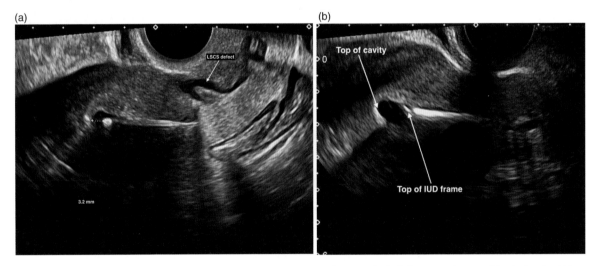

Figure 10.3 (a) Measurement of distance from the cavity fundus to the IUS frame. With ideal placement, the top of the device should be at the cavity fundus. (b) Image of distance from fundus to IUD frame.

the endometrial cavity should be documented. The transvaginal route is particularly useful when the uterus is retroverted or where the intrauterine device is not clearly seen. The proximal end of the IUC should be lying close to the fundal endometrium, the stem of the IUC should be lying parallel to the long axis of the cavity and ideally entirely within the endometrial cavity, proximal to the internal os of the cervix. The distance between the fundal endometrium and the proximal end of the IUC can be measured and

recorded if required (Figure 10.3). However, generally it is appropriate to comment that the device is correctly sited, or otherwise to describe the position of a suboptimal placement.

If the IUC is lying partially within the cervical canal then the IUC is placed sub-optimally and ideally it should be replaced (Figure 10.4). Where the IUC is partly or completely within the cervix, then its effectiveness may be reduced, although there is very limited evidence on this (Figure 10.5a, b). The option of

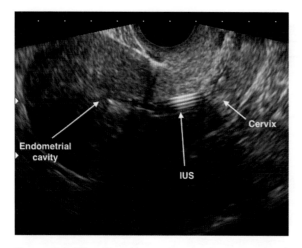

Figure 10.4 IUS positioned low, partly within the cervix and partly within the endometrial cavity.

replacing the device should be offered. However, if the woman is not inclined to do this then it can be left, as a sub-optimally placed device may be more effective than many alternative contraceptive options. Leaving the device but advising the option of an additional method should also be considered.

If partial placement within the cervix is found in relation to a recent insertion, the device may fundally seek and it is reasonable to rescan in 1–4 weeks. If the patient has had otherwise unprotected sexual intercourse within the last seven days, it is safer to leave the sub-optimally placed device than to remove it.

Copper containing IUCs show up clearly on ultrasound as the copper is highly reflective. Hormonal IUCs have a characteristic appearance with a dark hypoechoic shadow deep to the device (Figure 10.6a, b). A silver ring has been added to Jaydess (three-year hormonal

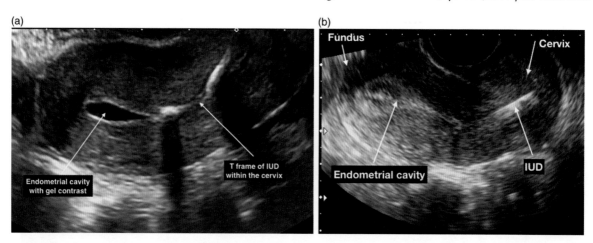

Figure 10.5 (a) A banded IUD frame within the cervix. (b) A non-banded IUD frame within the cervix.

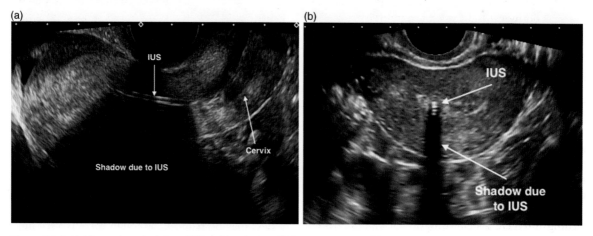

Figure 10.6 (a) A long axis sagittal view of IUS and the shadow. (b) A transverse view of the IUS and the shadow.

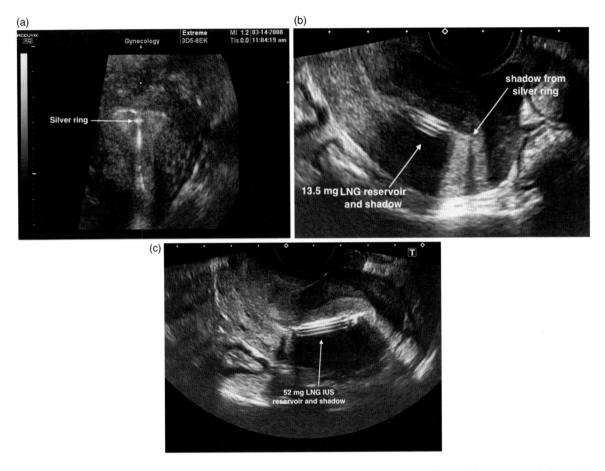

Figure 10.7 (a) A TV 3D image of the uterus showing the silver ring identifying Jaydess® (three-year licence). The ring is intended to assist it being distinguished from the five-year IUS with ultrasound (image courtesy of Bayer plc). (b, c) 2D TV long axis images showing the length of the reservoir in correctly sited devices. The reservoir is significantly shorter with Jaydess® (b) compared with the 52 mg IUS (c) Mirena®). This feature is also useful for differentiating between the two different sizes of IUS.

IUC) to assist allowing it to be distinguished from the five-year hormonal IUC on ultrasound (Figure 10.7a). The reservoir (parallel lines on scan) is also significantly shorter, and often this aspect is more obvious than the confidence that the silver ring is present or absent (Figure 10.7b, c).

10.4 Complications of IUC Fitting

10.4.1 Perforation

Perforation occurs in 1–2 per 1,000 IUC fittings[4] but is more likely to occur if an operator is inexperienced, the patient is post-natal (up to 36 weeks), is breastfeeding or if there is an unrecognised uterine infection (a contraindication to IUC insertion). On perforation, the IUC is forced through the uterine wall and into the pelvic cavity and on rare occasions can lead to haemorrhage and bowel/bladder perforation. If perforation is suspected, for example the sounding/fitting length is longer than expected or the fitting is perceived as difficult, then sonography is advised. In this circumstance the patient should be advised to use an alternative interim method of contraception or abstain from sexual intercourse until the position of the IUC is verified. If the IUC is not seen on ultrasound, then a plain abdominal and pelvic X-ray with sub-diaphragmatic views should be requested to clarify whether the device has perforated or been expelled (Figure 10.8).

All IUCs are radiopaque. If a complete perforation is diagnosed, the patient should be referred to gynaecology for removal of the device (usually done laparoscopically). In partial perforations, the device may be removed under local anaesthetic with ultrasound guidance or hysteroscopically, depending on the expertise of the operator. Partial perforation

occurs when the IUC enters the myometrium at the time of insertion, but is still within the uterus rather than the pelvic cavity (Figure 10.9). The patient may present with pain, irregular bleeding or this may be a coincidental finding on a scan organised for another indication.

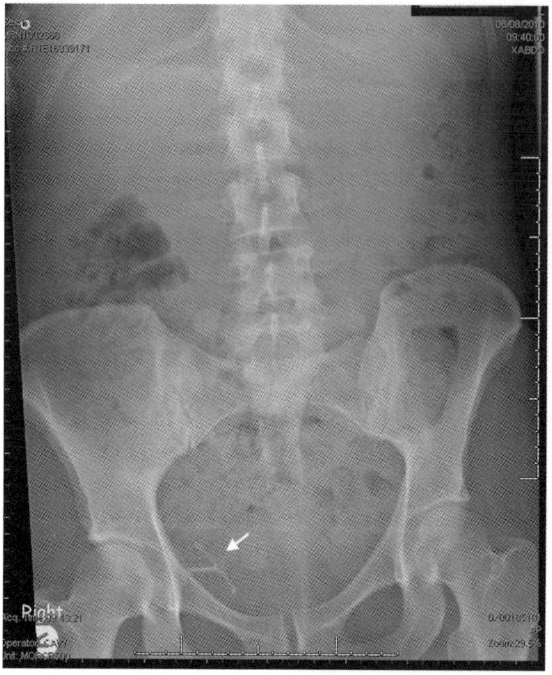

Where ultrasound is not routinely available, follow-up of the patient six weeks after an IUC insertion to verify the presence of the IUC threads has traditionally been recommended to exclude undiagnosed perforation or expulsion. However, the most recent clinical guidance advocates the woman should be encouraged to self-check her threads.[5]

10.4.2 Expulsion

Expulsion of the IUC occurs in 1 out of 20 insertions and is most likely to occur in the first three months post-insertion.[5] Risk factors for expulsion are heavy menstrual bleeding, insertion immediately post-partum, fibroids distorting the uterine cavity and any other uterine anomaly. At the time of the IUC fitting, the patient should be taught to feel for her threads, particularly with a copper IUC, after a period, as expulsion of the IUC is more likely in association with heavy bleeding. Patients should be advised to report to their local SRH service or GP if they are unable to feel their threads. If the threads are not found on speculum examination done for any indication, then

Figure 10.8 AXR showing a perforated device. The arrow points to an IUS lying outside the uterus but within the right side of the pelvis. The uterus itself cannot be seen on X-ray.

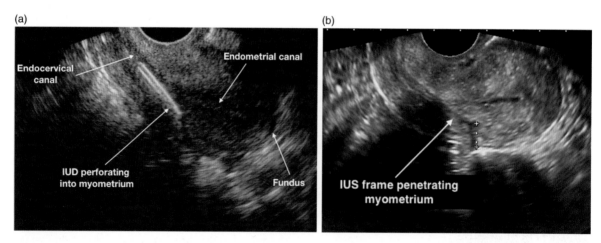

(a)   (b)

Endocervical canal

Endometrial canal

IUD perforating into myometrium

Fundus

IUS frame penetrating myometrium

Figure 10.9 (a) Image of myometrial perforation. The IUD frame is perforating at the level of the internal cervical os. The upper 2/3 of the device lies within myometrium. This occurs at the time of fitting and a clue apart from the resistance met at the level of the cervico-isthmic junction is that the IUC will often not readily release from the insertion tube. This perforation into the myometrium was diagnosed at the time of fitting (image courtesy of Dr A C Gazet). (b) Case referred following failed attempted IUS removal, which had been associated with severe pain when traction was applied to the threads. The point of penetration is also at the cervico-isthmic junction. This perforation into the myometrium was only diagnosed with investigation following a failed removal. The patient recollected that the fitting had been difficult and painful. The device had been in situ for several years.

an ultrasound scan should be performed to verify the position of the IUC. If no device is seen within the uterine cavity or the cervix, then the operator cannot assume that the device has been expelled, and an AXR is indicated.

10.4.3 Pregnancy with an IUC In Situ (Including Ectopic Pregnancy)

The risk of ectopic pregnancy occurring when an IUC is in situ (the absolute risk) is extremely low. If a woman conceives with an IUC in situ, the risk of this pregnancy being ectopic is higher than the background risk (that is, the risk, if she did not have an IUC in situ), and this risk appears highest with Jaydess.[6] If a woman using intrauterine contraception presents with symptoms of pregnancy, pain or unscheduled bleeding and a pregnancy test is positive, she should be managed as an ectopic pregnancy until proven otherwise. If there is no intrauterine pregnancy on scan, a careful evaluation of the adnexal regions should be performed together with a β-hCG level. The pregnancy should be presumed ectopic and the woman fast tracked to gynaecology for appropriate management of this potentially life-threatening condition.

Risk of pregnancy is greater if the IUC is sitting partially or completely in the cervical canal as there will be insufficient copper/hormone reaching the endometrium (Figure 10.10a).

If the pregnancy is intrauterine, then the risk of adverse pregnancy outcomes such as spontaneous abortion, preterm delivery, septic abortion and chorioamnionitis are higher if the device is left in situ. There is overwhelming evidence that removal of the device in early pregnancy reduces these risks.[5] Thus as soon as a pregnancy is diagnosed the cervix should be visualised and when the threads can be located, the 'IUC' removed. Any delay in the removal of the device increases the likelihood of the threads retracting due to the rapid growth of the uterus, with loss of the opportunity to reduce the risks to the pregnancy (Figure 10.10b).

When the woman chooses to continue with the pregnancy, she should be fully informed about the additional risks of an adverse outcome where an IUC is in the uterus.

10.4.4 Pain or Unscheduled Bleeding with an IUC

If a patient presents with pain or unscheduled bleeding with an IUC, then a history and examination needs to be performed prior to considering the need for ultrasound. Possible causes may be:

1. **Malposition** – The device can be found in a wide variety of different locations, other than within the endometrial cavity (Figures 10.11–10.12). The patient may experience pain on bimanual examination. Sometimes a partner may complain of feeling the device during sexual activity. Optimally both transabdominal and transvaginal ultrasound should be used to delineate the pelvis

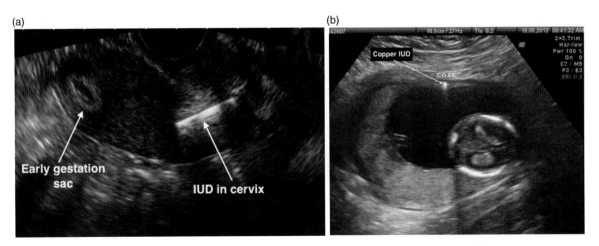

Figure 10.10 Pregnancy with IUCs. (a) An early pregnancy with an IUD in the cervix (this should be removed as soon as possible). (b) A mid-trimester pregnancy with an IUD (FlexiT 300) between the amniotic sac and the uterine wall (arrow).

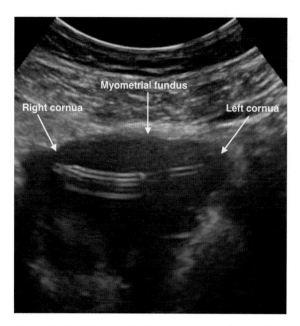

Figure 10.11 A 20-year-old nulliparous woman with an IUS frame dislocated within the endometrial cavity. This was fitted under GA as a management strategy for pelvic pain. She reported her pain was significantly worse since the fitting several months earlier, although she had become hypomenorrhoeic. It was retrieved with local anaesthetic gel to the cavity and an endocervical block using ultrasound guidance, as the thread had retracted.

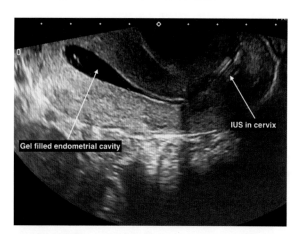

Figure 10.12 The patient had been amenorrhoeic with a previous IUS but her bleeding had returned since undergoing a routine removal and refit at five years. Her partner had also complained of being aware of something sharp in the vagina during sexual activity.

and the position of the IUC. This is particularly important if fibroids are present.

Women with an incorrectly positioned device may be asymptomatic; 10.4 per cent of ultrasound scans performed on women with IUC (having pelvic

ultrasound for another indication) showed malposition.[7] Ultrasound using a negative contrast or 3D ultrasound may be more sensitive in cases of malposition, particularly when looking for side arm embedment (Cases 1 and 4). It is important to understand that the endometrial cavity is a virtual space. In association with the use of an intrauterine system, the endometrium becomes thinned, such that the arms of a correctly sited frame may appear to be surrounded by myometrium, particularly towards the fundal and cornual regions of the cavity (Figure 10.13).

2. **Pelvic Infection** – The patient may present with complaints of a foul smelling vaginal discharge, irregular bleeding, pelvic pain, deep dyspareunia, and she may be pyrexial. Bimanual examination may reveal lower abdominal tenderness and cervical motion tenderness. A TV scan is less useful here unless the patient has a pelvic collection of pus or free fluid, which might be visualised or a tubo-ovarain mass – see Chapters 6 and 11. Diagnosis of pelvic infection should be based on clinical findings and is more likely if the patient is less than three weeks post-IUC insertion, post-instrumentation of the uterus or at higher risk of acquiring a sexually transmitted infection (under 25 years of age, multiple partners, recent partner change, etc.)

3. **Pregnancy** (including ectopic pregnancy)

Women need to be advised that irregular bleeding may occur within the first few months of IUC insertion and that this is normal within the first 3–6 months of a hormonal IUC insertion. It is therefore essential that any history of abnormal bleeding is established and appropriately investigated prior to or concomitantly with insertion of an IUC. It is especially important that the IUS is not used to treat abnormal bleeding in women with risk factors for endometrial cancer, without appropriate investigation.

10.5 Size of the Frame

Often the frame appears slightly large for the cavity dimensions, but in practice this does not matter as long as any discomfort experienced at the time of fitting settles. If it does not settle and the frame appears large (Figure 10.14) then it may be worth considering a device with a smaller frame or an IUD without a frame. The small frame (Flexi T 300 – Figure 10.15) and frameless IUDs all have a lower copper content with a shorter licenced duration and possibly higher failure rates.

(a) (b)

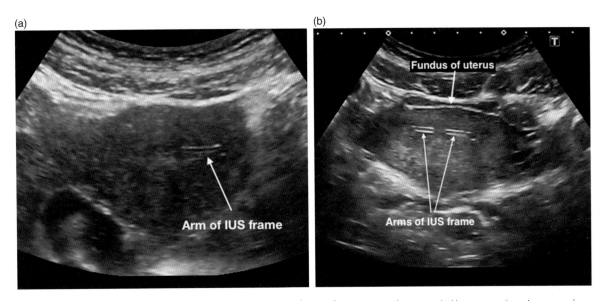

Figure 10.13 (a) Transverse TA view of the uterus shows one arm of an IUS frame apparently surrounded by myometrium. A sonographer had reported the frame appeared 'within the myometrium'. (b) This transverse view has imaged both arms of the IUS and they appear normally positioned relative to the uterine fundus. The endometrium does not image separately from the myometrium. The endometrial cavity is a virtual space. Where the endometrium is very thin (as with long-term use of IUS) endometrial tissue may not be distinguished separately from the myometrium (as in this case). The lack of brighter 'endometrium' around the IUS should not be mistaken for misplacement within the myometrium.

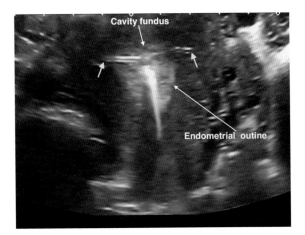

Figure 10.14 A TA transverse view of the uterus. The brighter endometrium outlines the endometrial borders of the cavity against the more hypoechoic myometrium. The ends of the T-arms (yellow arrows) of the correctly sited Nova-T frame appear wide for the cavity dimensions, and look to be protruding into the myometrium. The patient complained of pain since the time of fitting three months earlier, so it was changed for a smaller framed device (Figure 10.15).

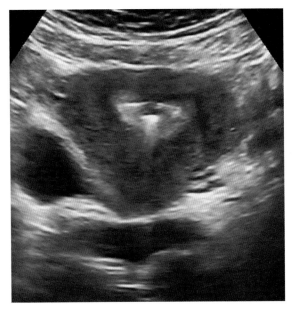

Figure 10.15 A TA transverse view of the uterus showing a FlexiT 300 correctly positioned within the endometrial cavity. The width of the frame is clearly less than the cavity.

10.6 Frameless IUCs

One brand of frameless IUC is currently marketed in the UK. GyneFix® is a frameless device consisting of six copper beads containing 330 mg copper on a polypropylene thread. There is also GyneFix 200 with four copper beads, although the only potential indication for this may be women who have had the cervix removed as a fertility sparing operation for cervical cancer (radical

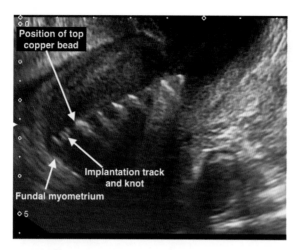

Figure 10.16 GyneFix® correctly implanted. Although it has six copper beads, seven bright bands show below the implantation knot. This implies it is the reflective ends of the beads that give the maximum echogenicity on ultrasound imaging.

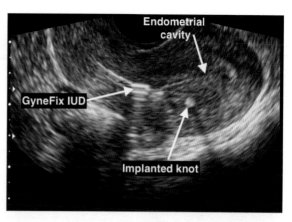

Figure 10.17 The acoustic shadow confirms the position of the implantation knot. The device has been implanted low due to the version angle between the cervical canal and the endometrial canal, even though this is a relatively small angle.

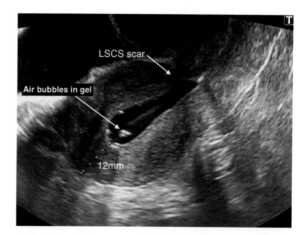

Figure 10.18 Patient post-natal and breastfeeding requested a frameless IUD owing to the pain experienced with a framed device. Measurement of the fundal myometrium is enhanced with gel contrast and clarifies there is sufficient thickness to allow safe insertion of GyneFix®.

tracelectomy). There is a knot at the proximal end of the thread that is embedded (8 mm depth) into the fundal myometrium at insertion. The device sits within the endometrial cavity, with a single thread protruding through the external os. (Figure 10.16)

GyneFix® is licenced for use for five years and it was hoped that the design would reduce dysmenorrhoea associated with framed devices. Certainly some women find it very satisfactory. It was also hoped that it would overcome the problem of expulsion, but in practice there is a significant expulsion rate as retention depends on the knot fibrosing into the myometrium and not being expelled. Safe insertion requires a relatively straight endocervical–endometrial canal as the insertion tube is not manoeuvrable in the way other IUCs are. Where the canal is not sufficiently straight this will result in low implantation (Figure 10.17).

GyneFix® has also been advocated for women with a small uterus. However, a minimum of 9 mm of myometrium is necessary for safe implantation. Those reproductive age women with the smallest uterine dimensions tend to be those who are relatively hypoestrogenic, for example amenorrhoea associated with breast feeding or Depo-Provera use or weight-related amenorrhoea. In these cases thinning of the myometrium may result in insufficient fundal myometrium for safe fitting. Therefore women with risk factors for hypoestrogenic status should have GyneFix fitted only where ultrasound assessment of the thickness of the myometrium and placement of the device can be performed.

Filling the cavity with Instillagel (local anaesthetic gel) may provide a dual benefit of enabling enhanced ultrasound assessment of the cavity and fundal myometrium (Figure 10.18), and also when left for approximately 20 minutes prior to instrumentation, some analgesic benefit. The implantation site is otherwise not accessible for local anaesthetic.

10.7 Difficult IUC Fittings

If an IUC fitting is difficult a simultaneous ultrasound scan should be performed. Information from the scan may reveal why there is difficulty.

(a)   (b)

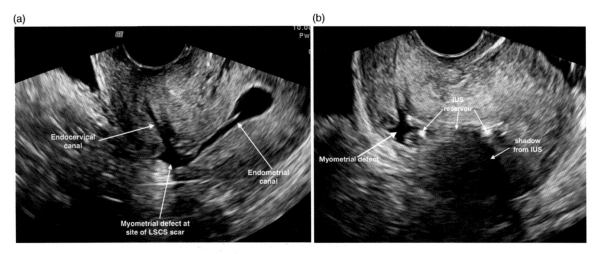

Figure 10.19 (a) Use of gel contrast helps to demonstrate an acute angle of retroflexion at the cervico-isthmic junction. A myometrial defect is also shown at the site of an old caesarean scar. Where this finding is associated with difficult IUC insertion, use of a tapered metal dilator enables the angle of insertion to be altered as the dilator tip reaches the junction and this allows passage into the endometrial cavity and straightening of the canal. The IUC insertion tube is generally too flexible to allow this change of direction during insertion, so insertion as the metal dilator is withdrawn is often key to success. (b) The sited IUS following correct insertion.

Normal uterine variants including acute ante or retroflexion or irregularity of the isthmic region may make IUC fitting more challenging and emphasises the need for effective local anaesthetic technique (Figure 10.19a, b).

The technique for ultrasound guidance requires use of the transabdominal probe and is therefore more limited in women with acute retroflexion, particularly when they are also obese.

From a sagittal view of the uterus, the probe is then tilted towards the pelvis to include the upper cervix. An assistant needs to hold the probe in position to maintain this view, and it is therefore important that the speculum is first in place. Routine use of Instillagel enhances visualisation, particularly identifying the retroverted cavity. The suprapubic pressure may also provide some 'distraction pain relief' and seems to facilitate opening the internal os. In the most difficult cases, use of a metal sound or dilator enables easy identification of its position during insertion and it is then often possible to see why resistance has been met. In most difficult cases this is usually because the angle of insertion needs to be altered at the level of the cervico-isthmic junction. (Figure 10.19a, b) In this circumstance previous 'blind' attempts may have created a false passage

Occasionally submucus fibroids may prevent instrumentation of the endometrial cavity (Figure 10.20). If an abnormal uterine shape/uterine septum is noted on ultrasound, then IUC insertion may be inappropriate,

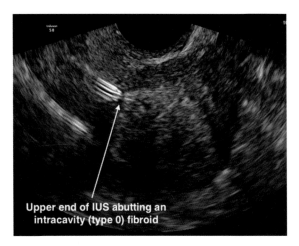

Upper end of IUS abutting an intracavity (type 0) fibroid

Figure 10.20 This case was referred with worsening bleeding despite a 52 mg IUS being in situ for 12 months. This TV long axis view of the uterus shows the upper end of the IUS in the cervix, abutting a fibroid that is filling the endometrial cavity.

although this does not mean that intrauterine contraception is absolutely contraindicated.

10.8 Conclusions

Ultrasound has a crucial role in the evaluation of IUC location as well as management of complications associated with the insertion and removal procedures. Availability of ultrasound at the time of fitting, particularly if the fitting is complex, is very useful and has a role in reassuring the patient and clinician.

10.9 IUC Case Studies
Mary Pillai

Case 1

A 37-year-old lady referred following attempts to remove the IUD had avulsed the threads. The patient reported she had experienced severe pain at the previous attempted removal and was very apprehensive about any further attempt.

(a)   (b)

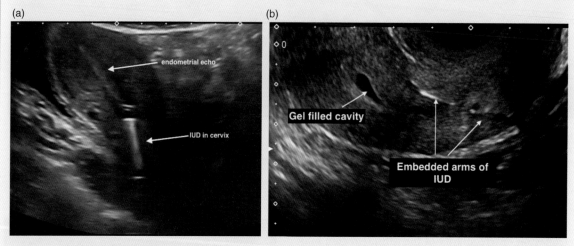

Case Figure 10.1 (a) The transabdominal view shows an anteverted uterus with the IUD stem lying within the cervical canal. (b) Local anaesthetic gel has outlined the endometrial cavity. This TV view shows the arms of the frame embedded in myometrium and cervical tissue at the level of the cervico-isthmic junction.

Topical 10 per cent Lidocaine spray was applied to the cervix and then a paracervical block inserted. Using TA USS guidance the stem of the frame was grasped by passing artery forceps into the endocervical canal. The frame was then initially pushed upwards into the endometrial canal to dislodge the arms before withdrawing the device.

Case 2

This 32-year-old lady was referred following a pelvic scan for pain. An IUS had been inserted under GA 18 months earlier, following two failed attempted IUC fittings.

(a)   (b)

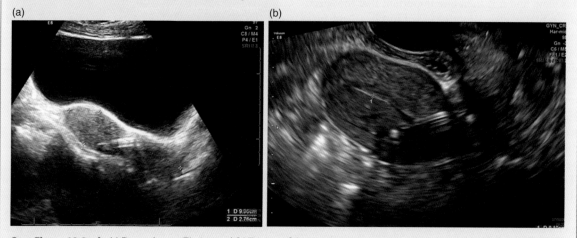

Case Figure 10.2a, b (a) Figure shows a TA view and (b) TV view of the IUS perforating the posterior myometrium at the level of the internal os.

The patient declined any local anaesthetic procedure for removal stating that she 'always had coils fitted with GA'. She was referred to gynaecology and waited several months to have the IUS removed under GA. She requested replacement of the IUS but hysteroscopy at the time of removal indicated the myometrium appeared very thin at the perforation site, so she was advised to allow several weeks for this to heal and then have a new device fitted using ultrasound guidance.

She was referred to the level 3 clinic for an ultrasound-guided fitting and initially declined stating she had to have a GA. After discussion that the previous perforation had occurred with a GA fitting and that good quality ultrasound for guidance was available in the clinic setting but not in theatre, she agreed to proceed with fitting in the clinic. Local anaesthetic was provided with 10 per cent Lidocaine spray to the cervix and filling the endometrial cavity with Instillagel. An IUS was then easily inserted into the endometrial cavity assisted with TA USS guidance.

Case 3

This 30-year-old lady had attended the GP practice for removal and refit of an IUS that had been in place for five years. The nurse noted the thread passing normally through the cervical os, but could also see thread separately to the left of the cervix. On opening the speculum fully the lower end of the IUS frame could be seen protruding through a fistula high on the left side of the cervix at the level of the vault.

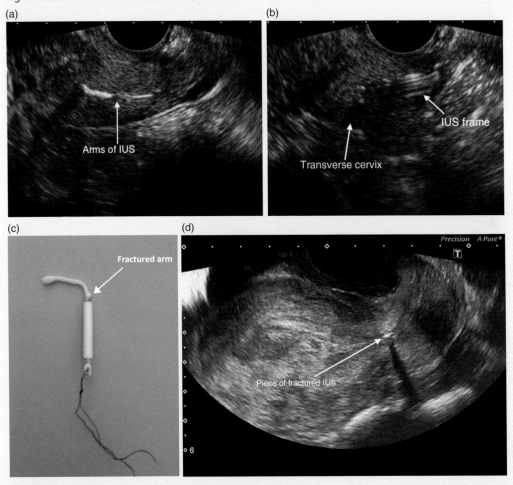

Case Figure 10.3 (a) This long axis view shows the arms of the IUS lying longitudinally in the endocervical canal. (b) Transverse view at the level of the upper cervix showing the IUS stem with reservoir penetrating the cervix. On speculum the thread attachment ring of the IUS frame was visible protruding through a fistula on the left side into the vault of the vagina. One thread ran back through the fistula and out of the cervical os, while the other thread was in the left fornix. (c) Topical and paracervical local anaesthetic was applied. The IUS was then removed by grasping the lower arm within the cervical canal and withdrawing it, so withdrawing the frame back through the fistula and out through the cervix. Unfortunately this fractured the device leaving a small piece of the frame in situ. (d) TV sagittal view of uterus showing the residual fragment located within the cervix.

Case 4

This 24-year-old lady was referred due to the threads having pulled off during attempted removal of an IUD.

(a)

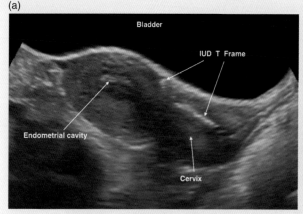

(b)

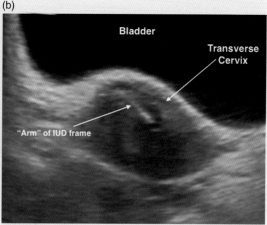

Case Figure 10.4a, b The longitudinal (a) and transverse (b) images show the arms of the frame embedded in cervical tissue at the cervico-isthmic level.

After inserting topical and paracervical local anaesthetic the lower end of the frame was grasped with Hartman forceps passed into the endocervical canal. The frame would not dislodge with moderate downwards traction so the frame was rotated to see if this would dislodge the arms. This manoeuvre resulted in fracture of the device, and further attempts at the removal of the residual embedded part of the frame with ultrasound and then hysteroscopic guidance was unsuccessful.

(c)

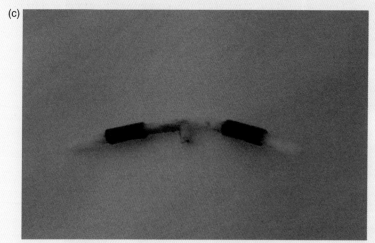

Case Figure 10.4c The residual fragment of the fractured IUD that was passed spontaneously 4 weeks after attempted removal.

Approximately four weeks later the patient contacted the service to report she had passed what she believed to be the remaining piece of the frame. She was asked if possible to provide a photo of the piece and this confirmed all of the fractured embedded part of the frame had been passed.

This case emphasises the importance that any device embedded at this level needs to be pushed upwards to disimpact the arms of the frame, using ultrasound guidance, before removal with downwards traction.

Case 5

This 28-year-old lady was referred for removal of IUD. Previous attempted removal resulted in severe pain when traction was applied to the threads.

(a)

(b)

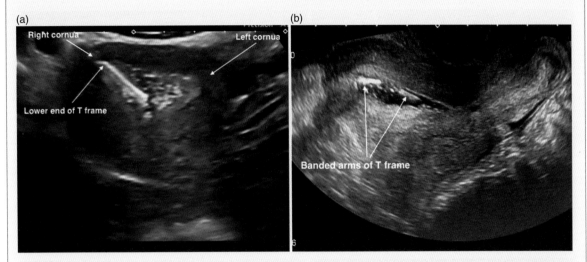

Case Figure 10.5a, b (a) Transverse transabdominal view of the uterus shows the stem of the frame lying obliquely on the right side of the cavity – the cavity has been filled with gel. (b) The longitudinal transvaginal view confirms the IUD was upside down with the banded arms lying longitudinally and in the lower part of the uterus. So what should normally be the lowest part of the frame (the thread attachment part) was positioned in the right cornual part of the cavity.

The device was removed after additional local anaesthetic (topical Lidocaine spray and a paracervical block) using Hartman forceps to directly grasp the frame.

Case 6

This 25-year-old was investigated for pelvic pain and was diagnosed with a uterine septum and endometriosis. Two LNG IUS devices were placed at the time of hysteroscopy and laparoscopy.

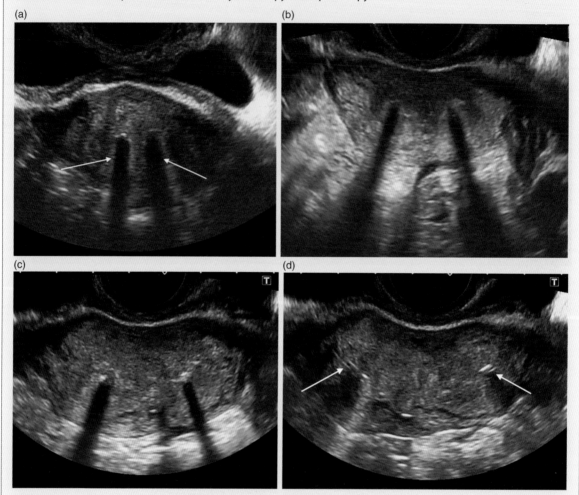

(a) (b) (c) (d)

Case Figure 10.6a–d Case Figures 10.6a–d are transverse views of the uterus, sequentially from the upper end of the cervix (a) to the fundus of the uterus (d). Two shadows can be seen from the two IUS devices in situ, lying on either side of the septum. At the fundus, just one of the arms of each device can be seen (arrows in Case Figure 10.6d).

Case 7

This 43-year-old lady had undergone surgical termination of pregnancy six years earlier. At the time of termination, an IUS was fitted. Subsequently a clinic had told her they were unable to remove the IUS.

She was referred for a scan to locate and date the pregnancy when a test was positive.

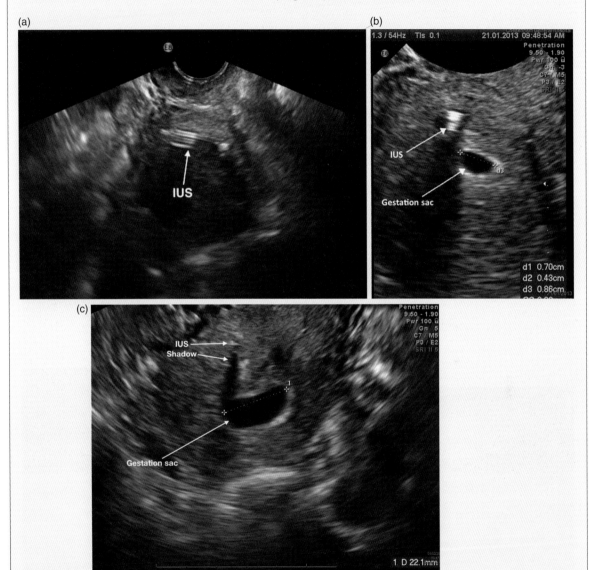

Case Figure 10.7a–c Case Figures 10.7a-c show the IUS lying within a false passage in the myometrium. There is a gestation sac in the endometrial cavity and no part of the IUS can be seen adjacent to the sac.

The pregnancy ended with an early miscarriage. At a subsequent hysteroscopy, no part of the frame or thread of the IUS was visible from inside the endometrial cavity. The lady was advised to leave the IUS as it would likely require hysterectomy for removal.

Case 8

This 51-year-old lady had an IUD in situ for 12 years and ALOs had been reported on a routine smear two years earlier. She had ignored letters from her GP requesting she make an appointment to discuss the smear report. She presented when she developed pelvic pain and fever. She had been experiencing intermenstrual bleeding for over 12 months.

(a)

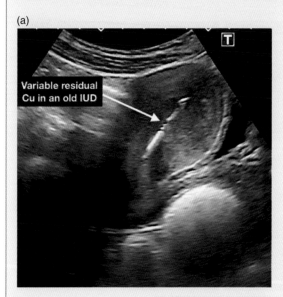

Variable residual Cu in an old IUD

Case Figure 10.8a A TA long axis view of the pelvis showing the uterus containing a copper IUD. The copper on the shaft of the IUD frame appears variable in amount, consistent with the device having been in situ for many years.

(b)

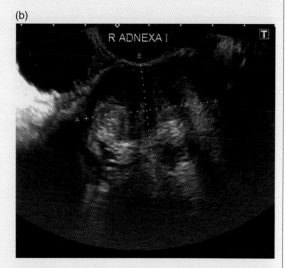

R ADNEXA I

Case Figure 10.8b A TV scan of the right adnexa showing a mass that appears very heterogenic, with shadowing and a poorly defined outline, consistent with an abscess.

(c)

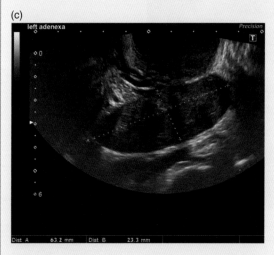

left adenexa

Dist A   63.2 mm   Dist B   23.3 mm

Case Figure 10.8c The mass in the left adnexa appears well circumscribed and solid.

(d)

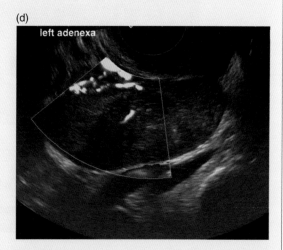

left adenexa

Case Figure 10.8d This shows moderate blood flow within the mass (colour score 3).

This shows some overlap with malignancy but some internal shadowing is demonstrated (B-feature) and with the clinical history and right adnexal finding it is most likely this is pelvic actinomycosis. Neither ovary could be identified separate to the right and left adnexal masses. Given the clinical history, this was managed as pelvic actinomycosis. The IUD was removed and her symptoms all resolved with removal of the IUD and a prolonged course of Penicillin.

References

1. United Nations, Department of Economic and Social Affairs. World contraceptive use 2011. www.un.org/esa/population/publications/contraceptive2011contraceptive2011.htm

2. Buhling KJ, Zite NB, Lotke P, Black K. INTRA Writing Group. Worldwide use of intrauterine contraception: a review. *Contraception* 2014;89:162–173.

3. NHS Contraceptive Services, England – 2012–13, Community contraceptive clinics. Health and Social Care Information Centre. www.hscic.gov.uk/catalogue/PUB12548

4. Heinemann K, Reed S, Moehner S, Minh T. Risk of uterine perforation with levonorgestrel-releasing and copper intrauterine devices in the European Active Surveillance Study on Intrauterine Devices. *Contraception* 2015;91:274–279.

5. Intrauterine Contraception. Clinical Effectiveness Unit FSRH October 2015. www.fsrh.org/pdfs/CEUGuidanceIntrauterineContraception.pdf

6. Jaydess 13.5 mg intrauterine delivery system. Summary of Product Characteristics, Bayer plc. Updated July 2015.

7. Braaten KP, Benson CB, Maurer R, Glodberg AB. Malpositioned intrauterine contraceptive devices: risk factors, outcomes, and future pregnancies. *Obstet Gynecol* 2011;118(5):1014–1020.

Chapter

11

The Role of Ultrasound Scanning in the Investigation and Management of Subfertility

Paula Briggs and Gab Kovacs

11.1 Introduction 182

11.2 Ultrasound and Subfertility 182

11.3 Baseline Investigation of the Male Reproductive System 183

11.4 Baseline Investigation of the Female Reproductive System 183

11.5 Investigating Ovulation 189

11.6 Assessment of the Pelvic Organs 190

11.7 Monitoring Ovulation Induction 191

11.8 Controlled Ovarian Hyperstimulation (COH) for In Vitro Fertilisation (IVF) 191

11.9 Monitoring the Endometrium 191

11.1 Introduction

Subfertility is defined as 'failure to conceive following regular unprotected sexual intercourse over a period of 12 months'.[1] Subfertility can be primary, where there has been no previous pregnancy, and secondary where the couple have previously conceived.

The three main fertility factors are:

1. The right number of **sperm** in the right place at the right time
2. Ovulation – healthy **ova**
3. The passages, including the cervix, uterine cavity and **tubes,** need to be normal and patent, so that the oocyte and sperm can unite and the developing embryo can be transported to the uterine cavity

Causes for subfertility include ovulatory disorders (25 per cent), male factor (30 per cent), tubal and utero-peritoneal causes (30 per cent) and unexplained in 25 per cent of cases. For women under 35 years, cumulative conception rates are around 75 per cent at 6 months, 90 per cent at 12 months and 95 per cent at 24 months. For women aged 35–39, the chance of natural conception is about half that of women aged 19–26 years.[2] While in a woman under 35 years of age, it is appropriate to delay investigations for 12 months, in an older woman earlier investigation/treatment is appropriate due not only to declining fertility but also to declining success rates of treatment with advancing age.

11.2 Ultrasound and Subfertility

Ultrasound is useful in the investigation of the three factors listed earlier, and also in the investigation of both male and female partners. When it comes to ART including ovulation induction and monitoring, ultrasound is essential and it is also useful for follicle tracking for artificial insemination. Care may be delivered in a community setting, in collaboration with fertility specialists. This allows women to be monitored locally, rather than travelling repeatedly to a specialist fertility unit. If there is a complication of COH with IVF, such as OHSS, scanning the ovaries and measuring ascites by ultrasound is an important tool which can be delivered in a community setting, as women often become unwell with OHSS several days after the IVF process is completed when they are back at home. The person doing the surveillance must have knowledge of National Guidance[3] and a good relationship with the fertility specialists to co-manage the patient under their guidance. In the early days of ovulation, induction[4] and IVF[5] ultrasound was not used because the technique became widely available only in the 1980s. With the development of transvaginal ultrasound scanning, providing greater clarity of imaging of pelvic structures, ultrasound became an integral part of ART. Ultrasound examination has become a dynamic extension of the bimanual pelvic examination. Colour Doppler is a useful addition, enabling blood flow to organs to be identified. Prior to this being available, it was possible to confuse vessels with structures such as ovaries.

11.3 Baseline Investigation of the Male Reproductive System

Ultrasound can be used to assist investigation of male infertility in the presence of azoospermia.

The male reproductive system is examined using a transrectal ultrasound probe. This allows visualisation of the prostate gland, the seminal vesicles, the urethra, vas deferens and ejaculatory ducts. Obstructive lesions of the duct system can be identified. These can be acquired or congenital. Congenital absence of the vas deferens is not uncommon, and may be associated with the carrier state for cystic fibrosis. Sometimes cysts can be seen in these tubular structures with ultrasound.

11.4 Baseline Investigation of the Female Reproductive System

Use of a transvaginal pelvic ultrasound scan allows various pathology to be identified (Box 11.1). The best time to perform a 'baseline scan' is early in the cycle

---

Box 11.1 Pelvic Pathology That Can Be Identified on Transvaginal Ultrasound Scanning – Modified from Hurley and Leoni[14]

Ovary

- PCO
- Endometriosis
- Cysts

Uterus

- Fibroids
- Endometrial /cervical polyps
- Congenital abnormalities – bicornuate/septate uterus
- Adenomyosis
- Endometrial thickness
- Ascherman's syndrome (intrauteriune synechiae)
- Endometritis
- IUD

Adnexae

- Hydrosalpinges
- Pelvic collections

---

when the ovaries are relatively inactive and the endometrium is thin.

The Uterus

It is estimated that 3 per cent of women have a congenital uterine abnormality.

Failure of development of the Mullerian ducts, resulting in agenesis or hypoplasia (Rokitansky (MRKH) syndrome) does not usually present as subfertility, as women with this condition generally present and are investigated and diagnosed during adolescence as a result of primary amenorrhoea. Other abnormalities including a bicornuate or septate uterus (Figures 11.1 a, b) are more likely to cause early or mid-trimester pregnancy loss rather than subfertility (see Chapter 6). The use of a negative contrast, such as instillagel, makes these abnormalities much easier to identify as seen in Figures 11.1 c, d.

Uterine Leiomyofibromata (Fibroids)

These become more common as women age, and are often an incidental finding during the investigation of a woman with subfertility. While subserosal (Figure 11.2a) and intramural fibroids (Figure 11.2b) are unlikely to cause subfertility, submucous fibroids (Figure 11.2c) may have a significant impact on fertility due to distortion of the cavity.[6] (See Chapters 6 and 13 for the classification of fibroids.)

Adenomyosis

This is also called *Endometriosis interna,* with endometrial tissue within the myometrium. It may be suspected when there is diffuse asymmetric enlargement of the uterus (Figure 11.3). The classical ultrasound appearance is described in Chapters 6 and 13. Its role in subfertility is poorly understood. The use of newer drugs such as Ulipristal Acetate, in a dose of 5 mg daily for three months, may be of benefit, although this is outside of the product licence. Other treatment options include GnRH analogues and long-term progestins.

The Endometrium

POLYPS (see Chapters 5, 6 and 13).

Endometrial polyps are not always easily seen on transvaginal ultrasound. The endometrium may appear thickened and only the introduction of a negative contrast such as saline (hydrosonography) or Instillagel® clearly outlines these lesions (Figure 11.4)

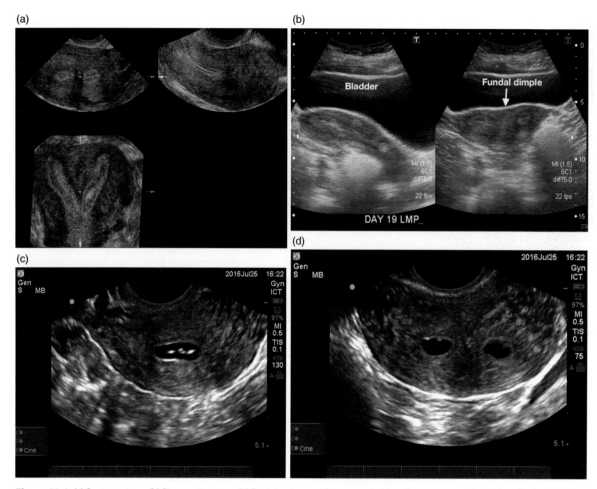

Figure 11.1 (a) Septate uterus. (b) Bicornuate uterus. (c) Septate uterus with contrast (mid-cavity- transverse view below the level of the septum). (d) Septate uterus with negative contrast, transverse view at fundus.

(Chapter 5). Sometimes blood in the endometrial cavity makes it easier to identify an endometrial polyp. There is some evidence that uterine receptivity is affected in women with endometrial polyps. Available evidence is insufficient to make a recommendation, although most clinicians perform polypectomy in subfertile women.

Asherman's Syndrome

This is a rare cause of secondary amenorrhoea, except where the endometrium has been ablated to treat menstrual problems and these women are advised not to become pregnant. In other circumstances it can follow surgical termination, curettage after miscarriage or management of morbid adherence of the placenta following a full-term pregnancy. The intrauterine synechiae caused by fibrotic scarring have a characteristic

appearance on ultrasound with loss of the cavity line and multiple echogenic foci.

Endometritis

The features of endometritis are not specific and include a tender and enlarged uterus identified with the transvaginal probe in association with a loss of definition of the uterine cavity, sometimes associated with intrauterine fluid.

The Ovaries

AFC

Currently combined measurement of AMH and ultrasound AFC provide the best guide to follicular ovarian reserve. Early follicular FSH is a less accurate marker. AFC consists of measuring follicles varying

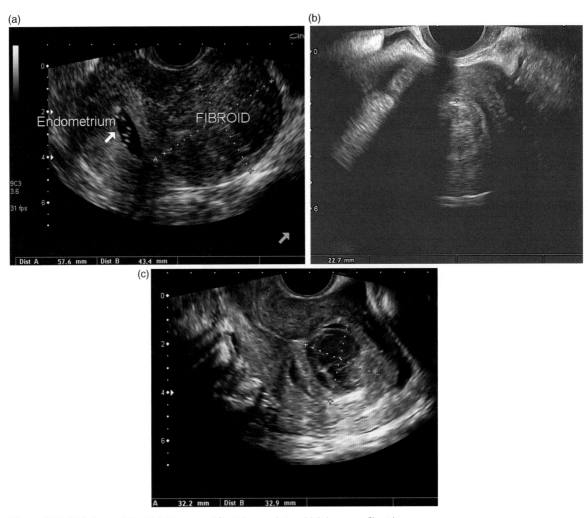

Figure 11.2 (a) Subserosal fibroid. (b) Intramural fibroid coronal view. (c) Submucous fibroid.

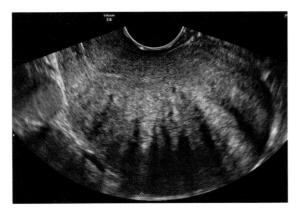

Figure 11.3 Uterine adenomyosis.

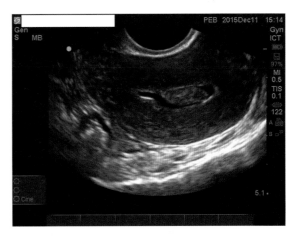

Figure 11.4 Uterine polyp with negative contrast.

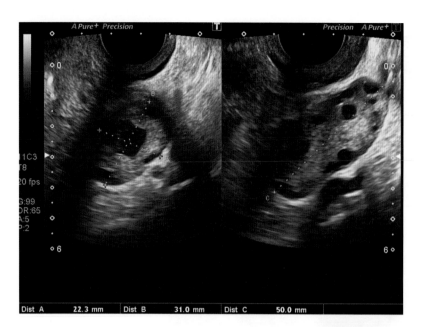

Figure 11.5 Ovary with several follicles –AFC.

| Dist A | 22.3 mm | Dist B | 31.0 mm | Dist C | 50.0 mm |

from 2–9 mm in diameter in both the ovaries done preferably between day 2–4 of a normal menstrual cycle (Figure 11.5). AFC is currently considered to be the second best predictor (after AMH) of ovarian response to stimulation in assisted reproduction.

PCO

PCO is an ultrasound diagnosis (see Chapter 12) and this type of ovary is found in about 20 per cent of reproductive age females. PCO is not synonymous with PCOS (see Chapter 12). The key features are 12 or more small (2–9 mm in diameter) peripheral cysts, with an enlarged ovarian volume (10 cc or more) and denser central stroma (Figure 11.6)

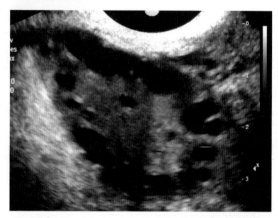

Figure 11.6 Polycystic ovary.

Ovarian Cysts

All ovulating women make functional cysts due to follicular development each cycle. If the dominant follicle does not ovulate, a follicular/functional (simple) cyst forms (Figure 11.7). These tend to be larger than the 20–22 mm 'mature' follicle size at the time of ovulatory rupture. The natural history of functional or simple cysts is spontaneous resolution. So a simple cyst under 5 cm diameter does not require any follow-up, but in the context of an abnormal cycle length it supports the concern that there is ovulatory dysfunction. Where a cyst is not simple, further assessment may be indicated (see Chapter 6).

The presence of a corpus luteum (Figure 11.8) confirms that ovulation has occurred and this would

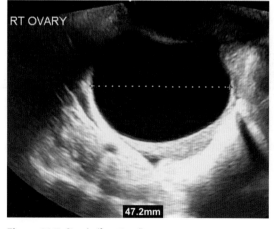

Figure 11.7 Simple (functional) cyst.

(a)

(b)

(c)

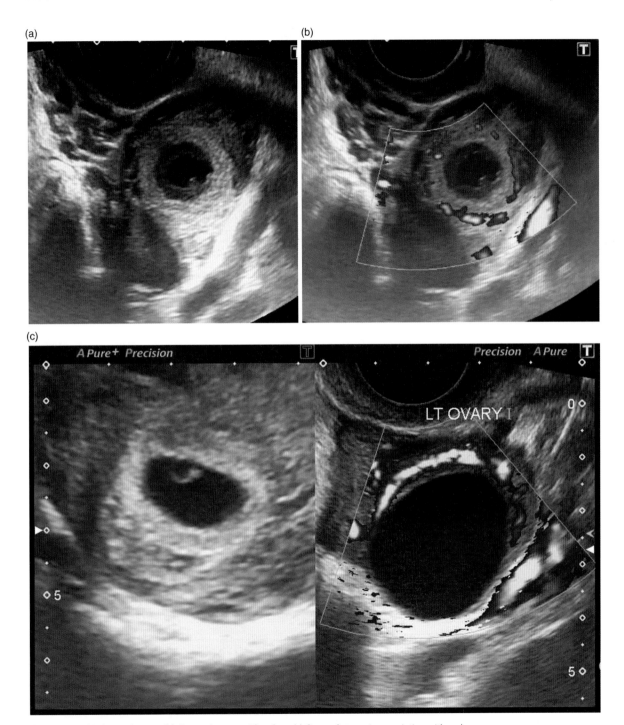

Figure 11.8 (a) Corpus luteum. (b) Corpus luteum with colour. (c) Corpus luteum in association with early pregnancy.

be corroborated by a progesterone level in mid-luteal phase consistent with ovulation – usually greater than 30 ng/ml.

Other ovarian pathology such as dermoid cysts or neoplastic cysts (mucinous or serous) may be detected on a baseline scan as an incidental finding, but are not covered in this chapter which focuses on subfertility investigation and management (see Chapters 6 and 15).

The Tubes

Normal fallopian tubes are not visible on ultrasound. However, if they are replaced by hydrosalpinges (Figure 11.9), or contain pus (Figure 11.10), they have a distinctive appearance, as a dilated cystic structure adjacent to the uterus. This is known as the 's sign'. The size of a fluid-filled tube can be very variable and does not correlate with the likelihood of symptoms. It is advisable to check chlamydial antibody titre levels in subfertility patients. The severity of tubal damage correlates with level of the titres.[7] Moreover, removal of hydrosalpinges is recommended prior to IVF, as it improves embryo implantation rates.[8] If removal of the damaged tube is not possible, then inserting an Essure device is an option.

Other Relevant Conditions

Endometriosis

Around 15–20 per cent of subfertile women have endometriosis. Although it may be a fertility factor that can impair ovarian and tubal function, it is also found in women who have conceived normally. Ovarian *endometriomata* have a classic 'ground glass appearance' (Figure 11.11). Small deposits of endometriosis are not usually detectable on ultrasound, but the possibility of resulting adhesions may be suspected when the adnexae appear fixed, with no movement in association with pressure applied to the probe. Mild/moderate endometriosis may not be detected with pelvic ultrasound, but more advanced stages may have features that can be detected (Chapter 6).

Pelvic Effusion

Collections of fluid, blood or pus can sometimes be detected in the pelvis with ultrasound (Figure 11.12 and Chapter 6). In women with OHSS after IVF, there is often a large volume of ascites, which can be measured.

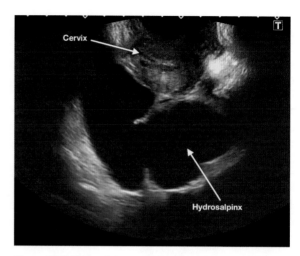

Figure 11.9 Hydrosalpinx.

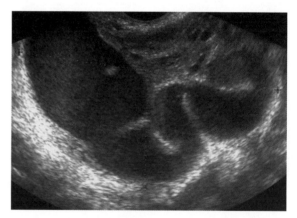

Figure 11.10 Pyosalpinx.

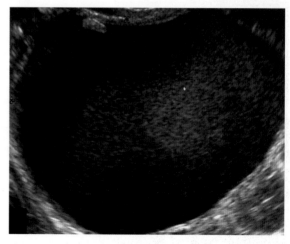

Figure 11.11 Ovarian endometrioma.

11.5 Investigating Ovulation

11.5.1 Follicle Tracking

The ovaries can be scanned throughout a natural cycle to observe follicular development, the occurrence and timing of ovulation and formation of the corpus luteum (follicle tracking). A number of antral follicles can be seen in the early follicular phase, but by about day 7 (in a 28-day cycle), the leading follicle, the one that is destined to mature and ovulate can be identified (Figure 11.13a, b). The dominant follicle grows at a rate of about 2 mm in diameter each day, and reaches a maximal pre-ovulatory diameter of around 18–25 mm, with a wide variation from cycle to cycle and woman to woman.

In addition to the follicle developing, the endometrium also undergoes changes. It thickens from a thin line post-menstrually to a characteristic triple layer, being 5–15 mm in thickness at the time of ovulation (Figure 11.14). The proliferation of the endometrium correlates directly with increasing serum estradiol levels.

Tracking follicular development with serial scanning will show the follicle disappear at ovulation, followed by the appearance of the corpus luteum with internal echoes and a thickened and vascular cyst wall. The triple echo disappears after ovulation and the endometrium appears more homogenous and echobright, as it continues to thicken due to secretory glandular proliferation. A small amount of fluid can sometimes be seen in the utero-rectal pouch (previously known as the 'Pouch of Douglas'), in association with ovulation.

11.5.2 Assessing the Corpus Luteum

If the features described cannot be identified, and a LH peak has been detected, but 36 hours later the follicle is still visible, malfunction of ovulation should be suspected. This is the 'unruptured luteinized follicle syndrome' which is a cause of unexplained subfertility.

This has a different appearance on ultrasound to a corpus luteum (Figure 11.15).

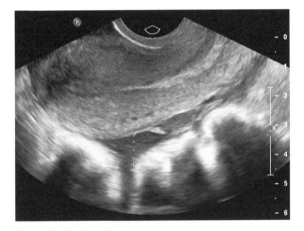

Figure 11.12 Pelvic fluid.

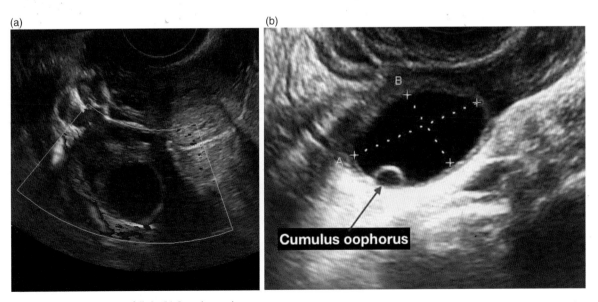

(a)

(b)

Cumulus oophorus

Figure 11.13 (a) Dominant follicle. (b) Cumulus oophorus.

11.6 Assessment of the Pelvic Organs

Baseline scanning of the pelvic structures is described earlier.

11.6.1 Assessment of Tubal Patency

Tubal patency has long been investigated using imaging as an alternative and less invasive modality when compared to laparoscopy. The most widely recognised test involves the use of radiological examination following injection of a contrast and observation, using fluroscopy, while taking still shots to show the

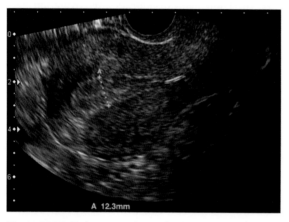

Figure 11.14 Endometrium day 12 of cycle (pre-ovulatory).

uterine outline, tubal flow and peritoneal spill – the HSG. The risks of HSG include exposure to radiation, which is small (500–1000 mrad), iodine allergy (in the contrast medium), and the risk of activating infection.

To remove the risk of radiation and the need for iodine-containing contrast, the technique of Hysterosalpingo-Contrast-Sonography (HyCoSy) has been developed. While plain ultrasound examination of the fallopian tubes is unrewarding, unless the tubes are blocked and filled with fluid (hydrosalpinges), introducing a fluid medium into the uterine cavity, while blocking exit of the contrast through the cervix using a special catheter, allows the patency of the Fallopian tubes to be tested by transvaginal ultrasound scanning. Initially a mixture of saline and air bubbles was used, but the technique has been refined using a variety of different contrast media. The bright echoes generated by the solution enable the tubes to be seen and patency is proven when the contrast can be seen spilling into the peritoneal cavity. HyCoSy has proved to be a reliable method for the assessment of tubal patency and uterine morphology and it is considered a safe and well-tolerated outpatient procedure.[9] Tubal spasm can give a false result, suggesting that the tube is blocked, and this might be an indication for a laparoscopy which is the gold standard. If there is a gross abnormality noted on the baseline scan, for example, S sign, laparoscopy is the first-line investigation.

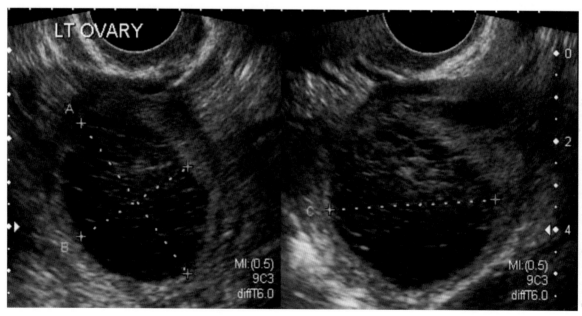

Figure 11.15 Unruptured luteinized follicle.

11.7 Monitoring Ovulation Induction

11.7.1 Clomiphene Citrate

One of the commonest causes of subfertility is anovulation. For women with an ovulation disorder, the first line of treatment is clomiphene citrate to induce ovulation. NICE guideline 1.5.2.3 recommends that women on clomiphene citrate should be offered ultrasound monitoring during at least the first cycle to ensure that they are taking a dose that minimises the risk of multiple pregnancy, that is, that there are not multiple follicles developing.[10] Ultrasound in a primary or secondary care setting where clomiphene citrate is prescribed has an important place in order to observe follicle development (ovulation induction monitoring).

11.7.2 FSH Injections

Women who are not suitable for clomiphene citrate or who have not responded may need injections of FSH to induce follicular maturation. The risk of OHSS is much higher for these women, and in line with the NICE guideline recommendation 1.5.4.2, ovarian ultrasound monitoring to measure follicle size and number should be an integral part of gonadotrophin therapy to reduce the risk of multiple pregnancy and OHSS.[10]

11.7.3 COH and IUI

The requirement for monitoring is the same as with FSH injections for anovulation, and ultrasound scanning is mandatory.

11.8 COH for IVF

The first IVF baby (Louise Brown, born 25 July 1978) was conceived in a natural cycle.[11] However, it took 102 embryo transfers for this to be achieved. In order to convert IVF into a realistic therapeutic process, stimulated cycles were then introduced.[12] As these cycles need monitoring to adjust the dosage to prevent OHSS (Figure 11.16a, b), ultrasound monitoring has become an integral part of IVF treatment. Each IVF clinic has its own protocol for how often this is performed. When hCG is used to trigger ovulation, ultrasound is used to estimate the best day to administer the hCG. In the twenty-first century many IVF units do no hormone assays, but depend solely on the ultrasound appearance of the number and size of follicles. This is currently not provided by community sexual and reproductive health services, but shared care could be offered in this setting in the future.

11.9 Monitoring the Endometrium

11.9.1 In Natural Cycles

There is little information on monitoring the endometrium to aid diagnosis of unexplained subfertility. The consensus is that implantation is unlikely if the endometrium is less than 4 mm thick, but this rarely occurs if there is ovulation. Consequently, monitoring the endometrium by ultrasound in natural cycles is not helpful.

11.9.2 For Stimulated cycle IVF

Again, the information that can be gained from ultrasound with regard to the endometrium in a stimulated

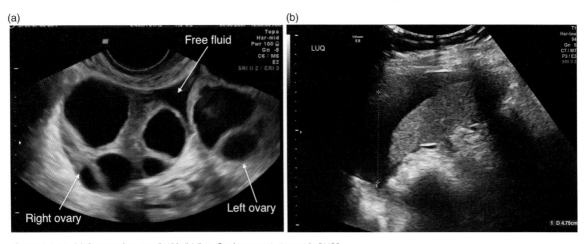

Figure 11.16 (a) Ovaries showing OHSS. (b) Free fluid in association with OHSS.

IVF cycle is minimal. If the endometrial thickness is 4 mm or less, implantation is unlikely, and freezing all the embryos is advised.

11.9.3 For Frozen Embryo Transfer – Hormone Replacement Cycles for IVF

Women who have frozen embryos and irregular cycles (< 25 or > 33 days) need to have an artificial cycle, where the endometrium is induced to proliferate by oestrogen administration. Endometrial thickness is then monitored by ultrasound, and when adequate, progesterone is used to achieve endometrial secretory changes. Consequently, ultrasound plays a vital part in the endometrial assessment for frozen embryo transfer.

11.9.4 For Embryo Transfer in IVF

The overall ease of embryo transfer is an important factor in a successful IVF cycle. There are now several studies which show that embryo transfer has a higher success rate when guided by ultrasound.[13] While the embryo is being transferred transvaginally, the cervical canal and uterine cavity are monitored by transabdominal ultrasound with a full bladder.

11.9.5 Early Pregnancy Diagnosis

The role of ultrasound in the assessment of early pregnancy is covered in Chapters 7 and 8. The surveillance of an early conception, especially after ART, is important to assess viability, to exclude multiple pregnancies and to rule out ectopic pregnancy.

An example of how ultrasound can be applied in a community sexual and reproductive health setting in the investigation and management of subfertility is described in the pages that follow.

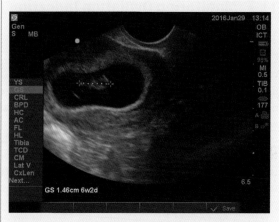

Figure 11.17 Early pregnancy at six weeks two days.

treatment with Clomiphene citrate once her BMI is below 30.

She and her partner are aware of the small risk of multiple pregnancy. He has had a normal semen analysis.

Betty continues to lose weight and is prescribed Clomiphene citrate when her BMI is 28. Prior to treatment she undergoes a HyCoSy which shows two patent tubes. Following one cycle of Clomiphene citrate (25 mg taken day 5–9) she has a scan on day 13, which demonstrates a single dominant follicle. One week later her progesterone is 36 mmol/l and, ten days later she has a positive pregnancy test.

Her next scan two weeks later shows a viable single intrauterine pregnancy with a gestation of six weeks, two days (Figure 11.17).

Case 1

Betty is 23 years old. She has infrequent periods and became pregnant recently, but this unfortunately was an ectopic pregnancy, which was managed conservatively.

She and her partner have decided that they would like a baby. She is Rubella immune and a sexually transmitted infection screen is negative.

Betty has polycystic ovaries on ultrasound scan and with her infrequent periods, she has been told that she has polycystic ovary syndrome. She has a BMI of 31, but is losing weight. She has been told that in view of her history, she will be eligible for

---

Case 2

Jayne is 29 and is undergoing IVF treatment. In her first cycle, she produced 5 embryos. One was transferred fresh, and two were frozen. Unfortunately she did not conceive, and she is now undergoing frozen embryo transfer. As her cycles are irregular, she is not suitable for a natural cycle transfer, and she is having a hormone replacement cycle. Before commencing HRT, she is given a GnRH Agonist to down-regulate her pituitary gland. A baseline ultrasound scan is then undertaken to exclude ovarian cyst formation and to confirm a thin endometrium.

She will now start taking oestrogen to proliferate the endometrium – oestradiol valerate 2 mg tds for 10–14 days. An ultrasound scan will be repeated at that time to ensure that the endometrium has responded. If the endometrial thickness is greater than 6–7 mm, she will commence progesterone pessaries to prepare the endometrium for embryo transfer.

It would be reasonable to undertake scans to check endometrial thickness in a community setting with constant liaison with the parent fertility unit to guide management at all times.

References

1. Practice Committee of the American Society for Reproductive Medicine. Definitions of infertility and recurrent pregnancy loss: a committee opinion. *Fertil Steril.* 2013;99:63.

2. Taylor A. ABC of subfertility: extent of the problem. *BMJ.* 2003;327:434–436.

3. *The management of Ovarian Hyperstimulation Syndrome.* Green-top Guideline No. 5, 3rd edn. RCOG February 2016.

4. Healy DL, Kovacs GT, Pepperell RJ, Burger HG. A normal cumulative conception rate after HPG. *Fertil Steril.*1980;34:341–345.

5. De Kretzer D, Dennis P, Hudson B, Leeton J, Lopata A, Outch K, Talbot J, Wood C. Transfer of a human zygote. *Lancet.* 1973 Sep 29;2(7831):728–729.

6. Kroon B, Hart R. The management of fibroids and polyps. In: Kovacs G, ed. *How to Improve Your ART Success Rates.* Cambridge University Press, 2011:P16–21.

7. Akande V, Hunt L, Cahill D et al. Tubal damage in infertile women: prediction using chlamydia serology. *Human Reprod.* 2003;18:1841–1847.

8. Surgical treatment for tubal disease in women due to undergo in vitro fertilisation. *Cochrane Database Syst Rev.* 2010 Jan 20(1):CD002125.

9. Lo Monte G, Capobianco G, Piva I, Caserta D, Dessole S, Marci R. Hysterosalpingo contrast sonography (HyCoSy): let's make the point! *Arch Gynecol Obstet.* 2015 Jan 291(1):19–30.

10. *NICE clinical guideline* 16. guidance.nice.uk/cg156.

11. Steptoe PC, Edwards RG. Birth after the reimplantation of a human embryo. *Lancet.* 1978 Aug 12;2(8085):366.

12. Trounson AO, Leeton JF, Wood C, Webb J, Wood J. Pregnancies in humans by fertilization in vitro and embryo transfer in the controlled ovulatory cycle. *Science.* 1981 May 8;212(4495):681–682.

13. Duran HE, VanVooris BJ. The role of ultrasound in embryo transfer. In: Kovacs G, ed. *How to Improve Your ART Success Rate.* Cambridge University Press: 161–164.

14. Hurley V, Leoni M. The role of ultrasound in subfertility. In: Kovacs G, ed. *The Subfertility Handbook. Cambridge University Press*, 1997:176–186.

Appendix
Ovulation Induction (OI) Using Clomiphene Citrate (CC) for Anovulatory/Oligo-Ovulation Sub-fertility

Objective

- To induce a single follicle in women with anovulatory/oligovulatory subfertility, minimising the risk of multiple pregnancy

The women who are suitable for treatment with CC include:

- Women with PCOS who have irregular cycles or cycles lasting longer than 33 days
- Women with secondary amenorrhoea, particularly those with post-pill amenorrhoea

Treatment with CC is not suitable for women with hypogonadotrophic hypogonadism (low FSH).

Ideally women should be of average weight (B.M.I. 19–25 kg/m^2), but a BMI <30 is acceptable.

Semen analysis should be performed and should be normal.

In a woman where it is obvious that conception is not possible due to amenorrhoea, tubal patency testing can be deferred, until she has experienced three ovulations without conception.

In women with oligomenorrhoea, tubal patency should be confirmed prior to treatment with CC. Recommended blood tests pre treatment:

- FSH
- TSH
- Prolactin
- Rubella immune status

Preparation for treatment:

1. A spontaneous bleed

   Or

2. An induced withdrawal bleed following a variety of regimes including:

   a. Medroxyprogesterone acetate 10 mg orally daily for ten days
   b. Norethisterone 5 mg orally daily for 5 days
   c. 21 days of a COC – recommended to give the endometrium a chance to build and shed in women with prolonged amenorrhoea

d. Pregnancy should be excluded by performing a urine pregnancy test or a serum progesterone level (P4) before commencing treatment; a low P4 is evidence of anovulation and a pregnancy is excluded

- Women are advised to 'phone-in' with the onset of bleeding
- Women with amenorrhoea, or very long cycles (> 42 days) should start on 50 mg CC
- Women with oligomenorrhoea should start with 25 mg CC
- CC is administered either day 2–6 or 5–9 depending on the preference of the clinician
- A transvaginal ultrasound scan is performed around day 10–12. If there are three or more developing follicles (> 14 mm), the cycle is abandoned and the couple are advised not to have sexual intercourse. If no preovulatory size follicles are present, the scan should be repeated in 3–5 days.

- Serum E2 can be measured to determine whether there is any follicular response
  - During the estimated luteal phase, measure both oestrogen (E2) and progesterone (P4) levels

Successful treatment with CC has two potential outcomes:

1. Best case scenario – pregnancy:

If no period three weeks after finishing CC, check a urine pregnancy test, or take blood for β-hCG

If β-hCG positive, follow up by ultrasound at six plus weeks for viability and to exclude a multiple pregnancy

2. Second best case scenario – good ovulation – determined by P4 levels (but no pregnancy). In this situation, the same regimen should be repeated.

If treatment is unsuccessful (no ovulation) the dose in the next cycle is increased by 25 mg (for women with oligomenorrhoea) and 50 mg (for women with amenorrhoea).

If there is no response/ovulation after CC 150 mg, then alternate treatment should be considered:

1. PCO:

    add Metformin

    consider ovarian cautery

    FSH OI

2. Non-PCO:

    FSH OI

- If ovulation occurs, three cycles of CC can be administered before further intervention. Cycles 2 and 3 do not have to be monitored by ultrasound (if unifollicular development on the CC dose that is being continued)
- If there are three ovulations, with well-timed intercourse with a fertile partner, and no pregnancy, then tubal assessment is mandatory
- After 3–6 ovulations, with patent tubes and a fertile partner, a diagnosis of unexplained subfertility is made and IVF considered.

Chapter 12

Polycystic Ovaries, Polycystic Ovary Syndrome and the Role of Ultrasound in Relation to This Condition

Paula Briggs and Gab Kovacs

12.1 Introduction 195
12.2 The Role of Ultrasound in the Management of Women with PCO/PCOS 195
12.3 The Ovary 196
12.4 The Uterus (Endometrium) 196
12.5 Understanding the Pathophysiology of PCOS 197
12.6 Management of PCOS 197
12.7 Clinical Cases 198
12.8 Take Home Messages 200

12.1 Introduction

Around 20 per cent of women are found to have a polycystic pattern on ultrasound examination of their ovaries, but only half of these women will have the syndrome, as defined by the Rotterdam Criteria.[1,2]

A PCO, when viewed by the naked eye, is seen to have an increased number of small antral follicles – fluid-filled 'pseudocysts'. The terminology is confusing for women, especially those without the syndrome, who then perceive their normal ovaries to be diseased.

This diagnostic criteria, agreed by concensus in 2003,[2] concluded that a diagnosis of PCOS could be made where features include any two of the following three characteristics:

1. Anovulation or oligo-ovulation (clinically manifesting in a woman not using hormonal contraception as amenorrhoea, oligo-menorrhoea or occasionally chaotic bleeding).
2. PCO on ultrasound.
3. Clinical and/or biochemical signs of hyperandrogenism (for example, acne or hirsuitism).

Therefore, an ultrasound scan is not mandatory in order to make the diagnosis, but is often easier and more reliable than biochemical tests. Ultrasound plays an important role in the assessment of the endometrium in women with PCOS, who have an increased risk of developing endometrial hyperplasia or cancer. The bleeding experienced by a woman with PCOS reflects ovarian function, with women who are not ovulating or who ovulate infrequently either not bleeding or bleeding infrequently, although the bleeding experienced can be heavy.

A diagnosis of PCOS should be made only when other possible causes of the clinical features described above have been excluded. This would include CAH. If this condition is suspected, particularly if there are signs of virilisation, such as cliteromegaly, a blood test to measure 17Hydroxyprogesterone should be done. In women who are amenorrhoeic, a prolactin level should be done to exclude a prolactinoma. In certain clinical situations, it may be relevant to measure thyroid function tests.

PCOS is a common endocrine condition, which can be associated with insulin resistance, dyslipidaemia, obesity, gestational diabetes, type 2 diabetes and cardiovascular disease, and therefore it is important to understand the diagnostic criteria, pathophysiology and potential management approaches for this condition.

12.2 The Role of Ultrasound in the Management of Women with PCO/PCOS

Ultrasound is not mandatory to make a diagnosis of PCOS. Its main role is in the assessment of the endometrium. Many radiology departments are struggling to manage their workload and therefore requests may be refused. The availability of ultrasound in community services enables its use as a diagnostic tool to support holistic care of women with PCOS.

Women with PCOS can be difficult to manage, and the management plan for any affected woman will be dependent upon her presenting problem, for example, infrequent but heavy bleeding, clinical symptoms associated with excess androgens (acne and/or hirsuitism) or subfertility.

If ultrasound is used to assess the ovaries, current-day practice promotes transvaginal ultrasound as the first-line investigation, unless the patient has never had penetrative sexual intercourse. Transabdominal ultrasound can be used, but it is less sensitive and is more likely to aid diagnosis in women with more extreme ovarian changes.[3]

12.3 The Ovary

A polycystic ovary has an increased number of antral follicles, with the classic definition suggesting 12 or more follicles measuring 2–9 mm in diameter, a dense central stoma and an increased ovarian volume (greater than 10 cm^3). The ovary may have a cartwheel appearance with the denser stroma giving the appearance of spokes. The classic appearance is usually recognisable without counting a distinct number of peripheral follicles. The follicles do not always have a peripheral distribution, depending on the plane of examination.

There are a couple of important caveats to highlight when considering ovarian volume. It is worth remembering that an increased ovarian volume can be seen in normal teenagers in association with the endocrine changes that occur at puberty. In addition, if there is a simple cyst in a polycystic ovary, measuring ovarian volume is not meaningful.

Ultrasound can be used only to diagnose PCO. PCOS is a clinical diagnosis, based currently on the Rotterdam Criteria as discussed earlier.

12.4 The Uterus (Endometrium)

Ultrasound features of the endometrium in women with PCOS may show a variety of appearances:

1. If there is unopposed oestrogen secretion, in the absence of ovulation, simple hyperplasia, atypical hyperplasia or even endometrial adenocarcinoma may develop. On transvaginal ultrasound, the endometrium may appear thickened, irregular and there may be loss of the endometrial–myometrial junction. It may also appear denser (Figures 12.1 and 12.2).

It is important to examine the whole of the endometrium in the long and short axis. In long axis the

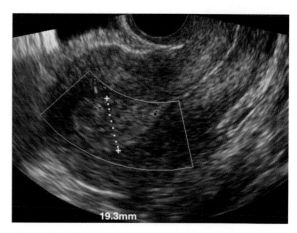

Figure 12.1 Thick endometrium – sagittal section.

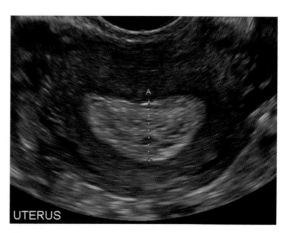

Figure 12.2 Thick endometrium – coronal section.

endometrium should be examined from side to side, ensuring that both cornua have been imaged in order to be certain that no focal lesion is missed. In short axis, the uterus should be examined from cervix to fundus by moving the probe up and down. The imaging can be further enhanced by the use of colour flow or the introduction of a negative contrast (gel or saline) (see Chapter 5). This will help differentiate between a thickened endometrium and a possible polyp.

The threshold to take a biopsy in women with PCOS, who have a thickened endometrium, should be lower than in unaffected women, as women with PCOS have an increase in the risk of developing endometrial hyperplasia and cancer.

2. Less commonly, if there is minimal ovarian activity, with low oestrogen levels, the

endometrium will appear thin and weakly proliferative.

12.5 Understanding the Pathophysiology of PCOS

The rest of this chapter is going to consider the role of ultrasound in the management of women with PCOS, yet understanding the pathophysiology of the condition is a prerequisite to the provision of optimal patient care.

The following information is based on an article by Colin Duncan regarding understanding polycystic ovary syndrome, published in the *Journal of Family Planning and Reproductive Healthcare*.[4]

All sex steroid hormones are derived from cholesterol. Androgens are produced from cholesterol by the theca cells, which are stimulated by LH. The granulosa cells make oestrogen from the androgen, and this process is controlled by FSH. These two gonadotrophins are normally balanced, but in women with PCOS, the basal level of LH is increased, resulting in an increase in androgen production. SHBG binds to androgens, reducing the level of freely available androgen. SHBG levels are inversely proportional to body weight, and as women with PCOS are often overweight, they frequently have a lower level of SHBG, with an increase in the amount of free or 'active' circulating androgens. This further exacerbates the clinical features of PCOS. Insulin resistance is common in women with PCOS, particularly those who are overweight and can be a precursor to impaired glucose tolerance. The effects of LH and androgens are augmented by insulin resistance. The ovary is sensitive to the growth factor effects of insulin, further increasing androgen production, exacerbating the condition in a vicious circle. Weight reduction will reduce the likelihood of insulin resistance occurring and also increase the level of SHBG, reducing free androgens. In the presence of higher insulin levels, even a normal LH can be associated with increased androgen production. In addition, as insulin is an anabolic steroid it is associated with weight gain, consequently reducing SHBG. Insulin also has a direct effect on hepatic synthesis of SHBG, further increasing the unbound circulating androgens.

In summary, the drivers for increased ovarian androgen production in women with PCOS include increased LH, hyperinsulinaemia and obesity, and affected women will have each of these to a varying degree.

For overweight women with PCOS, weight loss is the most important element of management. Once the body mass index is below 30, fertility improves, and contraception becomes essential.

12.6 Management of PCOS

This will depend on the presenting problem, and the information provided here is a simple guide to aid sexual and reproductive health clinicians:

1. All women with PCOS should be advised regarding diet and exercise.
2. Infrequent and/or heavy menstrual bleeding and symptoms of excess androgens:
   a. IUS for endometrial protection and contraception
   or
   b. Combined hormonal contraception – pill, patch or vaginal ring dependent upon individual preference
      - Women with clinical symptoms suggestive of excess androgens have the potential to benefit from the use of an antiandrogenic progestin, for example, cyproterone acetate (Dianette® or equivalent) or drosperinone (Yasmin® or equivalent)
   c. For those women who decline an IUS and who have contraindications to oestrogen, for example, a BMI > 40, a desogestrel only pill, (for example, Cerazette® or equivalent) can be provided both for endometrial protection and contraception. A progestogen only implant is another possible choice.

   Women with symptoms of hyperandrogenism can be prescribed cyproterone acetate in a dose of 50 mg bd for 10 days a month to reduce the level of free androgen. Cyproterone acetate can also be used in a longer regime, for example, 25 mg daily for 21 days out of 28, in conjunction with oestrogen, for example, oestradiol gel 1 mg for either 21 or 28 days. Cyproterone acetate is potentially teratogenic and this regime is not contraceptive; therefore it is essential that women comply with the contraceptive method provided. An IUS can be used in association with cyproterone acetate and oestradiol gel. Alternatively a progestogen only pill or implant could be provided.

3. Fertility: A common misconception among both women and clinicians is that women with PCOS

will not be able to conceive. This is not the case, and contraception is particularly important both for its non-contraceptive benefits as outlined and to control fertility/plan pregnancies appropriately.

4. Subfertility

   c. Ovulation induction with Clomiphene citrate – refer Chapter 11.

12.7 Clinical Cases

Case 1

- Jacqueline is 35 years old. She is overweight (BMI 39), hirsute and has infrequent heavy periods. She does not currently require contraception, but attends a community sexual health service as she finds the lack of predictable bleeding distressing and wonders whether there is anything that can be done to help.

- On the basis of her history alone, polycystic ovary syndrome can be diagnosed.

- A transvaginal ultrasound scan is done to assess her endometrium. Jacqueline had a bleed the week prior to attending; in fact this prompted the appointment as it was not expected and resulted in an embarrassing situation, requiring that she be sent home from work for a change of clothes.

   – The scan pictures show bilateral polycystic ovaries. Compare normal ovary (Figures 12.3) to PCO (Figure 12.4).

- The option of an intrauterine system is declined. Endometrial protection is delivered using a desogestrel progestogen only contraceptive pill and cyproterone acetate is provided twice daily, in a dose of 50 mg, on day 1–10 of every month. Jacqueline has dark facial hair and Vaniqa® is also prescribed, with a recommendation to apply it twice daily for eight weeks in the first instance, although it is likely that laser hair removal will be required for optimal results.

- She is supported to adopt lifestyle changes to help reduce her weight and reduce the risk of her becoming diabetic.

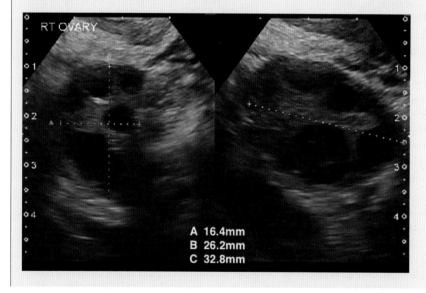

Figure 12.3 Normal ovaries.

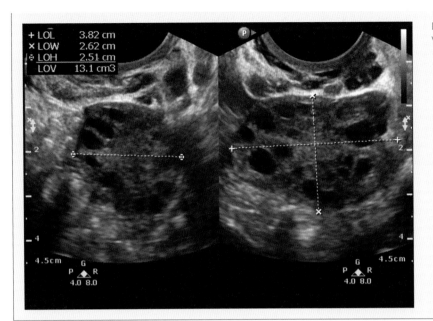

Figure 12.4 Ovarian volume – PCO.

Case 2

- Lucy is 31 years old. She is overweight (BMI 29), has infrequent periods and clinical symptoms of excess androgens – hirsuitism and acne. This is sufficient information to make a diagnosis of PCOS.
- She and her partner would like to conceive. Despite six months without contraception, this has not happened.
- They attend a community gynaecology service for advice.
- Baseline investigations include blood tests (FSH, prolactin, TFTs rubella immunity) and semen analysis.
- All investigations are within normal limits and Lucy is prescribed low dose Clomiphene citrate (25 mg day 5–9 following artificial induction of a withdrawal bleed using medroxy progesterone acetate 10 mg twice daily for 10 days).
- Her response is monitored with ultrasound to assess follicle size and number (if she makes several follicles she will be advised to avoid sexual intercourse because of the risk of a multiple pregnancy), and a progesterone level to assess ovulation, a week after anticipated ovulation.
- Four weeks after commencing Clomiphene Citrate, she has a positive pregnancy test.
- A dating scan at 6-weeks corresponds with her dates, and confirms a singleton pregnancy.

Case 3

- Alison is 21 years old. She has never had regular periods, with an infrequent pattern, bleeding 3–4 times a year on average. She has had lifelong acne, which has caused her considerable distress.
- She is under the care of a dermatologist who has prescribed Dianette® with good effect. It has given her regular withdrawal bleeds in association with a dramatic improvement in her acne.
- Her GP will not prescribe this for her as he is concerned about the potential increase in the risk of venous thromboembolism when compared to other combined pills.[5]
- She has no risk factors for combined hormonal contraception. She does not have focal migraine; there is no family history of venous thromboembolism; she does not smoke, takes no other medication, is not overweight and her BP is within normal limits.
- She will benefit from the use of a progestin which will block the androgen receptor. Cyproterone acetate is the most antiandrogenic progestin, with most potential benefit, as has already been proven and this can be prescribed in the longer term for its non-contraceptive benefits.

12.8 Take Home Messages

- PCO is an ultrasound diagnosis, whereas PCOS is a clinical syndrome.
  - These two abbreviations are not synonymous.
- Ultrasound is not essential for the diagnosis of PCOS.
- The main role of ultrasound in women with PCOS is for endometrial assessment.
- Subfertility associated with PCOS should first be treated with ovulation induction, not IVF.

References

1. Lowe P, Kovacs G, Howlett D. Incidence of polycystic ovaries and polycystic ovary syndrome amongst women in Melbourne, Australia. *Aust and N Z J of Obstet and Gynaecol.* 2005; 45:17–19.

2. Rotterdam ESHRE/ASRM-Sponsored PCOS Concensus Working Group. Revised 2003 concensus on diagnosis criteria and long-term health risks related to polycystic ovary syndrome. *Hum Reprod.* 2004;19:41–47.

3. Takahashi K, Nishigaki A, Eda Y, Yamasaki H, Yoshino K, Kitao M. Transvaginal ultrasound is an effective method for screening in polycystic ovarian disease: preliminary study. *Gynecol Obstet Invest.* 1990;30(1):34–36.

4. Duncan W C, A guide to understanding polycystic ovary syndrome (PCOS), *J FamPlann Reprod Healthcare*. http://jfprhc.bmj.com/, 25 August, 2015.

5. www.bnf.org/products/bnf-online.

Chapter 13

Ultrasound Imaging of Women with Abnormal Uterine Bleeding (AUB)

Jane Dickson

13.1 Introduction   201
13.2 Abnormal Uterine Bleeding in Non-pregnant Women of Reproductive Age: The PALM-COEIN Classification   201
13.3 Other Causes of Vaginal Bleeding   209
13.4 Assessment of Abnormal Uterine Bleeding   209

13.5 Problem Bleeding Associated with Contraception   211
13.6 Further Assessment   211
13.7 Management of Heavy Menstrual Bleeding   211
13.8 Ultrasound Applied Clinically for AUB   214

13.1 Introduction

AUB is a term used to describe uterine bleeding, primarily menstruation, which does not follow a 'normal' pattern.[1] There may be disturbances of regularity, frequency, heaviness of flow and duration.

Irregular menstrual bleeding is the term used to describe menstrual cycles that vary in length by more than 20 days (when observed over a one-year time frame).

Absent menstrual bleeding (amenorrhoea) is absent bleeding for > 90 days.

Infrequent menstrual bleeding (oligoamenorrhoea) is when there are one or two episodes of bleeding in a 90-day period. Frequent menstrual bleeding is when there are more than 4 episodes in a 90-day period.

Heavy menstrual bleeding is excessive menstrual blood loss, which interferes with a woman's physical, emotional, social and material quality of life, and which can occur alone or in combination with other symptoms.[2] **Prolonged menstrual bleeding** describes menstrual bleeding, which exceeds eight days on a regular basis.

Abnormal bleeding may also be non-menstrual as is the case with inter-menstrual and post-coital bleeding. This may occur as a regular event in 1–2 per cent of cycles, for example, around ovulation, but may often signify pathology such as infections or more serious conditions such as endometrial or cervical cancer.

Bleeding outside of reproductive age may also be considered as abnormal as is the case with precocious puberty or post-menopausal bleeding. Bleeding problems are the most common side effect of hormonal contraception and this is also important to consider, as it is essential that no significant pathology is missed.[3] When considering the differential diagnosis of abnormal uterine bleeding, it is also important to exclude other causes of vaginal bleeding.

13.2 Abnormal Uterine Bleeding in Non-pregnant Women of Reproductive Age: The PALM-COEIN Classification

Bleeding in non-pregnant women of reproductive age may be classified using the PALM-COEIN system. This is the FIGO classification system for non-pregnant women of reproductive age.[4] The PALM causes of abnormal bleeding are those that are structural and can be visualised using imaging, primarily ultrasound imaging. Transvaginal ultrasound imaging is usually the first choice, but transabdominal imaging should also be undertaken to ensure that no pathology is missed, such as a large fibroid uterus. The COEIN causes of abnormal uterine bleeding are those that were previously grouped together under the term 'dysfunctional uterine bleeding'.

13.2.1 Polyps

Endometrial polyps are epithelial projections arising within the endometrium and projecting into the cavity, which have a variable structure, but may contain vascular, glandular, fibromuscular and connective

Box 13.1 The PALM – COEIN System of Classification of AUB

PALM

P –Polyp

A –Adenomyosis

L –Leiomyoma (Fibroids)

M –Malignancy and hyperplasia

COEIN

C –Coagulopathy

O –Ovulatory dysfunction

E –Endometrial

I –Iatrogenic

N –Not yet classified

Usually adenomyosis is a generalised change, but occasionally it can present as a focal lesion, known as an 'adenomyoma'. The sonographic appearance of adenomyosis is partly related to endometrial tissue being present in the myometrium and partly related to a hypertrophic reaction in the myometrium. The classical ultrasound findings are demonstrated in Figures 13.4a–c and include the following:

1. Uterine enlargement – typically a 'globular' uterus
2. Cystic anechoic spaces in the myometrium
3. Asymmetric uterine wall thickening
4. Sub-endometrial linear striations
5. Heterogenous echotexture (the most predictive finding)
6. Obscure endometrial border
7. Thickening of the transition zone: a 'halo' around the endometrial layer. A thickness of 12 mm or more is associated with adenomyosis.

13.2.3 Leiomyomata (Fibroids)

Leiomyomata or fibroids are benign fibromuscular tumours of the myometrium. They are more prevalent in women of African ancestry and may be asymptomatic. The presenting clinical symptoms vary, depending on the position of the fibroid. Sub-mucosal fibroids are those which project into the endometrium, distorting the uterine cavity (Figures 13.5–13.7. See also Sections 5.5 and 6.3). In the PALM-COEIN classification system, fibroids are divided into sub-mucosal (SM) and other (O) (Table 13.1). Sub-mucosal fibroids are those which are most likely to cause AUB, HMB and dysmenorrhoea.

Occasionally sub-mucosal fibroids may be pedunculated. These can prolapse through the cervical canal and may cause acute pain because of torsion. They may also present with intermenstrual bleeding. Leiomyomata may be classified according to the leiomyoma sub-classification system.

On ultrasound examination, fibroids are usually well demarcated from the normal myometrium. They are dense and there may be acoustic shadowing behind the fibroid. Doppler may show classical vessels around the circumference of the fibroid.

A rare complication of leiomyomata is leiomyosarcoma when malignant change occurs. Peak incidence is 50–60 years and this is more common in women of Afro-Caribbean origin and those using tamoxifen. Lesions are very vascular with the loss of classical fibroid demarcation.

tissue elements (Figure 13.1a–c). Sometimes they are multiple but this can often be clarified only on ultrasound insertion of contrast into the cavity (Figure 13.2). They may be asymptomatic, but they may also contribute to abnormal or heavy menstrual bleeding. They are usually benign, but some may have atypical or malignant features, particularly in women with risk factors (Box 13.2). Endometrial polyps are common and are found in 10 per cent of women investigated for abnormal bleeding. Ultrasound appearances are similar to endometrium and they are usually hyperechoic and sometimes there are small cystic spaces (Figure 13.3). Sometimes a vascular feeding vessel can be seen if Doppler is used. If they are pedunculated, they may project into the cervical canal.

13.2.2 Adenomyosis

The term adenomyosis relates to the presence of endometrial tissue beneath the endometrial–myometrial interface. Ectopic endometrial glands and stroma are present within the myometrium and it is thought that this condition may affect up to 30 per cent women. It is thought that it is a variant of endometriosis and the two conditions may coexist in 20 per cent of patients. Typically patients with adenomyosis are older, often in their forties and typically present with heavy menstrual bleeding and dysmenorrhoea. There may be an association with previous Caesarean section or elevated oestrogen levels.[5]

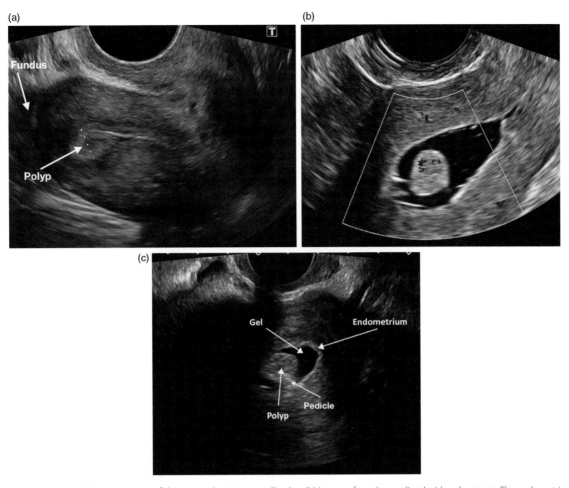

(a)

Fundus

Polyp

(b)

(c)

Gel   Endometrium

Polyp   Pedicle

Figure 13.1 (a) TV long axis view of the uterus showing a small polyp. (b) Image of a polyp outlined with gel contrast. The endometrium can be seen separate from the polyp and is uniformly thin. Colour flow is present within the polyp indicating one or two feeding vessels. (c) a small polyp outlined with gel in the cavity, outlining the width of the pedicle attachment. The gel enables the endometrium to be seen separate from the polyp and it appears uniform.

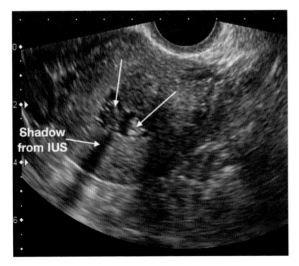

Shadow from IUS

Figure 13.2 Multiple polyps outlined with gel contrast (long arrows). The woman was referred for prolonged and heavy bleeding that was not resolving with a levonorgestrel IUS. This view does not show the IUS but its presence within the cavity is indicated by the shadow (short arrow).

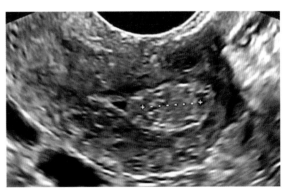

Figure 13.3 TV view – the outline of a polyp can be clearly seen without gel as it is hyperechoic with small cystic spaces that stand out against the surrounding myometrium. However, the endometrium and extent of attachment to the uterus cannot be judged.

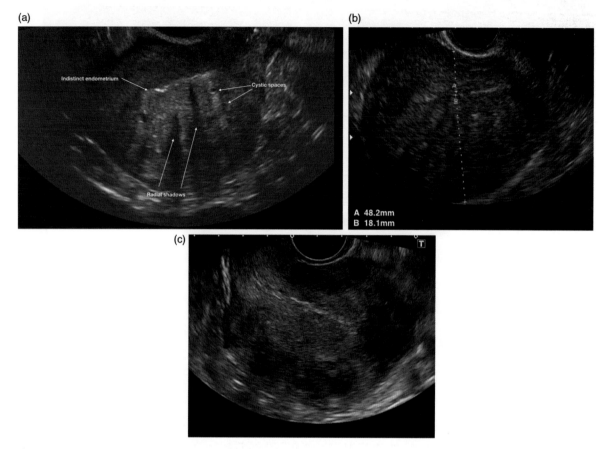

Figure 13.4 (a) Transvaginal view of the uterus showing multiple typical features of adenomyosis including heterogenous echotexture, linear acoustic shadows and cystic spaces in the myometrium (arrows), asymmetric thickening of the posterior myometrium and an obscure endometrial–myometrial border. (b) A TV long axis view of a uterus showing globular enlargement with marked asymmetric thickening and indistinct endometrium, typical of adenomyosis. (c) A TV long axis image showing a globular uterus with heterogenous echotexture, typical of adenomyosis.

Table 13.1 Leiomyoma Sub-classification System

Submucosal	0	Pedunculated with 100% intracavitary
	1	< 50% intramural with >50% intracavitary
	2	> 50%intramural with <50% intracavitary
Other	3	Contacts endometrium 100% intramural
	4	Intramural (Figure 13.8)
	5	Subserosal > 50% intramural
	6	Subserosal < 50% intramural
	7	Subserosal pedunculated
	8	Other, for example, cervical
Hybrid (impact on endometrium and serosa)		Graded according to position relative to endometrium and stroma

13.2.4 Malignancy and Hyperplasia

These are a relatively uncommon cause of AUB in women of reproductive age, but must be considered. These are more common causes of AUB in perimeno-pausal women and women who have higher exposure to oestrogen.

Endometrial hyperplasia is proliferation of the endometrial glands. There are four categories according to the World Health Organisation classification:

1. Simple hyperplasia without atypia –1 per cent risk of progression to endometrial carcinoma.
2. Complex hyperplasia without atypia – 3 per cent risk of progression.
3. Simple atypical hyperplasia – 8 per cent risk of progression.

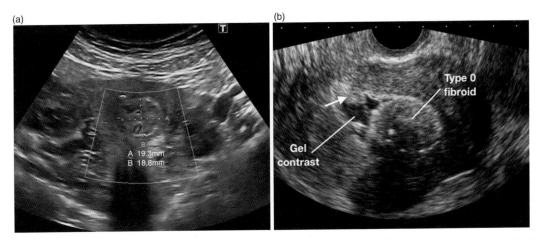

Figure 13.5 (a) A TA transverse view of an anteverted uterus showing a centrally placed fibroid which cannot be accurately classified with imaging alone. (b) A TV image following insertion of gel contrast shows this is a type 0 submucus fibroid filling the endometrial cavity and there is a smaller submucus fibroid projecting into the lower uterine cavity (arrow).

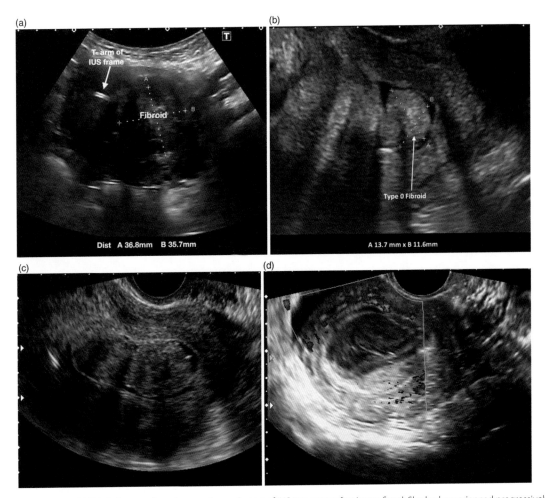

Figure 13.6 (a) This lady was referred requesting a change of IUS two years after it was fitted. She had experienced progressively heavier bleeding since the IUS was fitted. The TA image shows a fibroid close to the frame of the IUS, but its relationship to the endometrial cavity is not clear. (b) A TV image after instillation of gel demonstrates a smaller type 0 submucous fibroid filling the endometrial cavity. Multiple fibroids were present. (c) In this case instillation of gel outlines two type 0 fibroids filling the endometrial cavity. (d) Imaging this large type 0 fibroid filling, the endometrial cavity has been enhanced by a small rim of gel contrast around the fibroid.

(a)

(b)

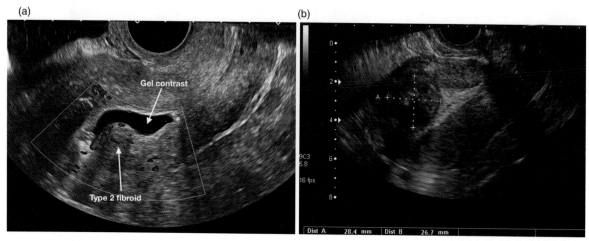

Figure 13.7 (a) Image of a small type 2 submucous fibroid. The cavity has been outlined by gel which shows less than 50 per cent of the fibroid is within the cavity. (b)This type 2 fibroid can be delineated without use of contrast.

(a)

(b)

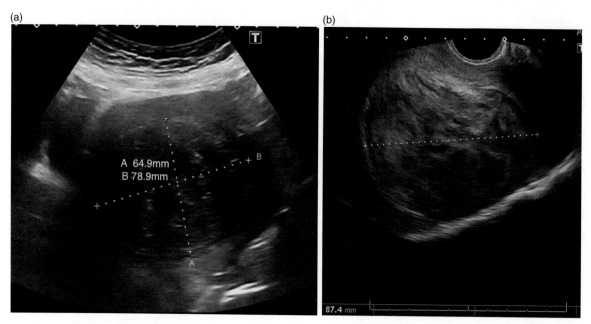

Figure 13.8 (a) TA image of a large fibroid. It is difficult to categorise the fibroid because the position of the endometrial cavity is obscured. (b) TV image of a large intramural fibroid.

4. Complex atypical hyperplasia – 29 per cent risk of progression (a proportion of women with severely atypical hyperplasia already have carcinoma on hysterectomy, because hyperplasia may be focal and a biopsy might be unrepresentative of the whole endometrium).

Diagnosis is based on histological examination and not by ultrasound, but there are ultrasound appearances that would be of concern particularly in high-risk women, including abnormally thick endometrium (Figure 13.9a), irregular endometrium (Figure 13.9b), turbid fluid within the cavity with irregular endometrium (Figure 13.9c), cystic endometrium (Figure 13.9d).

Endometrial cancer is the commonest female genital tract malignancy in the developed world, but it is

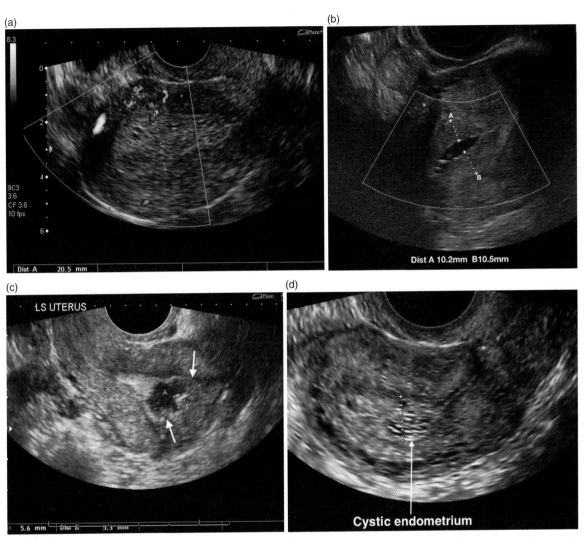

Figure 13.9 (a) Abnormally thick endometrium. (b) Instillation of gel excluded a polyp causing the thickened appearance, and just clarified the endometrium was regular and uniformly thick. (c) Spontaneous fluid outlining irregular endometrial with patchy loss of the endometrial–myometrial junction (arrows). (d) Cystic endometrium.

rarely seen before the menopause, with peak age incidence between 60 and 70 years. The main risk factor is unopposed excessive oestrogen stimulation, which occurs with anovulatory cycles preceding ovarian failure. Progesterone or long-term use of progestogen in any form of hormonal contraception is protective.

Type I (endometrioid) endometrial cancer accounts for 70–80 per cent of disease and relates to excess oestrogen exposure without progestogen opposition. Prognosis is better than with Type II (non-endometriod) endometrial cancers.

Endometrial hyperplasia usually needs to be diagnosed with endometrial biopsy as the measurement of endometrial thickness is not a reliable marker in pre-menopausal women.[6] Ultrasound findings related to endometrial cancer show a thickened endometrium, irregular endometrial–myometrial border and loss of homogeneity of the endometrium. The myometrium may also be asymmetrical and there is typically colour flow across the myometrial–endometrial border with high flow in 'endometrium' (Chapter 15, Figure 15.1a, b).

Box 13.2 Risk Factors for Endometrial Cancer

Endogenous unopposed oestrogen

- Chronic anovulation (unless hypothalamic, example – Weight related)
- PCOS
- Obesity

Exogenous oestrogen

- Oestrogen only preparations
- Tamoxifen

Age

Early menarche

Late menopause

Diabetes mellitus (especially non-insulin dependant)

Lynch syndrome

Long-term use of progestogens, including any form of hormonal contraception, is a strong protective factor against endometrial cancer.

13.2.5 Coagulopathy

Approximately 13 per cent of women with HMB may have a systemic disorder of haemostasis such as von Willebrand disease.[7] However, the mechanism of how these abnormalities contribute to problems is not clear.

13.2.6 Ovulatory Dysfunction

Ovulatory dysfunction may contribute to AUB because unpredictable progesterone production (linked to anovulatory cycles and lack of a corpus luteum) leads to unpredictable bleeding. Such disorders may be related to endocrine problems, for example, polycystic ovary syndrome, hypothyroidism and hyperprolactinaemia. In addition, problems relating to body mass index may impair ovulation, often anorexia, weight loss and extreme exercise.

13.2.7 Endometrial

Local factors within the endometrium may contribute to abnormal uterine bleeding in the absence of any structural abnormality. Factors that influence local haemostasis are important. There may be reduced local production of vasoconstrictors such as endothelin-1 and prostaglandin $F_{2\alpha}$ and increased factors which control vasodilatation, for example,

prostaglandin E_2 and prostacyclin. There may also be increased clot breakdown because of increased local production of plasminogen activator.

Inflammatory pathology of the endometrium may also contribute to abnormal uterine bleeding. This may be the situation with acute endometritis, which may occur post-instrumentation, post-termination or post-partum. The ultrasound appearances may show loss of the endometrial–myometrial borders and increased vascularity on Colour Doppler. There may also be associated signs of infection including tenderness and ultrasound features of tubo-ovarian infection (Chapter 6, Figure 6.36) or free fluid (Chapter 4, Figure 4.38).

13.2.8 Iatrogenic

This is bleeding caused by medical interventions or devices – the commonest cause being bleeding in relation to contraception. This classification includes 'breakthrough bleeding'. Some cases of breakthrough bleeding relate to reduced circulating steroid levels, for example, when contraceptive pills are missed. This leads to reduced suppression of FSH, allowing some ovarian activity. Endogenous oestradiol is produced which causes additional, irregular stimulation of the endometrium. Smoking and hepatic enzyme inducers such as carbamazepine may also trigger breakthrough bleeding by increasing the rate of hepatic metabolism of oestrogens and progestins, reducing circulating levels.

Unscheduled bleeding during the first 3–6 months of intrauterine system use is very common. For this reason it is particularly important that abnormal bleeding in women over 45 or those with risk factors for endometrial cancer is investigated prior to fitting an IUS, to avoid any presumption of bleeding due to the IUS and hence a delay in diagnosis.

Bleeding with the IUS is related to the fact that the intrauterine presence of levonorgestrel leads to the up-regulation of the enzyme 17β hydroxylase 2 which regulates conversion of oestradiol to the weaker oestrogen, oestrone. After several months the enzyme is down-regulated again leading to a more stable intrauterine environment.[8]

Medications which interfere with dopamine metabolism such as amitriptyline and phenothiazines may inhibit prolactin release. This can result in the disorder of the hypothalamic-pituitary-ovarian axis leading to irregular bleeding. Heavy menstrual bleeding may also be a consequence of anticoagulant use including warfarin and heparin.

13.2.9 Not Yet Classified

This group includes pathology which does not have a straightforward relationship with AUB, such as chronic endometritis and pelvic inflammatory disease.

13.3 Other Causes of Vaginal Bleeding

When considering abnormal uterine bleeding, it is important to remember that vaginal bleeding can originate from anywhere in the female genital tract. Generally, physical examination rather than ultrasound examination will be more important in elucidating the cause.

13.4 Assessment of Abnormal Uterine Bleeding

A full history should be taken including a full menstrual history counting cycle length and regularity. It must be identified whether the problem is with menstrual frequency, flow or both. Assessment of the impact of the bleeding problem on the patient must be made. Specific inquiry should be made about the presence of intermenstrual or post-coital bleeding and whether or not there is any associated pain.

When assessing abnormal bleeding, it is essential to eliminate the possibility of pregnancy, for example, by performing a sensitive pregnancy test. The PALM-COEIN classification applies to women who are not pregnant and are of reproductive age; note that pre-pubertal bleeding and post-menopausal bleeding are excluded from the criteria. More than one of the PALM–COEIN causes may co-exist.

Initial haematological investigations should include a full blood count, determination of ovulatory status, for example, by measuring luteal phase progesterone (if required) and screening for bleeding disorders in women who have had HMB since menarche or who have a personal or family history suggesting a coagulation disorder. Inspection and speculum examination allows assessment of the lower genital tract, and bimanual examination will identify cervical motion tenderness, uterine size and position and the presence of adnexal masses. Infection screening should be performed appropriately and cervical screening should be performed only if the patient is willing to undergo cervical

---

> **Box 13.3 Causes of Abnormal Vaginal Bleeding in Women of Reproductive Age**
>
> **Uterus**
>
> PALM_COEIN
> Pregnancy related
>
> **Cervix**
>
> Cervicitis
> Cervical polyp
> Ectropion
> Carcinoma
>
> **Vagina**
>
> Atrophic vaginitis
> Infection, example – candida
> Foreign body, for example, retained tampon
> Trauma
> Carcinoma
>
> **Vulva**
>
> Infection
> Carcinoma
> Melanoma
> Dermatological conditions, for example, lichen sclerosus
>
> **Other**
>
> Rectal bleeding
> Haematuria
> Bleeding disorders
> Iatrogenic, for example, related to medication such as heparin or warfarin

---

cytology testing according to the National Cervical Screening Programme.

Ultrasound is the first line investigation for suspected structural abnormalities, and endometrial biopsy should be undertaken if there are any factors which might suggest hyperplasia or cancer, such as persistent inter-menstrual bleeding, women aged 45 and over and treatment failure. Ultrasound with negative contrast has much greater diagnostic efficacy for endometrial pathology than just ordinary transvaginal ultrasound, as the infusion of fluid/gel better outlines the surface of the endometrium and improves visualisation of both endometrium and myometrium by acting as an acoustic window[9]; see Chapter 5.

13.4.1 The Use of Ultrasound for Assessment of Abnormal Uterine Bleeding

In the context of sexual and reproductive healthcare, it is best that clinician who performs the clinical assessment of a patient, that is, history taking, physical examination and performance of appropriate investigation, is the clinician who proceeds to perform the ultrasound examination. This means that the ultrasound examination can be interpreted immediately in the appropriate clinical context. The patient should be put at ease and the procedure should be explained. The patient's privacy and dignity should be respected and the offer of a chaperone should be made and recorded. The limitations of the procedure should be explained and it should be made clear to the patient, whether or not diagnosis and explanations will be given immediately or at a follow-up appointment. The patient's consent for the procedure should be sought and documented.

Transvaginal ultrasound is the approach of choice for the assessment of the pelvic organs. However, large masses may lie outside the transducer's field of view, so transabdominal scanning should be regarded as complementing the information. Transvaginal scanning allows assessment of the uterus and if the uterine cavity appears normal, hysteroscopic assessment would not usually be required. Coexisting pathology such as ovarian cysts or polycystic ovaries can also be identified.

Endometrial thickness varies during the menstrual cycle. It ranges from 4–8 mm in the proliferative phase to 10–14 mm in the secretory phase. In a post-menopausal patient, an endometrial thickness > 4 mm is considered abnormal, but in the reproductive years a thickness of up to 14 mm is considered normal. The endometrium should be of regular thickness and should be measured at the maximum double thickness on sagittal scan.

A thin endometrium may be related to the menstrual cycle or be associated with contraceptive therapy such as combined hormonal contraception, intrauterine system use. It may also be thin following any form of endometrial resection or ablation. A thickened endometrium may be suggestive of polyps, hyperplasia, malignancy or may be medication related (for example, hormone replacement therapy, Tamoxifen).

Introducing a negative contrast medium may aid diagnosis of polyps, submucous fibroids and focal endometrial thickening (see Chapter 5). Traditionally, saline is the contrast medium, but in sexual and reproductive healthcare, Instillagel® which is readily available can be used.[9] This is known as gel hysterosonography. Gel can be introduced into the uterine cavity with the use of the associated quill or catheter. Where the cervical os appears stenosed, application of intracervical Lidocaine and passage of a small dilator may be required before the introduction of the quill. Alternatively, lidocaine topical spray may be used, or just holding the end of the quill over the os and gentle pressure on the syringe may allow filling of the cavity and hydrodilatation of the os. In women with a normal cavity, only a small amount of gel may be required (2–3 ml). The gel must be introduced slowly; otherwise, intrauterine cramping may occur. Scanning transabdominally in sagittal plane while inserting the gel enables the gel filling the cavity to be imaged in real-time, and the suprapubic pressure from the transducer seems to facilitate successful filling of the endometrial cavity in many cases. The uterine cavity will be outlined and it may be possible to identify features not demonstrated by conventional ultrasound imaging alone. Filling the cavity with negative contrast also enhances imaging of the adnexae due to fluid, enhancing the ultrasound transmission, analogous to filling the bladder for TA imaging. (Figure 13.10)

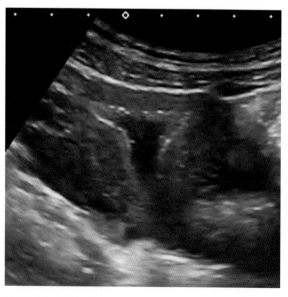

Figure 13.10 TA transverse view of a normal endometrial cavity filled with gel. Only 2–3 ml was required to fill the cavity.

13.5 Problematic Bleeding Associated with Contraception

Abnormal uterine bleeding is the commonest side effect related to hormonal contraception. The exact mechanisms of problematic bleeding are unknown, but it is thought to relate to increased endometrial blood vessel fragility in association with local angiogenic factors and loss of structural integrity. Oestradiol is responsible for endometrial proliferation and progesterone is anti-oestrogenic, inhibiting endometrial growth and glandular differentiation.

Bleeding associated with combined hormonal contraception is usually transient, settling after a couple of months of use. Bleeding associated with progestogen only methods can be more troublesome and may be irregular and prolonged. FSRH guidelines recommend that women with problematic bleeding, which is likely to be related to contraception, should have:

- a clinical history taken to ensure compliance and inquiry about related symptoms;
- sexually transmitted infections excluded;
- cervical screening if done according to the National Programme;
- a pregnancy test if necessary;
- underlying pathology excluded.

Examination should be performed if:

- there is persistent bleeding beyond the initial three months of use;
- new symptoms or change in bleeding pattern occur after three months of use;
- a cervical screening test is required according to the National Screening programme;
- requested by the woman;
- there is a failed trial of medical management;
- there are symptoms suggestive of pathology such as vaginal discharge, pain, dyspareunia or post-coital bleeding.

The management plan in Figure 13.11 may then be used.

Recommended medical therapy options for women using hormonal contraception when pathology has been excluded are shown in Figure 13.12.

13.6 Further Assessment

An endometrial biopsy with scan (preferably with contrast) should be considered in women 45 years and over, or in younger women (35–45 years) with risk factors for endometrial cancer and persistent problematic bleeding after the first 3 months of use of a method or a change of bleeding pattern.

A transvaginal ultrasound scan should be undertaken when structural abnormalities are suspected such as submucosal fibroids or endometrial polyps. It may also be a useful tool to ensure that intrauterine devices/systems are correctly sited. An intrauterine system, which is located low in the uterine cavity, may lead to more bleeding/spotting compared to fundally placed devices (Figure 13.13). A hysteroscopy may also be required in women with heavy menstrual bleeding for treatment or when ultrasound is inconclusive. Management will be dependant upon the pathology that is identified.

13.7 Management of Heavy Menstrual Bleeding

Intervention to improve heavy menstrual bleeding should focus on improving quality of life rather than focusing of volume of blood loss. Initially, a history and full blood count should be taken.[10] If the history does not suggest structural or histological abnormality, pharmaceutical treatment can be started without any prior examination or investigation.

Physical examination should always be undertaken before LNG-IUS insertion and before investigations for structural or histological abnormality. Ultrasound is the first-line diagnostic tool and should always be undertaken if the uterus is palpable abdominally, if vaginal examination reveals a pelvic mass or if pharmaceutical treatment fails. An endometrial biopsy should be undertaken if histological abnormality is suspected. Any woman who has risk factors for endometrial carcinoma (for example, age over 45 or past history of prolonged oligo/amenorrhoea) must have endometrial assessment before treatment, including treatment with an IUS. The IUS insertion can be undertaken at the time but an endometrial biopsy should be sent for histological assessment (Figure 13.14).

Pharmaceutical treatment should be considered where there is no structural or histological abnormality and for fibroids < 3 cm when there is no distortion of the uterine cavity. However, even when there is distortion of the cavity, a more experienced clinician may opt to try insertion of an IUS with the proviso that the risk of expulsion is higher or that it may not control bleeding.

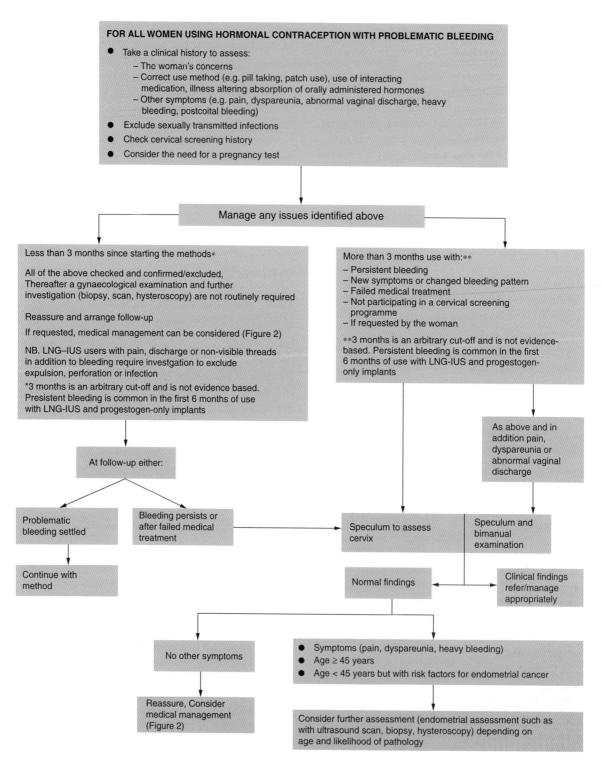

Figure 13.11 Suggested management plan for a woman using hormonal contraception with unscheduled bleeding (reproduced with kind permission from the Clinical Effectiveness Unit of the Faculty of Sexual and Reproductive Healthcare).

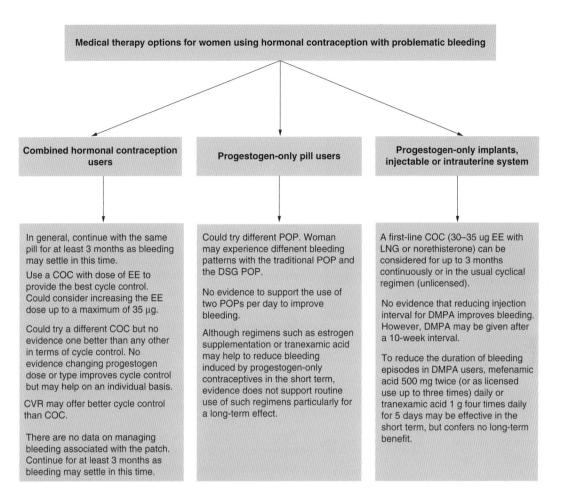

Medical therapy options for women using hormonal contraception with problematic bleeding

Combined hormonal contraception users	Progestogen-only pill users	Progestogen-only implants, injectable or intrauterine system
In general, continue with the same pill for at least 3 months as bleeding may settle in this time.	Could try different POP. Woman may experience different bleeding patterns with the traditional POP and the DSG POP.	A first-line COC (30–35 ug EE with LNG or norethisterone) can be considered for up to 3 months continuously or in the usual cyclical regimen (unlicensed).
Use a COC with dose of EE to provide the best cycle control. Could consider increasing the EE dose up to a maximum of 35 µg.	No evidence to support the use of two POPs per day to improve bleeding.	No evidence that reducing injection interval for DMPA improves bleeding. However, DMPA may be given after a 10-week interval.
Could try a different COC but no evidence one better than any other in terms of cycle control. No evidence changing progestogen dose or type improves cycle control but may help on an individual basis.	Although regimens such as estrogen supplementation or tranexamic acid may help to reduce bleeding induced by progestogen-only contraceptives in the short term, evidence does not support routine use of such regimens particularly for a long-term effect.	To reduce the duration of bleeding episodes in DMPA users, mefenamic acid 500 mg twice (or as licensed use up to three times) daily or tranexamic acid 1 g four times daily for 5 days may be effective in the short term, but confers no long-term benefit.
CVR may offer better cycle control than COC.		
There are no data on managing bleeding associated with the patch. Continue for at least 3 months as bleeding may settle in this time.		

Medical therapy options for women using hormonal contraception with problematic bleeding. COC, combined oral contraceptive pill; CVR, combined vaginal ring; DMPA, depot medroxyprogesterone acetate; DSG, desogestrel; EE, ethinylestradiol; LNG, levonorgestrel; POP, progestogen-only pill.

Figure 13.12 Medical treatment options for problematic bleeding related to hormonal contraception (reproduced with kind permission from the Clinical Effectiveness Unit of the Faculty of Sexual and Reproductive Healthcare).

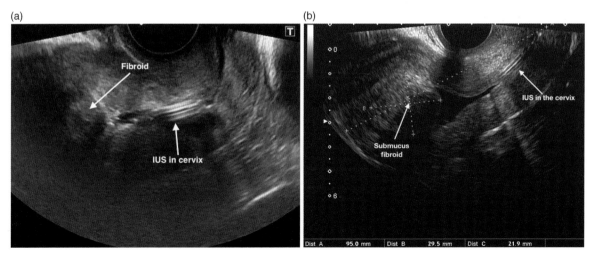

Figure 13.13 Images of submucous fibroids with IUS devices positioned in the cervix.

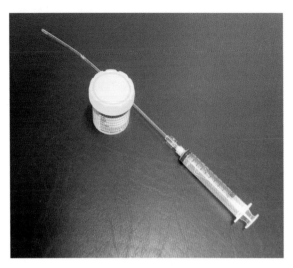

Figure 13.14 An endometrial sampling system with histology pot. This system is ideal where contrast has been infused since the 10 ml syringe will enable aspiration of the contrast and endometrial sample without need for repeated removal and insertion of the sampler.

The treatments should be considered in the following order:

- **First line** – Intrauterine system which acts by suppressing endometrial growth and causing endometrial atrophy (79–97 per cent improvement in symptoms at one year).
- **Second line** – Anti-fibrinolytics: example – Tranexamic acid 1g tds (34–59 per cent improvement at one year), non-steroidal anti-inflammatories: for example, Mefenamic acid 500mg tds (20–49 per cent improvement at 1 year).

- **Third line** – Progestogens: for example, Norethisterone 5mg tds, day 5–26 of cycle or injected long-acting progestogens.

The ECLIPSE study (2013) demonstrated that when an IUS was used to treat heavy menstrual bleeding, compared to standard medical treatment, there was greater improvement in symptoms and patients were twice as likely to continue with treatment.[11] There are some pharmaceutical treatments, such as gonadotropin-releasing hormone analogues and ulipristal acetate, that can be used to shrink fibroids, particularly prior to surgical treatment. These help by reducing the endometrium and reducing the size and vascularity of fibroids. The updated NICE guideline on management of heavy menstrual bleeding states that women with fibroids 3 cm or more in diameter can be offered up to four three month courses of ulipristal acetate 5 mg per day.[2]

When pharmaceutical treatment has failed, further intervention can be considered. Endometrial ablation can be considered in women who have no desire for subsequent pregnancy with a uterus no bigger than a ten-week pregnancy. Methods include impedance – controlled bipolar radiofrequency, fluid-filled thermal balloon and microwave endometrial ablation. Further treatments for uterine fibroids include: hysteroscopic resection for type 0 or type 1 submucus fibroids that are smaller than 5 cms (these can be pre-treated with GNRH analogues to reduce size), uterine artery embolisation or more definitive surgery such as myomectomy or hysterectomy.

13.8 Ultrasound Applied Clinically for AUB

Cases

Case 1

A 48-year-old obese Caucasian woman presents with a history of erratic vaginal bleeding for 3 years. She has had four children and suffers from asthma and non-insulin-dependant diabetes. She works in a supermarket and has been finding that she often feels tired and breathless, but has attributed this to her asthma. She has been married for 27 years and had a laparoscopic sterilisation when she was 35 years old. She went to her general practitioner who advised that she should attend the local Sexual and Reproductive Health Service to have an intrauterine system inserted.

She attended the local SRH service and said that her periods are heavy and last 5–6 days, but she often experiences some brown blood loss between her periods. She also occasionally experiences brown blood loss after sexual intercourse. During her period, she often notices blood clots. She has no symptoms suggestive of the menopause or hypothyroidism. She had her last cervical screening test a year previously and there had been no abnormalities. She is advised to have some initial investigations including a full blood count and an ultrasound scan.

Investigations show haemoglobin level of 98 g/l and the following images are obtained on transvaginal scan. A transvaginal scan with gel contrast demonstrates a polyp (arrow) (Figures 13.15a, b). Although initially the endometrium appears thin and regular, on evaluation of the whole cavity, an area of irregular thickening is found (Figure 13.15c).

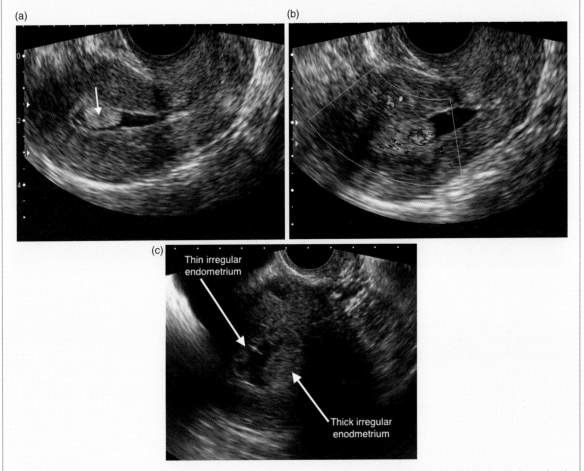

(a)

(b)

(c) Thin irregular endometrium

Thick irregular enodmetrium

Figure 13.15 (a) An endometrial polyp outlined by gel contrast instilled into the cavity. (b) Thin regular endometrium is also outlined separate from the polyp. (c) Complete visualisation of the cavity and endometrium reveals areas of irregular endometrial thickening (arrows) and therefore the need for further evaluation.

The appropriate management would be to refer on for a hysteroscopy, targeted endometrial biopsy and polypectomy. It would be appropriate to offer the fitting of an IUS at the procedure as removal of the polyp alone may not resolve the heaviness of her bleeding and the anaemia. The IUS will also provide protection from endometrial hyperplasia in the longer term, which she has risk factors for, as well as suppression of her bleeding. If the scan had only demonstrated uniform endometrial thickening rather than a polyp, it would be appropriate to take an endometrial biopsy and fit an IUS in the community setting, and then where indicated alter this management in accordance with the histology result.

Case 2

A 33-year-old Afro-Caribbean woman, who has had three normal vaginal deliveries, attends an SRH clinic for contraception. Her youngest child is one year old. This woman is having regular periods. Her periods have become much heavier since delivery of her children and she bleeds for eight days every month. She needs to use two sanitary towels at a time and often uses a tampon in addition. A recent haemoglobin level was 108 g/l. The images from transvaginal scan are shown (Figures 13.16a and 13.16b).

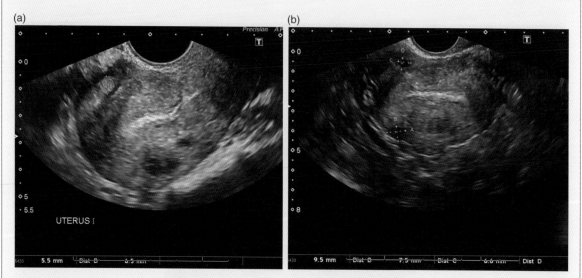

Figure 13.16 (a) A TV longitudinal (long axis) view of the uterus showing several small intramural fibroids. (b) A transverse (short axis) view of the same uterus.

The images demonstrate some small intramural fibroids. There are no submucosal fibroids and the endometrium is not distorted. The options were discussed and the patient opted to have an intrauterine system inserted. Her bleeding was reduced and acceptable within three months.

Case 3

A 45-year-old Caucasian woman was referred to a community gynaecology clinic because of heavy bleeding which has not improved since an IUS was fitted 10 months ago. She has a BMI of 37 kg/m² and is nulliparous. She is not currently sexually active. She has no other medical history of note. She had no inter-menstrual bleeding prior to the IUS but now has more days with bleeding although the heaviest days are reduced. A recent haemoglobin level is 100 g/l. A transabdominal scan shows a 35 mm central fibroid within her uterus (Figure 13.17a).

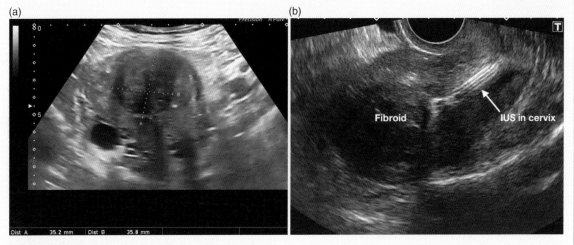

(a)   (b)

Figure 13.17 (a) TA view showing a central 35 mm fibroid. The IUS is not clearly demonstrated but a shadow below the fibroid may indicate its position below the cavity. (b) TV view showing the IUS in the cervix and the upper frame adjacent to a fibroid clarifying the fibroid lies within the endometrial cavity. The extent of fibroid within the myometrium and hence the FIGO classification and suitability for fibroid resection cannot be ascertained from the TV image alone.

References

1. Fraser IS, Critchley HO, Broder M, Munro MG. The FIGO recommendations on terminologies and definitions for normal and abnormal uterine bleeding. *Semin Reprod Med.* 2011;29:383–390.

2. Heavy menstrual bleeding: assessment and management. *NICE Clinical Guideline.* 2007;CG 44, updated August 2016.

3. Problematic Bleeding with Hormonal Contraception. Clinical Effectiveness Unit. Faculty of Sexual and Reproductive Healthcare. July 2015.

4. Munro MG, Critchley HO, Broder MS, Fraser IS. FIGO classification system (PALM-COEIN) for causes of abnormal bleeding in non-gravid women of reproductive age. *Int J Gynaecol Obstet.* 2011;113:3–13.

5. Sakhel K, Abuhamad A J. Sonography of adenomyosis. *J Ultrasound Med.*2012;31:805–808.

6. Turnbull H, Glover A, Morris EP, Duncan TJ, Nieto JJ, Burbos N. Investigation and management of abnormal peri-menopausal bleeding. *Menopause International.*2013;19; 147–154.

7. Shankar M, Lee CA, Sabin CA, Economides DL, Kadir RA. Von Willebrand disease in women with menorrhagia: a systemic review. *BJOG.* 2004;111:734–740.

8. Guttinger A, Critchley HO. Endometrial effects of intrauterine levonorgestrel. *Contraception.* 2007;75(6 Suppl):S93–S98.

9. Pillai M, Shefras J. Experience with Instillagel® for hysterosonography and analgesia in a complex contraception clinic: a QIPP initiative. *J Fam Plann Reprod Health Care.* 2012;38:110–116.

10. Heavy menstrual bleeding. *NICE Quality Standard;* September 2013;QS47.

11. Gupta J, Kai J, Middleton L, Pattison H, Gray R, Daniels J. Levonorgestrel intrauterine system versus medical therapy for menorrhagia. *N Eng J Med.* 2013;368:128–137.

The Use of Ultrasound in the Perimenopausal Patient

Steven R. Goldstein

14.1 Introduction   218
14.2 Basic Histology   219
14.3 Clinical Use of Ultrasound in Perimenopausal
     Endometrium   220

14.4 Pitfalls and Pearls   222
14.5 Summary   223

14.1 Introduction

The term 'perimenopause' is somewhat confusing not only to patients, but also to some healthcare providers. Menopause is defined as the final menstrual period. The ovary is no longer capable of responding to follicle-stimulating hormone (FSH) produced from the pituitary. Thus, no ovarian oestrogen is produced and there is a depletion of ovarian follicles. This results in no epithelial stimulation of the uterus by oestradiol. How this manifests on ultrasound will be discussed in this chapter.

In 2012, a consensus conference known as 'STRAW + 10' defined reproductive aging in women and categorised 'perimenopause' as 'early' and 'late' menopausal transition.[1] The 'early' menopause transition is characterised by variable duration cycle length, which is variable and persistently greater than seven days difference in the length of consecutive cycles. FSH values are variable. Anti-Mullerian Hormone (AMH) will be low as will inhibin B. Antral follicle count on ultrasound will also be low.

In the 'late' menopausal transition, the interval of amenorrhea will be greater than or equal to 60 days. It may last one to two years. Follicle stimulating hormone will be elevated. AMH and inhibin B levels will be low. In addition, vasomotor symptoms (hot flashes, night sweats) are likely.

The clinical sequelae of the perimenopause are a phase characterised by oligo ovulation. The hallmark of ovulation is regular predictable cyclic menses. The hallmark of anovulation/oligo ovulation is irregular timing and length of uterine bleeding. As the follicular reserve becomes increasingly low, the regularity of ovulation may be lost and this is the most likely cause of irregular or chaotic bleeding among women of perimenopausal age.

Clinically, one should realise that a true menses is a uterine bleed preceded two weeks earlier by ovulation. Dysfunctional uterine bleeding, which to many patients is their 'period', results from erratic oestrogen production without ovulation, which can result in unpredictable bleeding. Such bleeding is associated with oligo or anovulation and is characterised by its irregular nature (can be heavy or light, with or without cramps, in longer or shorter intervals). The continued production of oestrogen without ovulation results in unopposed oestrogen stimulation of the endometrium. This increases the risk of development of endometrial hyperplasias and carcinoma. Endometrial cancer is the most common gynaecological malignancy in the Western world and endometrial hyperplasia is its precursor. The WHO classification of hyperplasia has been simplified into two types, with and without atypia.[2] Atypical endometrial hyperplasia has a high risk of progression to endometrial cancer.

Abnormal uterine bleeding in the perimenopausal women mandates evaluation to rule out endometrial hyperplasia and cancer.[3] Laboratory tests such as a full blood count, targeted screening for bleeding disorders, pregnancy, thyroid stimulating hormone and chlamydia nucleic acid testing should be considered. The ACOG Practice Bulletin goes on to recommend, 'When indicated, diagnostic or imaging tests can include transvaginal ultrasonography, saline infusion sonohysterography, and/or hysteroscopy, which would preferably be office based'.[3]

14.2 Basic Histology

The endometrium consists of the basalis and a functionalis. Oestrogen causes the functionalis to proliferate. Proliferative endometrium is characterised by abundant mitoses (Figure 14.1). In the late proliferative phase of a normal cycle, this will appear as a multilayered endometrial echo (Figure 14.2) with sonolucencies extending from the central midline echo to the basalis. Progesterone after ovulation (or progestogen in sequential hormone therapy) will convert an oestrogen-primed endometrial functionalis to a secretory phase (Figure 14.3). Sonographically, this will appear as an echogenic, homogeneous, thickened central midline echo (Figure 14.4). After shedding of the functionalis, the basal endometrium that remains is quite thin and appears as a thin echogenic line on transvaginal ultrasound (Figure 14.5). In the perimenopause, follicular reserve is low and this is often reflected in anovulation. The lack of progesterone over time, while there are still follicles and variable oestrogen production may result in hyperplasia. Hyperplasia is a histologial diagnosis and requires careful follow-up.[4]

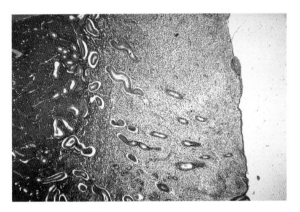

Figure 14.1 H and E staining of a hysterectomy specimen done in the proliferative phase, showing glands with abundant mitoses

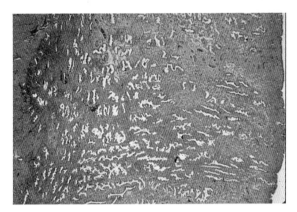

Figure 14.3 H and E stain from a hysterectomy specimen showing secretory endometrium, and glands lining in a linear fashion.

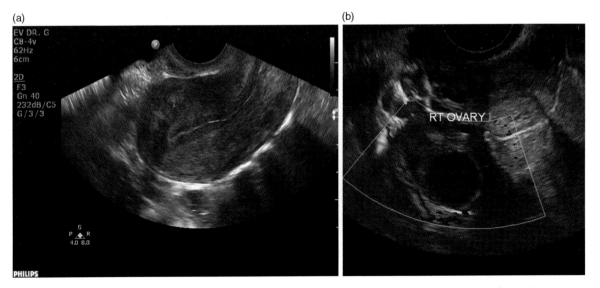

Figure 14.2 (a) Transvaginal ultrasonography showing a multilayered preovulatory endometrial echo in the late proliferative phase. (b) A grey scale view with colour Doppler of a dominant follicle in the right ovary of the patient whose endometrium is depicted in 2a.

219

(a)

(b)

(c)

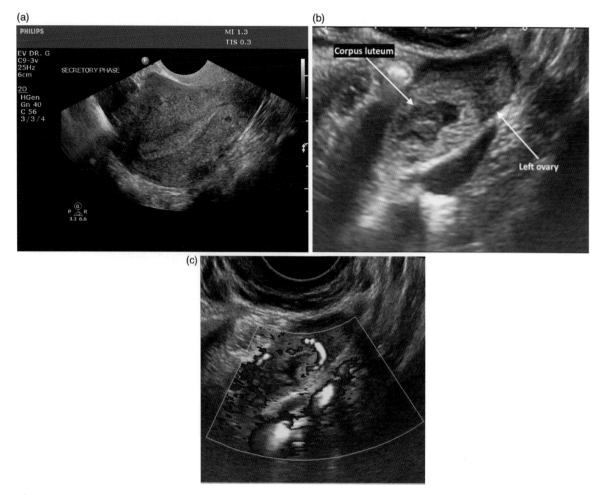

Figure 14.4 (a) Transvaginal ultrasonography showing an homogenous endometrial echo in the secretory phase. (b) A grey scale view of a corpus luteum in the left ovary. (c) Colour Doppler applied to the corpus luteum showing its peripheral vascularity within the ovary.

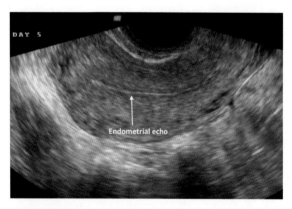

Figure 14.5 Transvaginal ultrasonography immediately post-menstrual displaying a thin distinct endometrial echo. This is the interface between two sides of basalis, now devoid of any functionalis.

14.3 Clinical Use of Ultrasound in Perimenopausal Endometrium

There is no 'normal' width of endometrial thickness in perimenopausal patients. The uterus grows with childbearing, and endometrial thickness will depend on hormonal status as well as uterine size. The proper use of the endometrial echo clinically relies on the high negative predictive value of a thin, distinct echo in patients with abnormal uterine bleeding, when the transvaginal ultrasound is performed just as the bleeding ends. This will prevent misinterpretation of heterogeneity that can result as the endometrium proliferates and thickens. These have been referred to as endometrial 'moguls' (Figure 14.6). Perimenopausal women with this finding have often had numerous uterine procedures (childbirth, curettage or uterine evacuation, caesarean sections, myomectomies), all of which can result in topographic irregularities to the surface of the endometrial cavity as tissue proliferates under the influence of oestrogen.

It is essential to realise that not all uteri lend themselves to a meaningful ultrasound examination. Certain factors such as an axial uterus, coexisting fibroids, previous uterine surgery, adenomyosis and marked obesity can all result in an inability to adequately visualise an endometrial echo (Figure 14.7). In such cases, saline infusion (or other contrast) sonohysterography will better delineate the endometrial cavity (See Chapter 5). This procedure involves the installation of sterile saline (or other negative contrast) into the uterine cavity through a sterile catheter or cannula under direct ultrasound visualisation. This has the effect of distending the cavity and allowing better visualisation of endometrial contents (Figures 14.8–14.11).

Thus, saline infusion (or other contrast) sonohysterography should be thought of as a subset of transvaginal ultrasound when the endometrial echo is not visualised adequately to exclude pathology or the endometrial echo is not sufficiently thin to exclude pathology.

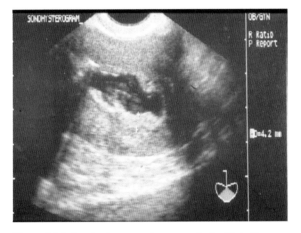

Figure 14.6 Sonohysterogram done on cycle day 17. As the endometrium proliferates, it is not always topographically homogenous and can produce these irregularities that have been characterised as 'moguls'.

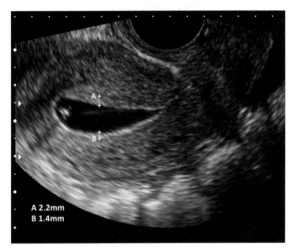

Figure 14.8 Sonohysterography in a perimenopausal patient showing no anatomic abnormality and thus diagnosing dysfunctional anovulatory bleeding.

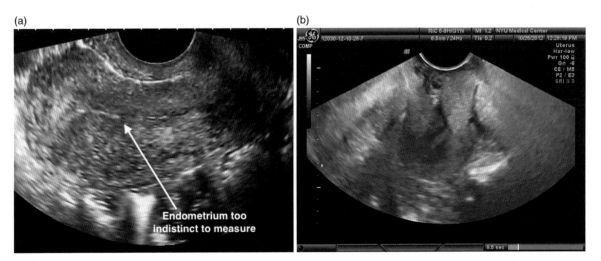

Figure 14.7 (a) Transvaginal ultrasonography in which the endometrial echo cannot be characterised secondary to adenomyosis. (b) Transvaginal ultrasound of an axial uterus in which the endometrial echo is too indistinct to be evaluated.

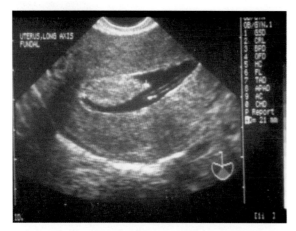

Figure 14.9 Sonohysterography in a perimenopausal patient showing an obvious 21 mm polyp. The rest of the cavity is thin indicative of early proliferative stage.

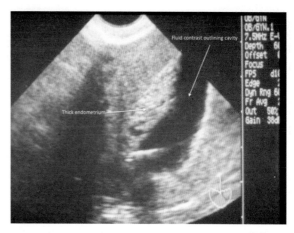

Figure 14.11 Sonohysterography in a perimenopausal patient displaying endometrial hyperplasia that occupied only the anterior wall while the posterior wall is thin. This underscores the fact that endometrial pathologies are often not global.

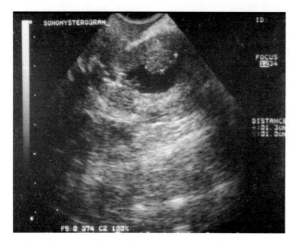

Figure 14.10 Sonohysterography in a perimenopausal patient reveals a 13 × 10 mm type 1 submucous myoma protruding about 75 per cent into the cavity. If this finding is associated with abnormal uterine bleeding, she would be an excellent candidate for hysteroscopic resection of this small fibroid.

In a large prospective trial of perimenopausal patients with abnormal uterine bleeding, 433 perimenopausal patients with menorrhagia, metrorrhagia or both were studied.[5] Of these, 280 had a thin, distinct endometrial echo ≤ 5 mm on day 4–6 of the cycle and no further workup was undertaken; 153 patients underwent saline infusion sonohysterography of which 44 (29 per cent) were for non-visualisation of the endometrial echo and 109 (71 per cent) were for an endometrial echo > 5 mm. Their results demonstrated dysfunctional anovulatory bleeding in 79 per cent of patients; 5.3 per cent had submucus myomas. Although 33 per cent had fibroid uteri, only 5.3 per cent had a submucous component; 13 per cent had endometrial polyps and 3.5 per cent of the cohort had hyperplasias. The advantage of this approach, utilising transvaginal ultrasound and then sonohysterography when necessary, allowed 65 per cent of the patients to be thoroughly evaluated with transvaginal ultrasound only; 17 per cent required sonohysterography for better visualisation; 2.3 per cent had global lesions and, thus, were candidates for blind endometrial sampling; 16 per cent underwent operative hysteroscopy but for proven endoluminal masses.

14.4 Pitfalls and Pearls

Any two-dimensional frozen ultrasound image is a 'snapshot.' Thus, a single long axis view of a seemingly normal endometrium does not rule out pathology (Figures 14.12a, b, c and d). The entire endometrial cavity must be observed and three-dimensional anatomy reconstructed in one's mind.

Contrast sonohysterography does not require any anesthesia or analgesia. Sometimes it will be difficult to distend the endometrial cavity. However, unlike hysteroscopy, even a small amount of fluid will allow diagnostic capability (Figure 14.13). The main purpose of sonohysterography is to ensure that the whole endometrial cavity has been evaluated and that any biopsy is appropriately representative. In most cases where perimenopausal bleeding is being investigated, endometrial biopsy will follow sonography, and where

(a)
(b)
(c)
(d)

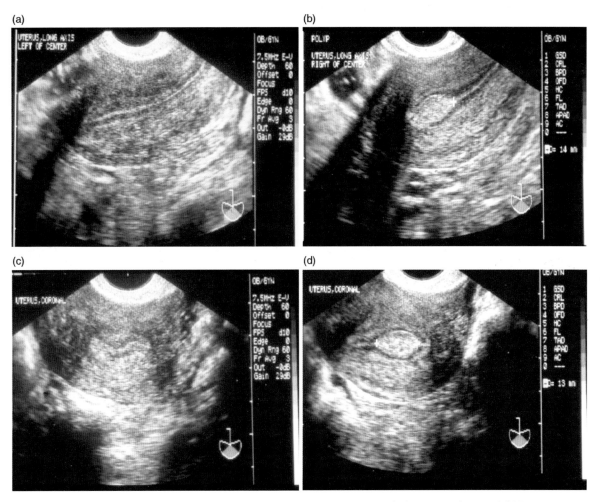

Figure 14.12 (a) Transvaginal ultrasound in a perimenopausal patient in a long axis view, which appears to be normal. (b) Same patient as 12A slightly to the right of midline displaying an obvious 14 mm polyp. (c) Transverse view of same patient in the lower uterine segment which appears normal. (d) Transverse view of the same patient at the fundal region clearly showing the polyp to the left of midline.

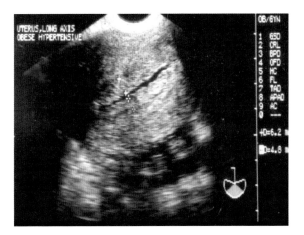

Figure 14.13 Sonohysterogram in an obese patient in which only a small ribbon of fluid was able to be infused. This still allowed adequate visualisation to see symmetrically thickened tissue that ultimately proved to be simple hyperplasia.

hyperplasia is confirmed histologically, further management is essential.[4]

Contrast sonohysterography should be avoided during heavy bleeding. Sometimes a clot of blood may appear to be polypoid-like in the endometrial cavity. Clinicians should consider an empiric course of a progestogen as a 'medical curettage' to thoroughly evacuate the uterine contents and then perform a transvaginal ultrasound examination at the end of the withdrawal bleed, when the endometrium will be thinnest.

14.5 Summary

In summary, understanding the hormonal fluctuations of the perimenopause and the effect on the endometrial histology is paramount to successful clinical evaluation. Transvaginal ultrasound and sonohysterography, when indicated, are excellent tools for excluding organic pathologies such as polyps, myomas, hyperplasias and even carcinoma from the majority of patients. They will distinguish pathology from dysfunctional anovulatory bleeding which may be treated expectantly or hormonally, avoiding surgical intervention.

References

1. Harlow SD, Gass M, Hall JE, Lobo R, Maki P, Rebar RW et al. STRAW + 10 Collaborative Group. Executive summary of the Stages of Reproductive Aging Workshop + 10: addressing the unfinished agenda of staging reproductive aging. *Climacteric.* 2012;15(2):105–114.

2. Kurman RJ, Carcangiu ML, Herrington CS, Young RH, eds. *WHO Classification of Tumours of Female Reproductive Organs.* 4th ed. [Lyon]: IARC, 2014.

3. American College of Obstetricians and Gynecologists. Practice Bulletin no.128: Diagnosis of abnormal uterine bleeding in reproductive age women. *Obstet Gynecol.* 2012;120(1):197–206.

4. Endometrial Hyperplasia, Management of (Green-top Guideline No. 67) RCOG/BSGE Joint Guideline/February 2016.

5. Goldstein SR, Zeltser I, Horan CK, Snyder JR, Schwartz LB. Ultrasonography-based triage for perimenopausal patients with abnormal uterine bleeding. *Am J Obstet Gynecol.* 1997;177(1):102–108.

Chapter 15

Recognition of Possible Gynaecological Cancer

Kathryn Hillaby

15.1 Background   225
15.2 Endometrial Pathology   225
15.3 Myometrial Pathology   227
15.4 Ovarian Pathology   227
15.5 International Ovarian Tumour Analysis (IOTA)   228

15.6 Borderline Ovarian Tumours   228
15.7 Invasive Epithelial Ovarian Malignances   229
15.8 Non-epithelial Ovarian Malignancies   231
15.9 Fallopian Tube Pathology   232
15.10 Non-gynaecological Pathology   233

15.1 Background

Ultrasound scanning is a key investigation in the detection of gynaecological malignancy. A significant number of gynaecological malignancies are not diagnosed through the two-week wait urgent cancer pathways, but instead are found during investigations for other symptoms.

The majority of gynaecological cancers affect women outside of reproductive age. However, the number of women being diagnosed with endometrial cancer at an earlier age is increasing, due to obesity.

Ultrasound has a key role to play in the diagnosis of endometrial cancer and ovarian cancer, but has no role in the diagnosis of vulval carcinoma, unless an obvious lesion is noted on introduction of the transvaginal probe, and has a very limited role in the diagnosis of the majority of cervical cancers.

It is always important to make a full assessment of the pelvis, as occasionally other abnormal findings may lead to an early diagnosis of a non-gynaecological malignancy.

15.2 Endometrial Pathology

When assessing the endometrium, it is important that the endometrial thickness is measured at its widest part perpendicular to the endometrium, and care should be taken that the whole of the endometrial echo can be visualised when the measurement is taken (see Chapter 4, Figure 4.20d).

Sometimes fluid may be found within the endometrial cavity, and when measuring the endometrial thickness in such women, the thickness from the outer aspects of the endometrium should be measured, as well as the fluid, and the fluid measurement then subtracted from the endometrial thickness measurement. Alternatively, two single thicknesses (excluding the fluid) are measured and added together (Figure 4.27).

In most benign conditions, except adenomyosis, there should be a clear interface between the endometrium and myometrium. In malignancy this may be blurred, and on ultrasound scanning it may be possible to see the tumour invading into the myometrium. A disrupted endo-myometrial border is strongly associated with an endometrial malignancy in retrospective studies.[1] Failure to visualise a clear endometrial–myometrial margin precludes measurement and should be regarded as an abnormality requiring further investigation.

In a post-menopausal woman with bleeding, a cut off of 4 mm is used for endometrial thickness, above which an endometrial biopsy is mandated to exclude an endometrial malignancy. In a post-menopausal woman who is not bleeding, the upper limit for normal endometrial thickness is 8.8 mm (Map of Medicine), above which endometrial sampling must be undertaken. In women taking Tamoxifen, the same cut offs are used, but hysteroscopic assessment of the endometrium must be undertaken as opposed to blind endometrial biopsy with just a Pipelle, as these women are subject to a higher rate of endometrial malignancies and endometrial polyps than the general population (Figure 15.1).

(a)

(b)

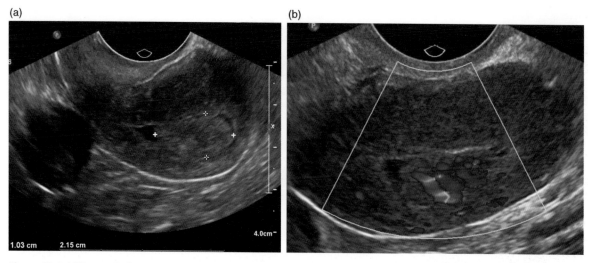

Figure 15.1 (a) Transvaginal scan in a woman taking Tamoxifen, demonstrating a small amount of fluid outlining a polypoid lesion measuring 10.3 mm × 21.5 mm. (b) Colour flow demonstrating multiple vessels feeding the lesion, consistent with a high likelihood of malignancy.

(a)

(b)

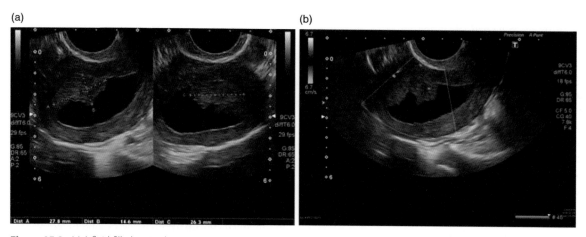

Figure 15.2 (a) A fluid-filled cavity demonstrating an irregular endometrial lesion with loss of the endo-myometrial margin. (b) Colour Doppler demonstrating multiple vessels within the lesion.

In pre-menopausal women, abnormal endometrial thickness is more difficult to judge, and a note should be made as to where in her menstrual cycle the patient is, with the endometrium typically measuring < 4 mm immediately after cessation of menstruation, 5–7 mm in the early proliferative phase (day 6–14), up to 11 mm in the late proliferative – preovulatory phase, and up to 16 mm in the secretory phase (day 15–28). Depending on their age and risk factors, women with endometrial thicknesses greater than these measurements at the appropriate phase in their cycle should be referred for endometrial sampling, ideally with hysteroscopy or sonohysteroscopy,

to exclude an endometrial malignancy. Endometrial cancer is still rare in pre-menopausal women, but is becoming increasingly common with rising rates of obesity, and 4 per cent of cases of endometrial cancer are diagnosed in women < 40 years of age.[2]

Case 1: A 69-year-old who presented with post-menopausal bleeding. Pelvic ultrasound investigation showed a fluid-filled endometrial cavity with an irregular endometrial lesion (Figure 15.2).

Hysteroscopy and biopsy confirmed endometrial cancer. In this case, spontaneous fluid in the cavity enhanced the images of the lesion. In other

(a)   (b)

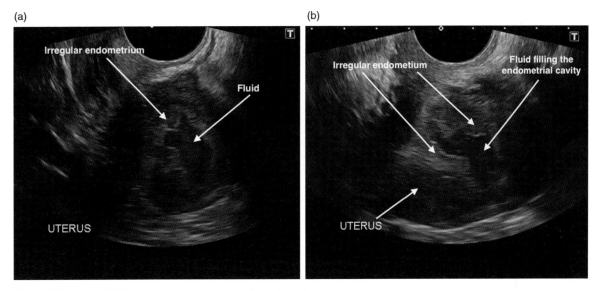

Figure 15.3 (a and b) Gel infusion demonstrating irregular endometrium.

circumstances gel infusion sonography, where gel (typically containing local anaesthetic) is infused into the endometrial cavity, allows the best morphological assessment of the endometrium (Chapter 5), but is not always possible. It is especially useful in pre-menopausal women to diagnose the presence of endometrial polyps. Endometrial polyps are most commonly benign; the use of Doppler ultrasound is also useful in differentiating benign from malignant polyps. Benign polyps typically have a single feeding blood vessel, whereas malignant polyps/endometrial pathology typically can be seen to have multiple feeding vessels and demonstrate Doppler flow patterns suggestive of low resistance, but high flow (Figure 15.1b). Gel infusion sonography demonstrating an irregular endometrium should also prompt biopsy, as this finding is strongly associated with malignancy[1] (Figure 15.3 a, b).

15.3 Myometrial Pathology

Uterine sarcomas are uncommon tumours, and are notoriously difficult to diagnose using imaging pre-operatively. They typically appear as solid masses within the myometrium, of a similar echogenicity as fibroids, but with evidence of degeneration and are difficult to differentiate from benign degenerating fibroids. Features cited as suggestive of a sarcomatous lesion include a clinical history of a rapidly increasing size pelvic mass, weight loss and pyrexia of unknown

origin; however, retrospective studies have shown that even women with this clear history have an incidence of sarcoma of <1 per cent when hysterectomy is undertaken.[3] Large fibroid masses with a cystic central area, or other features suggestive of degeneration along with a history of abdominal pain, or a rapidly increasing size pelvic mass, should prompt referral under the 2WW criteria to a gynaecologist, and further imaging with MRI or CT should be undertaken prior to any surgery.

15.4 Ovarian Pathology

A full inspection of both ovaries should always be made when undertaking imaging of the pelvis. The ovaries should be scanned in their entirety in two planes, and measurements taken in three planes of each ovary. Any ovarian pathology should be measured again in three planes, and described in accordance with the IOTA (International Ovarian Tumour Analysis) protocol.[4]

Case 2: This 77-year-old lady presented with abdominal pain. Ultrasound findings demonstrated a complex solid/cystic ovarian tumour with thick, irregular septae (arrows) (Figure 15.4).

The final histology was a high-grade serous ovarian cancer.

Ovarian cysts are frequently encountered and cause considerable anxiety in both the patient and

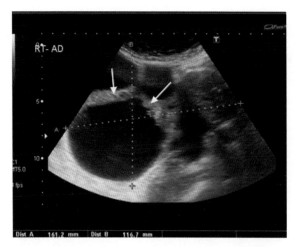

Figure 15.4 A complex solid/cystic ovarian tumour with thick, irregular septae (arrows).

the investigator, with 6.6 per cent of pre-menopausal women having a functional ovarian cyst at any point in time,[5] the majority of which will resolve spontaneously within two cycles.[6] Increasing complexity of an ovarian cyst is associated with an increased suspicion of ovarian malignancy, and the aim of any investigation is to allow accurate discrimination between benign and malignant lesions, to allow rapid reassurance of the majority of women, with expeditious referral for further investigation and treatment in those women whose cysts have features suggestive of an ovarian malignancy.

15.5 International Ovarian Tumour Analysis (IOTA)

A lack of standardisation in the characterisation and descriptions of ovarian lesions led a multinational group of gynaecologists to propose standard definitions of tumours. These have been widely adopted and allow all clinicians to clearly understand what is meant when ultrasound findings are reported, as well as allowing accurate discrimination between benign and malignant ovarian tumours (see Chapter 6). The importance of preoperative characterisation plays a key role in the timing and type of surgery and whether surgery is performed by a specialist gynaecological oncologist, a benign gynaecological surgeon or a general surgeon. Correct preoperative assessment correlates strongly with survival times.

An adnexal *lesion* is defined as part of the ovary or adnexal mass that is not consistent with normal

physiological findings.[4] The lesion should then be further described as unilocular, with or without a solid component, or papillary proliferation, multilocular, with or without a solid component, or papillary proliferation, or solid (where ≥ 80 per cent of the tumour is solid).[7] The assessor should then also judge if the lesion has a smooth inner wall, or an irregular inner wall (Chapter 6 and Figures 6.26–6.33).

A more detailed assessment of the morphology of the tumour should be undertaken, focusing on the characteristics listed in Chapter 6, p. 108, including whether the tumour contains a septum, or an incomplete septum (Figure 15.5a). A measurement perpendicular to the long axis of the septum allows description of whether this is thin, or thick, and regular, or irregular.

An assessment of any papillary proliferation or solid areas should also be undertaken (a papillary proliferation being defined as any solid area arising from the inner surface of the ovarian tumour and measuring > 3 mm) (Figure 15.5b). Finally, an assessment of the vascularity of the tumour should be made, recording the PI (pulsatility index), RI (resistance index), PSV (peak systolic velocity) and TAMXV (Time-averaged maximum end-diastolic velocity). At the time of writing the ADNEX model does not include these objective Doppler indices but a subjective visual colour assessment (score 1–4). It is important to understand the use of Pulsed Repetition Frequency (PRF) which can drastically alter the appearance of flow (Chapter 2, p 24).

Multiple studies were undertaken using this standard set of descriptions of ovarian tumours and two models proposed to discriminate benign from malignant ovarian tumours that performed almost as well as that of pattern recognition by an expert.[8] The IOTA classification system (Figure 15.6) was based on outcome data for 1,066 cases by ultrasound morphologic classification showed the risk of malignancy was 0.6 per cent for a unilocular cyst, 10 per cent for a multilocular cyst, 33 per cent for a unilocular solid cyst, 41 per cent for a multilocular solid tumour and 62 per cent for a solid tumour.[9]

15.6 Borderline Ovarian Tumours

These are an intermediate group between benign and invasive malignant tumours, and are also referred to as tumours of low malignant potential. They are predominantly of mucinous and serous type, and on ultrasound are found to have some quite characteristic features.

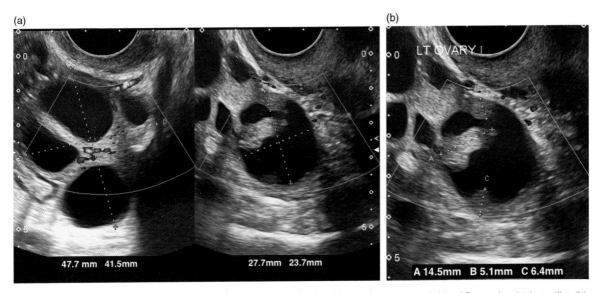

Figure 15.5 (a) A multilocular solid ovarian mass demonstrating multiple thick complete septae with blood flow and multiple papillae. (b) Same lesion demonstrating multiple papillae. Despite the presence of 'M' features (> 4 papillae), the histology was ultimately benign.

The majority of borderline mucinous tumours are multilocular in nature, with a smooth outer surface (Figure 15.7). They can be large, typically larger than borderline serous tumours, and 25–50 per cent of these tumours have papillary proliferations on their internal surfaces.[10] This group are divided into gastrointestinal type, which is the commonest, and these have a distinctive ultrasound appearance with the presence of a 'honeycomb' within the tumour.[11]

These are rarely bilateral (< 5 per cent), but the less common type of endocervical borderline mucinous tumours are more commonly (40 per cent) bilateral. If spread occurs from these types of tumours it may present as pseudomxyoma peritoneii, which is a thick, gelatinous type of ascites. On ultrasound this appears as free fluid in the pelvis, and abdomen, that typically has low-level echogenicity, as opposed to being anechoic, or blood stained, which most ascites is.

Borderline serous tumours (Figure 15.8) are more common than borderline mucinous tumours, and account for approximately 15 per cent of epithelial cancers. They are more frequently bilateral, and the majority contain papillary proliferations.

Borderline tumours tend to occur in younger women and are often diagnosed incidentally on ultrasound imaging of the pelvis, often in pregnancy. Any woman found to have such a tumour should be referred on for further investigation by a cancer lead, or gynaecological oncologist. CA125 should be measured, although it is frequently not elevated in borderline tumours. Accurate diagnosis is key, as these tumours have a good prognosis, with a 95 per cent 10-year survival rate. Fertility sparing surgery can be used in most cases where future pregnancy may be desired.

15.7 Invasive Epithelial Ovarian Malignancies

Ovarian malignancies affect 1 in 50 women in their lifetime. They are, however, notoriously difficult to diagnose at an early stage, with the majority presenting at FIGO stage 3 (indicating spread within the peritoneal cavity), and earning them the unfortunate label of 'the silent killer'. Ultrasonographically they have quite distinct features. Characteristically they have complex architecture, and are usually multilocular with solid areas and papillary proliferations (Figure 15.9).

They are frequently bilateral, and ascites may be present, along with tumour deposits at other sites within the pelvis and abdomen, and the tumours may be fixed to the uterus, pelvic sidewall, or rectum, suggesting direct invasion. Doppler blood flow patterns are those of neovascularisation, with high flow and vessels with low resistivity (low Resistance index RI) (Figure 15.10).

Owing to the importance of detecting these tumours at an early stage and accurately identifying

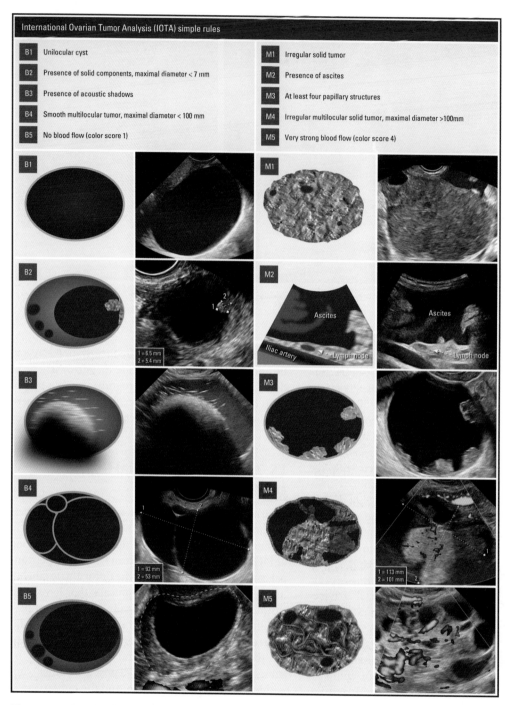

Figure 15.6 IOTA classification (reproduced with permission of the IOTA group; www.iotagroup.org/uploads/images/educational_material/
EN_TableOfLesionsIOTA_12APR2015.jpg.)

(a)

(b)

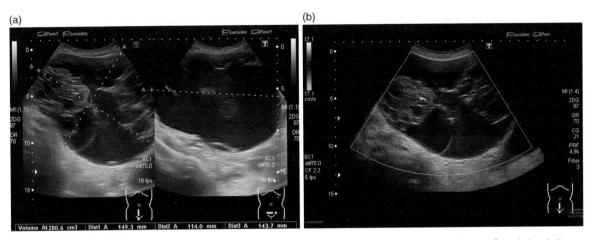

Figure 15.7 Multilocular 15 × 11.5 × 14 cm mass with thick mucus and a solid peripheral component. Histology confirmed a borderline mucinous tumor, FIGO stage 1a.

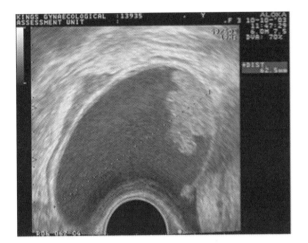

Figure 15.8 Borderline serous ovarian tumour (unilocular with large papillary proliferation).

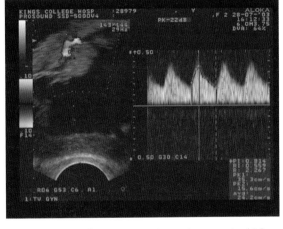

Figure 15.10 Papillary ovarian carcinoma demonstrating high flow with low resistance.

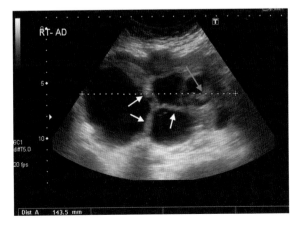

Figure 15.9 Serous papillary ovarian carcinoma, demonstrating a multilocular solid and cystic tumour, with thick septae (white arrows) and papillary proliferations (blue arrow).

these as malignant as opposed to benign, to allow the most appropriate surgery to be undertaken, a large body of work has been undertaken to improve pre-operative discrimination. Multiple logistic regression, and neural network models have been proposed, incorporating morphological features, Doppler indices and serum tumour marker results; however, to date the best discrimination has been demonstrated by pattern recognition.[12]

15.8 Non-epithelial Ovarian Malignancies

These are rarer than epithelial ovarian tumours, but are most commonly found in the younger population, and are broadly divided into tumours of sex cord and stromal origin, and those of germ cell origin.

Granulosa cell tumours are the commonest, and also typically behave in a similar fashion to that of low malignant potential ovarian tumours. On ultrasound these appear as solid lesions, sometimes with a central cystic area, related to necrosis or haemorrhage. They are rarely bilateral (1–2 per cent), and tend to be well vascularised on Doppler examination. They frequently secrete oestrogen, and so these women may present with irregular vaginal bleeding, or post-menopausal bleeding due to endometrial hyperplasia, which is associated with adenocarcinoma of the endometrium in 5 per cent of cases.

Theca cell tumours and Sertoli-Leydig tumours are much less common, and difficult to diagnose ultra-sonographicaly. Theca cell tumours are morphologically identical to granulosa cell tumours (predominantly solid, and unilateral). Sertoli Leydig are small and solid, but do demonstrate an extremely high blood supply.

Dysgerminomas are most commonly found in adolescence or early adulthood; they appear as solid tumours. Ten–fifteen per cent of germ cell tumours are bilateral, and tend to grow rapidly.

Teratomas are among the most common ovarian tumours, > 95 per cent are mature, and as such benign (Dermoid cysts – Chapter 6). Very occasionally these can be composed of immature material. These typically present between the ages of 10 and 20 years, and behave in an aggressive fashion, implanting on to the peritoneum within the pelvis, metastasising to pelvic and para-aortic lymph nodes, and to the liver and lungs.

Six percent of ovarian tumours are metastases from a distant primary, most commonly from the uterus, breast or gastro-intestinal tract. These are usually bilateral, solid and demonstrate increased vascularity on Doppler studies.

Case 3: A 63-year-old presented with a 6-month history of abdominal discomfort, and more recently had noticed a mass in her abdomen as well as urinary frequency. Abdominal ultrasound demonstrated extensive ascites (Figure 15.11).

Following referral to gynae oncology, she had image-guided omental biopsy and was treated with neoadjuvant chemotherapy and then surgery.

Case 4: A 48-year-old presented with acute urinary retention. She had a history of menorrhagia, and

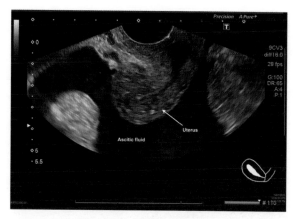

Figure 15.11 Malignant ascites. Extensive free fluid in the pelvis outlines the uterus. Cytology was consistent with a high-grade serous carcinoma of ovarian, tubal or peritoneal origin.

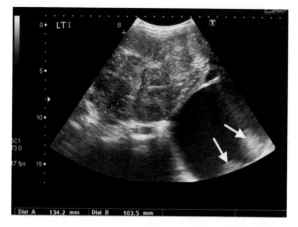

Figure 15.12 A transabdominal longitudinal view to the left of the midline shows a solid mass measuring 134 mm by 103 mm lying anteriorly and the cystic mass with solid areas (arrows) more posteriorly.

Hb=87g/l. Once catheterised, she was noted to have a pelvic mass (Figures 15.12 and 15.13).

15.9 Fallopian Tube Pathology

A large number of what were previously thought to be ovarian malignancies are now being recognised as being of primary fallopian tube origin. These are usually high-grade serous malignancies. Unfortunately, these are usually asymptomatic until they have spread, and the primary lesions are often microscopic, so ultrasound diagnosis of these at an early stage is incredibly difficult. Any solid or cystic mass adjacent to an ovary should be fully characterised. Features suggestive of malignancy would be a thickened wall,

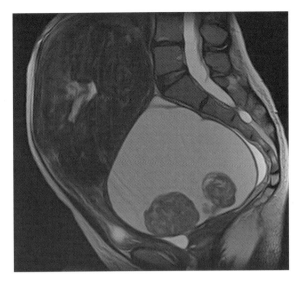

Figure 15.13 MRI of the same patient. Underwent TAH BSO, omentectomy, appendicectomy, pelvic and para-aortic lymph node sampling. Final histology revealed a grade 3 stage 1a clear cell ovarian cancer, as well as a grade 1 stage 1a endometrial cancer. She went on to have further treatment with chemotherapy.

papillary proliferations or other solid areas within the mass, as well as Doppler indices suggestive of neovascularisation. Ascites is often present at diagnosis. Any of these features should mandate urgent referral for further investigation, as well as serum biochemistry for CA125, which is usually elevated in such lesions.

15.10 Non-gynaecological Pathology

If transabdominal scanning is undertaken, a full bladder is used as an acoustic window through which to view the pelvic organs, and a note of any abnormal features within the bladder should be made. These are rare; however, a polypoid mass should prompt urgent referral to a urologist for further imaging, or direct imaging with cystoscopy.

Transvaginal scanning should ideally be undertaken with an empty bladder; however often there is urine within the bladder allowing the internal bladder wall to be studied, and again, any abnormal masses within the bladder should warrant rapid referral for further investigation.

Ascites not associated with ovarian tumours should lead to further investigations as to the cause. A careful clinical history should be taken looking for hepatic-related causes, or symptoms of other malignancies such as pancreatic cancer that may also present with ascites. A small volume of free fluid is more typically associated with inflammation or infection.

References

1. Dueholm M, Møller C, Rydberg S, Hansen ES, Ørtoft G. An ultrasound algorithm for identification of endometrial cancer. *Ultrasound Obstet Gynecol.* 2014;43: 557–568.

2. Duska LR, Garrett A, Rueda BR, Haas J, Chang Y, Fuller AF. Endometrial cancer in women 40 years old or younger. *Gynecol. Oncol.* 2001;83(2):388–393.

3. Parker WH, Fu YS, Berek JS. Uterine sarcoma in patients operated on for presumed Leiomyoma and rapidly growing Leiomyoma. *Obstet Gynaecol.* 1994;8(3):414–418.

4. Timmerman D, Valentin L, Bourne TH, Collins WP, Verrelst H, Vergote I. Terms, definitions and measurements to describe the sonographic features of adnexal tumours: a consensus opinion from the International Ovarian Tumour Analysis (IOTA) group. *Ultrasound Obstet Gynecol.* 2000;16:500–505.

5. Borgfeldt C, Andolf E. Transvaginal sonographic ovarian findings in a random sample of 25–40 years old. *Ultrasound Obstet Gynecol.* 1999;13:345–350.

6. MacKenna A, Fabres C, Alam V, Morales V. Clinical management of functional ovarian cysts: a prospective and randomized study. *Human Reprod.* 2000;15:2567–2569.

7. IOTAgroup.org eductational material (2016).

8. Kaijser J, Bourne T, Valentin L, Sayasneh A, Van Holsbeke C, Vergote I, Testa AC, Franchi A, Van Calster B, Timmerman D. Improving strategies for diagnosing ovarian cancer: a summary of the International Ovarian Tumor Analysis (IOTA) studies. *Ultrasound Obstet Gynecol.*2013;41:9–20.

9. Timmerman D, Testa AC, Bourne T, Ferrazzi E, Ameye L, Konstantinovic ML, Van Calster B, Collins WP, Vergote I, Van Huffel S, Valentin L. Logistic regression model to distinguish between the benign and malignant adnexal mass before surgery: a multicenter study by the International Ovarian Tumor Analysis Group. *J Clin Oncol.*2005;23:8794–8801.

10. Exacoustos C, Romanini ME, Rinaldo D, Amoroso C, Szabolcs B, Zupi E, Arduini D. Preoperative sonographic features of borderline ovarian tumours. *Ultrasound Obstet Gynecol.* 2005;25:50–59.

11. Yazbeck J, Raju KS, Ben-Nagi J, Holland T, Hillaby K, Jurkovic D. Accuracy of ultrasound subjective 'pattern recognition' for the diagnosis of borderline ovarian tumours. *Ultrasound Obstet Gynecol.*2007;29:489–495.

12. Valentin L, Hagen B, Tingulstad S, Eik-Nes S. Comparison of 'Pattern recognition' and logistic regression models for discrimination between benign and malignant pelvic masses: a prospective cross validation. *Ultrasound Obstet Gynecol.*2001;18:357–365.

Chapter

16

Quality in SRH Ultrasound Service Provision

Julie-Michelle Bridson

16.1 Context 234

16.2 A Quality Service? 234

16.1 Context

Those clinicians undertaking ultrasound examinations in SRH will often be working in a community setting, remote from the traditional radiology-based ultrasound service. However, the same principles of governance and quality standards must also apply in SRH, to safeguard patients and to ensure a high quality, monitored service. There are many organisations to which SRH practitioners can look for publications on standards of ultrasound practice, and clinicians are encouraged to visit the websites of the British Medical Ultrasound Society, the Society of Radiographers, the Royal College of Radiologists and the Royal College of Obstetrics and Gynaecology. These organisations are the leaders in the field of ultrasound imaging and professional quality standards. The principles from their documents can easily be exported and applied to SRH applications to promote best practice.[1–4]

Ultrasound service providers are encouraged to seek advice from the Imaging Services Accreditation Scheme (ISAS).[2] This accredits high-quality ultrasound services offered within a robust and compliant framework, using a quality metric, the principles of which could be applied again to SRH applications.

In addition, it is a legal requirement that all providers of diagnostic services, as is the case with SRH examinations, are registered with the Care Quality Commission (CQC).[5]

16.2 A Quality Service?

There are many factors that influence the setup, delivery and monitoring of a quality diagnostic service. As a minimum, this should include governance initiatives for all aspects of the ultrasound service.

16.2.1 Training and Updating

1. The operator must be 'appropriately trained' as evidenced by a robust competence evaluation in accordance with guidance set out by a recognised professional body/higher education qualification. However, the definition of what constitutes 'proper training' in ultrasound is difficult to define. In SRH service provision, ultrasound examinations are performed within a clinical consultation and the scan outcome is used to inform clinical decision making and patient management. This is different from the traditional role of a sonographer or radiologist who may be performing scans in a more isolated dedicated image department.

    Traditionally, a logbook has been used to record ultrasound experience in SRH. However, a logbook in isolation does not provide any evidence of competence, rather it is a record of clinical experience.[6] Assessment of competence in ultrasound is complex, but typically utilises work-based assessment using a robust and validated competence tool.[7] Many examples of these can be found in Higher Education Institutions which run accredited ultrasound training programmes.[8]

2. All those performing ultrasound in an SRH setting should have a mentor, a clinician with appropriate qualifications and expertise who can offer help, support and give guidance on individual cases or on the service provision. This is essential for new ultrasound users, who should undergo a period of preceptorship (3–6 months) once deemed first post 'competent'.

3. All operators performing ultrasound examinations should have firmly established roles

and boundaries, which clearly reflect their own personal competence and capability. Applications undertaken in SRH can be considered to be 'focused ultrasound' for which standards are set down in *Focused Ultrasound Training Standards* published by the Royal College of Radiologists.[4]

Here, levels of ultrasound training are defined (levels 1–3), and these provide useful advice on training, roles and boundaries, which can be applied to SRH.

4. The ultrasound evidence base changes quite rapidly, not least in the areas of reproductive medicine. Therefore, the operator has a professional responsibility to ensure that their ultrasound practice (knowledge and skills) remains up to date and is evidence based. The clinician's practice and governance framework should evolve dynamically as the evidence base evolves and with increasing experience. Maintenance of CPD activity, evidenced through the professional portfolio, is essential.

5. Those working in ultrasound services for SRH will normally be doctors and nurses who are registered with the General Medical Council and the Nursing and Midwifery Council respectively. There are a small number of ultrasound operators who do not have a base qualification allowing entry to a statutory register. Those personnel should be aware that there is a managed voluntary register to which they can apply.[8] This is to be encouraged.

6. Critical reflection on one's own practice is an important skill to engender in all healthcare staff. In this context, all ultrasound practitioners must be able to recognise their self-limitations, particularly when to refer a patient on to a more expert-imaging practitioner. A typical example in SRH is where a complex adnexal cyst is found at a dating scan in a pregnancy advisory clinic. Appropriate processes need to be in place to ensure timely further referral. In general, this will be either a referral to non-urgent gynaecology or a referral to the gynaecology two-week waiting list, if a malignancy is suspected. The main challenge for the SRH clinician is ensuring that the patient is assigned correctly to either a 'benign' gynaecologist or the two-week wait service.[10]

7. Those working in SRH ultrasound services must also understand the merits and limitations of ultrasound imaging in their practice, particularly the diagnostic limitations. SRH clinicians need to have a wider contextual knowledge and understanding of the role of other interventions such as blood tests, MRI and CT scanning which may be required once the patient has been referred for specialist gynaecological assessment.[2,3,10]

8. The SRH service should have a clearly defined leader who assumes overall responsibility for the quality and efficacy of the ultrasound service provision within the wider context of the SRH services. This should include, for example, robust and effective organisational and operational frameworks, audit of performance/outcome and triggers for adverse event reporting. The designated lead should offer a peer review process for their colleagues, negotiated through their job plan, with time specifically allocated.[2,3]

16.2.2 Ultrasound Systems and Image Archiving: 'Fitness for Purpose'

Purchase of ultrasound equipment, which is 'fit for purpose' and is suited to the clinical task, is essential for optimum diagnostics/interventions.

16.2.2.1 Choosing an Ultrasound System

When you find yourself 'in the market' for purchasing/leasing an ultrasound system, it is essential that you obtain one which is 'fit for purpose' for SRH applications. Many systems are marketed for particular applications such as obstetrics, gynaecology, general medicine and so on.

First, you should draw up a specification that defines the scope of clinical practice that the system is to be used for. In SRH, you will be undertaking transabdominal and transvaginal ultrasound scanning; but will you be offering an implant service? Latter will require an additional superficial linear array transducer. It is also appropriate to consider that all services are experiencing increasing numbers of patients with elevated BMIs and so the ability of a machine to achieve good quality images across a wide range of BMIs is important.

You will no doubt have a budget allocated and after defining the scope of the service to be provided and the available monies, you should draw up a technical specification. It is worth seeking advice from colleagues in dedicated imaging departments at this stage. Research the systems available on the market that meet your criteria and invite the company to demonstrate the equipment. You must also use and evaluate the equipment in your own clinical setting, considering factors such as image quality and ease of use. After all, you would not buy a car without road-testing!

These basic, simple steps will enhance your diagnostic capability and confidence. Further detail of standards for the commissioning and replacement of ultrasound equipment are clearly set out in the document *Standards for the Provision of an Ultrasound Service*.[2]

16.2.2.2 'Adopting' Ultrasound Equipment

It is often the case that equipment that is no longer of use in one department is offered to another service provider. While this might seem an efficient way to obtain ultrasound equipment within the financial constraints of the NHS, it is not necessarily in the best interests of the patients. In fact, use of an 'acquired' piece of ultrasound equipment may give rise to sub-quality images, which can adversely affect patient outcomes. Ultrasound equipment is typically produced with specific applications in mind, and both the software and hardware are usually tailored beyond a generic specification to specifics such as SRH. If 'adopting' ultrasound equipment, then it must meet the specification that you would set down for your dedicated service if you were commissioning from new and must have the requisite service history and contracts normally required.

16.2.2.3 Transducers for SRH

Ultrasound systems suitable for SRH female pelvic scanning will require a curved linear transducer for transabdominal scanning and a transvaginal probe for intracavity imaging. For those offering a deep subdermal implant service, a high frequency linear transducer for implant location and removal will be required (Figure 16.1).

16.2.2.4 Image Archiving and Reporting in SRH

Some portable scanners are difficult to link to PACS systems and in fact PACS is often not an option readily available to those performing ultrasound examinations in an SRH setting. However, it should be noted that all ultrasound images should be archived and be available for future review and should be linked to the image report through an Image Management System (IMS). However, this remains a challenge to

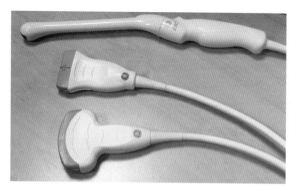

Figure 16.1 Photograph showing transvaginal probe (E8C), linear array (12L) and curved array (3C) transducers.

SRH clinicians due to a lack of both PACS and IMS in this specific clinical setting. Images tend to be stored as thermal prints, which have poor diagnostic quality and longevity (Figures 16.2a, b).[1-3] This is clearly disadvantageous when image review is required, for example, in audit and litigation. SRH service providers should evolve a strategy for satisfactory image recording.

16.2.3 The Scanning Environment

Ultrasound examinations in SRH are usually performed in a clinical room, set up for consultation including history taking and examination, with the availability of an ultrasound system as an adjunct tool. Consequently, the scanning environment may not be optimum. For example, there may be no air conditioning, a lack of ambient lighting and suitable ergonomic environment to limit work-related musculo-skeletal disorders. However, where possible, the ideal standards (as expected in a dedicated ultrasound service) should be fulfilled. Yet, there are significant benefits to the patient of scanning in a clinical setting, in general, which outweigh the possible disadvantages; notably to provide a 'one stop' patient service, holistic and expedited care.

There are some general principles that should be considered when setting up or reviewing a SRH service.[1-3]

1. The examination room size should be large enough to accommodate the facilities for the clinical consultation, physical examination/ interventions and the ultrasound equipment. There should be sufficient space to safely allow movement of staff, patients and attendants around

(a)

(b)

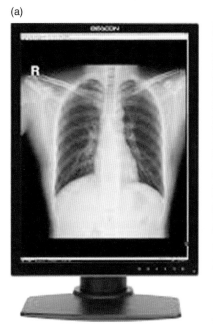
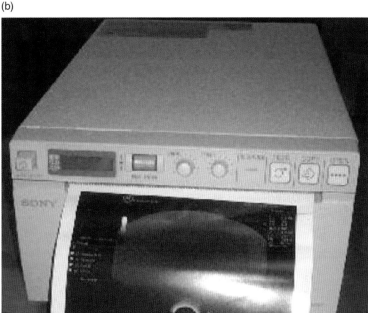

Figure 16.2 (a) PACS monitor; (b) thermal printer with print.

the room, ensuring no trip hazards (for example, transducer cables) and safe access to areas such as private changing, examination couch and so on.

2. There have been reports of work-related musculo-skeletal injury disorders (WRMSD) in staff repeatedly performing ultrasound examinations. The ergonomic set-up including seating, the console, foot-rest, display monitor and transducer must be considered as well as workload issues, scanning technique and posture. There are detailed publications on this subject which can be used to inform practice.[11] It is essential that SRH ultrasound operators familiarise themselves with this literature.

3. Patient privacy and dignity should be considered when locating the position of examination couch and curtains and so on relative to room entrances.

4. Ultrasound systems generate heat and without air conditioning, room temperature can become excessive and cause operator fatigue. Air conditioning is recommended in all rooms where ultrasound systems are permanently located.

5. Low ambient lighting should be available to aid visual acuity, with awareness that it is not so dark that there is a safety hazard.

16.2.4 Standard Operating Procedures/Protocols/Guidelines

SRH services should have Standard Operating Procedures (SOPs)/guidelines in place that clearly detail what is expected at each stage of the patient journey. In SRH clinical practice, this is likely to be in the context of a pregnancy advisory service, a community gynaecology service or to assist in dealing with intrauterine device and implant problems (Level 3 sexual health service). There should be a clear operational policy for the patient pathway. With regard to the use of ultrasound within the pathway, this will include the indication for the scan and recording and dissemination of the findings. If a pregnancy advisory service is part of the SRH service, a range of views exist as to whether guidelines should be very detailed/prescriptive or left vague, to allow flexibility and some professional autonomy in their application. It is advised that such guidelines are current, evidence based, regularly reviewed and adhered to by all staff to support service provision.

16.2.5 Request for Ultrasound Examinations and Justification

Ultrasound examinations must be performed only when there is a valid and justified clinical reason. The situation in SRH is different from traditional radiology; in the latter, requests for examinations are submitted to trigger an examination. However, in SRH, ultrasound scanning becomes an extension of the consultation and physical examination and is conducted at the discretion of the clinician. Sometimes it is an integral part of a procedure, for example, to guide removal of a lost intrauterine device or non-palpable implant, or to guide uterine instrumentation where this is not straightforward. However, there should be clearly established local guidelines, which set out when and how an ultrasound examination should be performed to standardise practice for patients.

16.2.6 Infection Control[12]

Ultrasound equipment has the potential to transmit infection, and the following guidance should be adopted in SRH ultrasound services:

1. Transducers should be cleaned in accordance with the manufacturer's specification and this should also be compliant with the service provider's local policy on infection control. First, all gel should be removed from the transducer with soft tissue and then chemical cleaners applied as recommended by the manufacturer.

Endovaginal transducers used in TVUS have specific published guidance for their cleaning, and use of disposable covers is essential (Figure 16.3).

Where ultrasound is used during deep implant removal (for example, to guide needle lift of the implant) the transducer should be placed in a sterile bag which is part of the sterile field during the procedure and single use sterile gel sachets used (Chapter 9).

2. The console, cart and display screen must be kept clean and only the manufacturers-recommended proprietary cleaning products should be used.

There is published literature on gel bottles and the risk of spread of infection from ultrasound transmission gel, and these are frequently overlooked (Figure 16.4). There are studies that have reported the transmission of bacterial infection to patients via the gel. All those users of ultrasound gel must be aware of the potential risk of infection, despite the label that these gels are bacteriostatic. In fact, Pseudomonas aeruginosa, Escherichia coli and Staphylococcus aureus have all been grown in ultrasound transmission gel. Departments should have an evidence-based infection control policy to avoid putting patients at risk.[12]

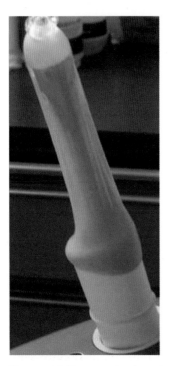

Figure 16.3 Transvaginal probe with disposable cover.

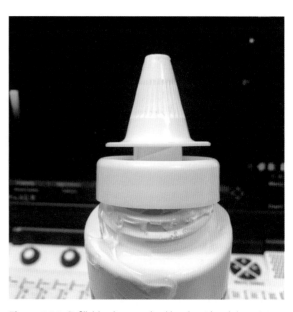

Figure 16.4 Refillable ultrasound gel bottle with gel deposits around neck; potential infection risk.

16.2.7 Intimate Examinations, Informed Consent and Chaperones

Pelvic ultrasound is usually classified as an intimate procedure. Privacy, dignity, courtesy and respect are paramount in such sensitive examinations and patient's specific requests should be accommodated as far as possible.

Valid consent is required for all gynaecological examinations and this includes the offer of a chaperone. The purpose of a chaperone must be explained to the patient. Acceptance of a chaperone (including name and designation) or when the offer is declined must be documented in the medical records. In the case of TVUS examinations, the patient must be made aware of the need for the movement of the endovaginal transducer in situ when performing the scan.[1,13]

16.2.8 Ultrasound Examination Techniques

A systematic scanning technique is invaluable to ensure that a thorough examination is performed to answer the clinical question, with extension of the ultrasound examination as appropriate (see Chapter 4). This approach should be detailed in scan protocols that are current, evidence based and are reviewed and updated regularly in accordance with local practice.[1,2,3]

16.2.9 Ultrasound Safety

Ultrasound has been widely used in medicine for four decades and there have been no reported significant bio-effects causing harm. All personnel who operate ultrasound equipment have a duty to ensure that they are using it properly, in accordance with published guidance, to produce optimum diagnostic image quality with the minimum 'ultrasound dose'.[14]

Compliance with safety guidance is a requirement for all those undertaking ultrasound examinations, including in focused applications such as SRH.

There are some key principles to be aware of:

1. Ultrasound examinations should be performed only when there is a valid reason that can be justified.
2. The operator must ensure that previous medical records have been scrutinised to ensure that a repeat unnecessary examination is not performed.
3. The scan time must be kept to a minimum to keep the 'dose' to a minimum, consistent with achieving a diagnostic result.

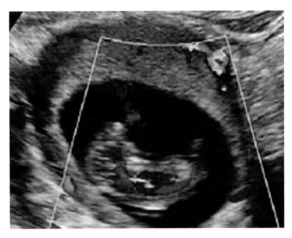

Figure 16.5 Sagittal section of embryo showing the use of Colour Doppler, not recommended in early pregnancy for safety reasons.

4. Use optimum set-up of the equipment to keep the 'dose' low, for example, overriding the power setting in the preset to reduce the power output.
5. Utilise the ALARA principle – that is use of the equipment in a manner which keeps the dose to the patient As Low As Reasonably Achievable.
6. Monitor the MI and TI on screen in accordance with published data (see Chapter 2).
7. Avoid the use of Doppler in early pregnancy scanning services (Figure 16.5).

16.2.10 Image Quality and Quality Assurance

Ultrasound is a diagnostic imaging modality that influences clinical decisions affecting patient care. As such, image quality should be monitored regularly and there should be a Quality Assurance (QA) process in place to support this. The purpose of a QA programme is to detect changes in the performance of the ultrasound machine and imaging archiving systems. Any faults can then be addressed prior to them having an adverse impact on patient outcome. Effective QA must be performed by a highly experienced ultrasound practitioner, with robust knowledge and understanding of the ultrasound and ancillary equipment.[2] It is advised that clinicians from SRH liaise with senior colleagues in their dedicated ultrasound service, since these personnel understand the professional requirements for QA and are used to undertaking such monitoring, which is outwith the scope of this book.

References

1. Guidelines for Professional Ultrasound Standards. Society of Radiographers and British Medical Ultrasound Society December 2015. www.sor.org/sites/default/files/document-versions/ultrasound_guidance.pdf

2. Standards for the provision of an Ultrasound Service. Society and College of Radiographers and the Royal College of Radiologists December 2014. www.sor.org/sites/default/files/document.../bfcr1417_standards_ultrasound.pdf.

3. *Ultrasound training recommendations for medical and surgical specialties.* 2nd Edition. Ref No. BFCR(12)17 the Royal College of Radiologists December 2012. www.rcr.ac.uk/sites/default/files/.../BFCR(12)17_ultrasound_training.pdf.

4. Focused Ultrasound training standards. Ref No. BFCR(12)18. The Royal College of Radiologists December 2012. www.rcr.ac.uk/sites/default/files/.../BFCR(12)18_focused_training.pdf

5. Care Quality Commission. www.cqc.org.uk/

6. Careers and Training. The Faculty of Sexual and Reproductive Healthcare of the Royal College of Obstetricians and Gynaecologists. www.fsrh.org/careers-and-training/

7. Englander R, Cameron T, Ballard AJ, Dodge J, Bull J. Aschenbrener CA. Toward a common taxonomy of competency domains for the health professions and competencies for physicians. *Acad Med.* 2013;88:1088–1094.

8. Consortium for the Accreditation of Sonographic Education. www.case-uk.org/

9. The Public Voluntary Register of Sonographers, Society of Radiographers. www.sor.org/practice/ultrasound/public-voluntary-register-sonographers-application-form

10. Jayatilleke N, Mackie A. Reflection as part of continuous professional development for public health professionals: a literature review. *J Public Health.* 2012. doi: 10.1093/pubmed/fds083 First published online: 17 October 2012.

11. Work Related Musculo-Skeletal Disorders (Sonographers) Society and College of Radiographers 2014

12. Oleszkowicz C, Chittick P, Russo V, Sims M, Band J. Infections associated with use of ultrasound transmission gel. Proposed guidelines to minimize risk. *J Infect Control Hosp Epidemiol.* 2012;33(12):1235–1237.

13. Obtaining Valid Consent (Clinical Governance Advice No. 6). Royal College of Obstetricians and Gynecologists. London 2015. www.rcog.org.uk/en/guidelines-research.../clinical-governance-advice-6/

14. Safety Statements British Medical Ultrasound Society 2015. www.bmus.org/policies-statements-guidelines/safety-statements/.

Annotation, Archiving, Reporting and Audit

Julie-Michelle Bridson

17.1 Image Labeling   241
17.2 Image Archiving   241
17.3 Reporting/Recording the Outcome of an
     Ultrasound Examination   242

17.4 Governance and Auditable Standards   246
17.5 Further Interventions and Appropriate
     Actions   246
17.6 Summary   246

17.1 Image Labeling

It is the responsibility of the professional performing the ultrasound examination to ensure that the correct patient data is entered before commencing the examination. In an ideal assessment, images to be stored should be annotated (Figure 17.1) including:

- Appropriate body marker (pictogram) showing patient position or body part and related transducer position; the latter gives an indication of the scan plane.

- Text annotation stating which organ/structure is shown and the anatomical section. For example, *long axis uterus, short axis of right ovary, oblique section left adnexae.*

This is considered best practice and all staff undertaking ultrasound examinations should aspire to this. It is acknowledged, however, that this can be time consuming and cumbersome when undertaking ultrasound in a busy SRH clinic. However, the minimum annotation must enable a third-party observer to interpret the image.

All images should include:

- patient identification (including DOB and Service/NHS Number)
- service provider identification
- date
- time
- preset and core system settings, for example, gain, frame rate
- safety indices (MI and TI).

17.2 Image Archiving

17.2.1 Why?

Representative images should be archived for every ultrasound examination. Archived images are a useful adjunct to the ultrasound report as they reflect the 'quality' of the examination. The evidence they can provide to an independent reviewer is shown in Box 17.1.

Archived images are also useful for audit purposes.[1-3]

17.2.2 How?

- Images archived should be of high quality and representative of all normal anatomy, anatomical variants, measurements and any pathology.
- Ideally, archiving should be to PACS. However, it is recognised that in SRH settings PACS is not normally available. In addition, there are considerations around patient confidentiality since some patients may not wish their appointment within a sexual health service being accessible to other health services and providers, for example, attendance at a pregnancy advisory service to discuss termination of pregnancy. In such situations, exporting data to an external hard drive can be useful; however, back up, patient confidentiality and secure data storage must be considered.
- Many SRH practitioners have the option only to archive images by thermal printing facilitating

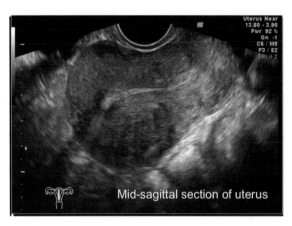

Figure 17.1 Good practice image annotation: transvaginal scan, midline sagittal section of the uterus showing body marker/pictogram and descriptive text.

Box 17.1 Traits That Can Be Established from Expert Review of Archived Images

Date of examination

Was the ultrasound equipment used appropriate, providing adequate image quality? Was it fit for purpose and in good working order?

Was the correct system pre-set used?

Was the transducer type and frequency used appropriately?

Were the equipment settings optimised throughout the scan?

Gives an overall 'impression' of scan 'quality'

Gives an indication as to whether the operator adhered to local protocol in terms of technique, measuring and archiving

May highlight any omissions/variance from local protocol

Provides pictorial review to allow images to be assessed with the reported findings and how that aligned with the patient's clinical presentation

Indication of the duration of scan

Compliance with safety recommendations (MI/TI)

---

storage in the medical records. While this is better than no image archiving it is not ideal since the longevity of thermal prints is poor and may not be of diagnostic quality if called upon for review some years down the line. The printer must be set up carefully so that the prints are a good representation of the on-screen image, and this should be checked regularly. This can be done by generating a high-quality image on the US system screen and then printing to thermal paper. The print is then compared to the on-screen image and is appraised to assess whether it is a realistic copy of the on-screen image. If not, then the printer controls can be adjusted systematically and resultant images compared to the on-screen image until adequate reproduction is achieved.

- It is essential that the representative images archived afford a comprehensive pictorial summary of the examination, including normal and abnormal findings and any measurements.[1-3]

17.3 Reporting/Recording the Outcome of an Ultrasound Examination

A report is defined as

> a specialist interpretation of images relating the findings, both anticipated and unexpected, to the patient's current clinical symptoms and signs in order to diagnose or contribute to the understanding of their medical condition or clinical state. It often incorporates advice to the referring clinician on appropriate further investigation or management.[4]

The report is the legal record of the examination and it is imperative that it is accurate and if possible answers the clinical question. The responsibility for verifying that the 'report' or record of the examination is accurate normally lies with the person who performed the scan. It is recommended that this be done immediately on completion of a patient consultation.

In SRH applications, ultrasound is an adjunct to the wider consultation and typically, the examination findings are recorded in the medical records as part of that process. Hence, the issue of a formal 'report' in the wider radiological sense is not normally adhered to in such focused settings. In an SRH clinic setting, patient correspondence to the referring GP would include the findings of the scan and explanation of any influence this had on the agreed management and the relevance to any future management. In this context, production of a separate report is redundant. In a Pregnancy Advisory Service (PAS) there will be no routine correspondence to the GP or any other medical professional, as many women self-refer and do not consent to sharing information about the pregnancy. However, in the event of non-routine findings, for example, ectopic pregnancy, which require referral to another service, it is essential that there is an agreed process for providing the scan findings and other essential information.

There is some clear guidance set out by the Royal College of Radiologists on *Standards for the Reporting and Interpretation of Imaging Investigations,* from which SRH practitioners can adopt some useful quality standards to their own practice.[4] Suggestions are set out here.

1. **Patient identification**
   - It is imperative that the clinician checks that the record is being noted in the correct medical records for the correct patient.

2. **Staff identification**
   - The clinician performing and documenting the scan must be clearly recorded, including his or her name, status and registration number (if required locally).
   - Where a second party has been involved in the scan (for example, a trainee), his or her name and role in the scan should also be documented.
   - The name of any chaperone present should also be recorded. If the patient declines a chaperone, this must be documented.

3. **Date**
   - The date and time of the scan should be recorded and must align with the images archived for that patient episode.

4. **Clinical indication and nature of the examination**
   - The reason for performing the ultrasound scan should be recorded together with the nature of the examination. For example,
     - Transvaginal ultrasound examination to evaluate the position of an intrauterine device.
     - Transcutaneous ultrasound examination to evaluate the location of a subdermal implant.
     - TA and TV ultrasound to assess location of IUC and pelvic anatomy in a patient with presenting complaint of pelvic pain.
     - TA, TV ultrasound and contrast sonohysterography to investigate abnormal bleeding, followed by endometrial biopsy and IUS fitting.

5. **Menstrual/reproductive/hormonal status/parity**
   - In women of reproductive age, it is important to report timing in the menstrual cycle or to refer to relevant hormonal treatment. Gravida, parity status should be noted.
   - It is equally important to document use of any hormonal treatment in women of post-reproductive age.

This reflects awareness of an understanding of the impact of the menstrual cycle and hormonal medication on the pelvic ultrasound appearances.

6. **Description of findings including anatomical variants**
   - The **S**ize, **S**hape, **O**utline, **T**exture of all structures assessed should be noted, together with clinically relevant **M**easurements (SSOTM).
   - Where structures are 'normal', it is preferable to record that rather than provide a lengthy technical description with measurements. This can be confusing for a second party reading the medical records, particularly as a non-ultrasound user is unlikely to know the normal ranges for pelvic structures.
   - The use of acoustic terminology is discouraged (for example, anechoic, transonic, echogenic). Such terms can be ambiguous and confusing. Describing findings as 'normal' or explaining what is seen and the range of possible interpretations is recommended (Box 17.1).

Probably the best example to reinforce this principle comes from an abdominal scan on a patient with right upper quadrant pain. The report read: 'There

---

Box 17.1 Examples

'The uterus appears normal for patient's age, parity and reproductive status'.

This shows understanding of the wider clinical picture in SRH.

'The uterus measures 7 × 2.5 × 3 cm and appears normal in size, shape, outline and texture. The myometrium is of normal echogenicity. The endometrial stripe is echogenic centrally, with some evidence of hypoechoic tissue around the cavity'.

This is confusing to a second party as the outcome is not clear and ambiguity introduced by use of acoustic terms.

(a)   (b)

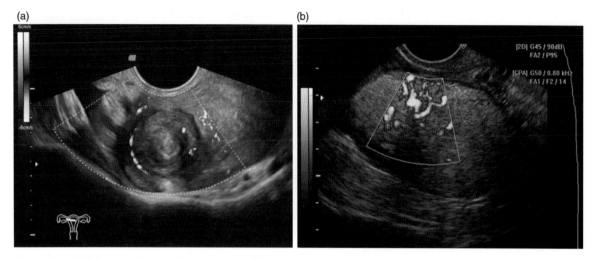

Figure 17.2 (a) Colour Doppler applied to uterine mass. (b) Power Doppler image showing internal vascularity in solid ovarian mass.

are multiple echogenic foci in the gall bladder with distal acoustic shadowing'. When asked by a surgeon what this meant, the answer was 'gallstones'; to which the retort was 'Why didn't you put that in the first place?'

In SRH, it is common to identify anatomical variants notably:

– Congenital uterine malformations – the type should be noted (see Chapter 6).

– Pelvic kidney – this is often mistaken for a solid pelvic mass, but is easily identified by a trained ultrasound practitioner by scanning the renal fossae to establish whether the kidneys are present and in their expected position. If this is outside the practitioner's scope of practice, then referral for further imaging is required.

7. **Abnormal findings**

In the presence of any abnormal findings, SSOTM should be applied to describe and quantify the anomaly and the origin of the pathology (where possible).

For example – 1.0 cm submucosal uterine fibroid, 2.4 cm functional cyst right ovary.

- Thorough assessment of pathology will often require use of other modalities on the ultrasound system such as Colour/Power Doppler to inform a diagnosis (Figure 17.2).

- Knowledge and understanding of when to extend an ultrasound examination to assess other structures is important, for example, to

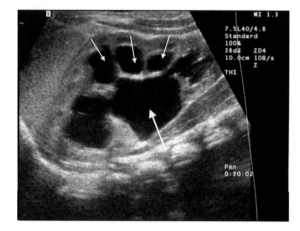

Figure 17.3 Ultrasound image of right kidney showing obstruction of the collecting system (hydronephrosis) due to pressure on ureter from pelvic mass. (The small arrows point to dilated renal calyces and the larger arrow points to the dilated renal pelvis.)

assess the kidneys for obstruction, if there is a large pelvic mass (Figure 17.3).

All practitioners need to be aware of their roles and boundaries and must be able to recognise when onward referral for a further, more expert opinion is recommended.

Onward referral should be accurately documented in the medical records.

8. **Technically limited examination**

Where an examination is technically limited, details must be recorded in the medical records. Examples include:

- High Body Mass Index (BMI)
- Excess bowel gas affecting visualisation of anatomy.

9. **Conclusion**

   There should be a clear conclusion to the ultrasound examination with any differential(s) which reflect the clinical presentation.

10. **Summary – examples of good and poor reports**

    A good report should:
    - State that consent was obtained for intimate procedures
    - Include the demographics of all personnel involved (ultrasound practitioner, trainee, chaperone, etc.)
    - Include the date of the examination
    - State the nature of the ultrasound examination: TVUS only, TAUS only, TAUS progressing to TVUS.
    - LMP, reproductive/hormonal status, relevant medication(s)
    - Summarise the clinical history to contextualise the case
    - Be clear, succinct and free from acoustic terminology to avoid ambiguity and misinterpretation
    - Avoid use of abbreviations which may be misinterpreted
    - Include details of any extension of the examination, for example, imaging of the kidneys/liver/abdomen
    - Include any technical limitations (for example, high BMI, excessive bowel gas)
    - Include any appropriate actions (for example, urgent referral)
    - Answer the clinical question

- Always include a conclusion, which summarises the important findings and any actions.

You should now critically review the reports that follow against the content of this chapter to identify which reports fulfill the required criteria (good) and those that do not (poor), and be able to justify your response. Remember, simplicity will avoid misinterpretation (Boxes 17.2 and 17.3).

Box 17.2 Case 1

35-year-old female (G2, P2), referred for location of IUS.

Transvaginal ultrasound with verbal consent.

Normal anteverted uterus. IUS in satisfactory position.

Both ovaries and adnexae appear normal.

No further imaging required.

Chaperone present: (name and designation)

Ultrasound practitioner: (name, role, status and statutory regulatory registration number)

Box 17.3 Case 2

56-year-old female, referral for PMB.

Transvaginal ultrasound.

Uterus measures 5.0 × 2.5 × 3 cm. The endometrial cavity measures 6 mm and is echogenic with small cystic areas within.

The right ovary measures 3.0 × 2.0 × 2.0 cm.

Left ovary wasn't seen due to overlying bowel gas.

Conclusion: endometrial hyperplasia.

(Answers given in a footnote)[‡§]

[‡] Case 1: Good, reflecting principles set out in this chapter.

[§] Case 2: poor, ambiguous and not founded on good clinical reasoning to get to the conclusion. Specifically:

- No reference to parity, consent, chaperone or ultrasound practitioner.
- It does not clarify whether any HRT medication is being administered.
- The size of the uterus is consistent with postmenopausal status, and this comment would be more helpful than the actual uterine measurements. If measurements are included, the normal range should be put in brackets to contextualize the size for referring clinician. Easier to say normal in size for this age and status!
- The right ovary is surprisingly large for a post menopausal woman, but if the appearance was normal then the report should state this.
- The endometrial appearance and measurement is abnormal for the clinical history and the report should conclude with this and recommendation that further assessment of the endometrium is indicated, including recommended further interventions.
- Endometrial hyperplasia is a histological diagnosis, NOT an imaging diagnosis.

Table 17.1 Recommendations for Minimum Auditable Standards for Ultrasound in SRH

Standard	How and Why?
Performance characteristics of the ultrasound equipment	Monitored through regular QA testing, to identify problems prior to affecting patient outcomes
Reproducibility of measurements	If measurements are to be used to inform clinical decisions, it is essential that they are audited to ensure that all staff are measuring in a similar way. Typically linear measures should be within +/− 1 mm maximum difference within and between operators. Intra- and interoperator repeatability studies should be undertaken to minimise impact of measurement errors.[5]
Staff performance	This is essential but can be controversial as it may highlight issues with a member of staff's clinical competence and capability. This requires sensitive handling and a supportive, remedial action plan to be put into place to update/upskill.
Assessment of ultrasound image quality	Retrospective review of image quality as shown on archived images is a well-established method for assessing staff 'performance' (Box 17.1). This is normally undertaken by expert peers and is best performed randomly to avoid any clinician change in performance during a known period of audit.
Assessment of documentation of findings in medical records	In SRH, there is seldom a formal ultrasound report; rather the ultrasound findings are included in the medical notes. Retrospective review of medical records can yield useful information such as style, language used, accuracy, etc. with the aim of standardisation.
Comparison of ultrasound diagnosis to other interventions	Where a patient has undergone additional interventions, for example, MRI, it is useful to audit the results from both imaging modalities and to discuss any issues in an MDT setting.
Patient outcome measures compared to ultrasound clinical contribution to a case	Both negative and positive ultrasound findings should be evaluated and the impact of the outcome on the case evaluated.

17.4 Governance and Auditable Standards

It is useful to audit the ultrasound service provision holistically. However, the increasing use of ultrasound outside a traditional radiology setting makes this difficult since it is increasingly being used as a clinical 'tool'. There are well-established auditable standards, which can be adapted and applied to SRH (Table 17.1). In addition, some examples are shown in the RCR document *Standards for the Provision of Ultrasound Services.*[2]

17.5 Further Interventions and Appropriate Actions

Understanding of the role of further interventions which may be carried out in an SRH setting is important. In some SRH services this might include:

- Sonohysterography
- HyCoSy

These may be carried out at the time of an initial clinic attendance if there are staff who are trained in these procedures. Alternatively, the patient will need to be rebooked.

The SRH clinician has a duty of care to the patient to ensure that when immediate or urgent action is required, that this information is documented and

the referral made in accordance with local policy, for example, through appropriate 'alert mechanisms'.[6]

17.6 Summary

This chapter highlights the importance of the basic principles of labelling, archiving, documentation of scan findings and governance of equipment, staff and services in the SRH setting. The aim of adopting these best practice minimum standards in the SRH setting is to ensure early recognition of any problems and ensure timely intervention to minimise the risk of adverse patient outcomes, thereby enhancing your service provision.

References

1. Guidelines for Professional Ultrasound Standards. Society of Radiographers and British Medical Ultrasound Society. December 2015. www.sor.org/sites/default/files/document-versions/ultrasound_guidance.pdf.

2. Standards for the Provision of an Ultrasound Service Society and College of Radiographers and the Royal College of Radiologists. December 2014. www.sor.org/sites/default/files/document.../bfcr1417_standards_ultrasound.pdf

3. Ultrasound Training Recommendations for Medical and Surgical Specialties. 2nd edn. Ref No. BFCR(12)17

the Royal College of Radiologists. December 2012. www.rcr.ac.uk/sites/default/files/…/BFCR(12)17_ultrasound_training.pdf

4. Standards for the Reporting and Interpreting of Imaging Investigations BFCR(06)1 RCR Updated. September 2015. www.rcr.ac.uk/publication/standards-reporting-and-interpretation-imaging-investigations

5. Epstein E, Valentin L. Intraobserver and interobserver reproducibility of ultrasound measurements of endometrial thickness in postmenopausal women. *Ultrasound Obstet Gynecol*. 2002;20:486–491. doi:10.1046/j.1469-0705.2002.00841.x

6. *Standards for the Communication of Critical, Urgent and Expected Significant Radiological Findings*, 2nd edn, Royal College of Radiologists. London. 2012. www.rcr.ac.uk/sites/default/files/docs/radiology/pdf/BFCR(12)11_urgent.pdf

Glossary of Abbreviations and Terms

AC. Abdominal Circumference

AFC. Antral Follicular Count

AIUM. American Institute of Ultrasound in Medicine

ALARA. As Low as Reasonably Achievable – the principle that governs the "dose" of ultrasound delivered during examinations

ALIASING –. an effect that causes different signals to become indistinguishable (or aliases of one another) when sampled

ALOs. Actinomycosis-Like Organisms

AMH. Anti-Müllerian Hormone

AP. Axis and Anteroposterior

ART. Assisted Reproductive Technology

AUB. Abnormal Uterine Bleeding

BIOMETRIC. Measurements (typically fetal measurements for estimating size and dating)

β-hCG. Beta Human Chorionic Gonadotropin

BMUS. British Medical Ultrasound Society

BPD. Bi-parietal Diameter

CAH. Congenital Adrenal Hyperplasia

CEA. Carcinoembryonic Antigen

CFI. Colour Flow Imaging

CL. Corpus Luteum

COH. Controlled Ovarian Hyperstimulation

CPD. Continuing Professional Development

CRL. Crown Rump Length

DCDA. Dichorionic Diamniotic (type of twinning)

D & E. Dilatation Evacuation

EH. Endometrial Hyperplasia

FL. Femur Length

FH. Fetal Heartbeat

FIGO. Federation International in Obstetrics & Gynaecology

FIS. Fluid Infusion Sonography

FL. Femur Length

FOV. Field of View

FR. Frame Rate

FSH. Follicle Stimulating Hormone

GA. General Anaesthesia

GIS. Gel Infusion Sonography

HC. Head Circumference

HMB. Heavy Menstrual Bleeding

HRT. Hormone replacement therapy

HSG. Hysterosalpingogram

HyCoSy. Hysterosalpingo-Contrast-Sonography

Hyperechoic –. tissue reflecting a bright image (typically bone)

Hypoechoic –. dark areas in a reflected image (typically fluid)

IETA. International Endometrial Tumour Analysis

IMS. Image Management System

IOTA. International Ovarian Tumour Analysis

ISAS. Imaging Services Accreditation Scheme

Isoechoic –. area of tissue having the same brightness as surrounding structures and therefore difficult to distinguish

ISUOG. International Society of Ultrasound in Obstetrics & Gynecology

IUC. Intrauterine Contraception

IUD. Intrauterine Device

IUI. Intrauterine Insemination

IUS. Intrauterine System

IVF. In Vitro Fertilisation

LH. Luteinising Hormone

LMP. Last Menstrual Period

MCDA. Monochorionic Diamniotic (type of twinning)

MHz. Megahertz – the frequency of ultrasound in cycles per second

MI. Mechanical Index

MSD. Mean Sac Diameter

MTOP. Medical Termination of Pregnancy

NICE. National Institute Health and Care Excellence

OHSS. Ovarian Hyper Stimulation Syndrome

PACS. Picture Archiving and Communication System

PAS. Pregnancy Advisory Service

PCE. Post-cystic Enhancement

PCO. Polycystic Ovaries

PCOS. Polycystic Ovary Syndrome

PE. Piezo-Electric – crystals located at the front face of the transducer which generate ultrasound waves

PERT. Pulse-Echo Return Time

PI. Pulsatility Index

PID. Pelvic Inflammatory Disease

PMB. Post-menopausal Bleeding

PPV. Positive Predictive Value

PRF. Pulse Repetition Frequency

PSV. Peak Systolic Velocity

PT. Pregnancy Test

PUL. Pregnancy of Unknown Location

PUV. Pregnancy of Uncertain Viability

PV. Per Vaginum

PW. Pulsed Wave Doppler

QA. Quality Assurance

RADAR. Radio Detection and Ranging

RBC. Red Blood Cells

RI. Resistance Index

RIS. Radiology Information System

RMI. Risk of Malignancy Index

ROI. Region of Interest

RPC. Retained Products of Conception

SHBG. Sex Hormone Binding Globulin

SIS. Saline Infusion Sonography

SONAR. Sound Navigation and Ranging

SONOHYSTEROGRAPHY. Filling the endometrial cavity with fluid contrast to enhance ultrasound examination of the uterus

SRH. Sexual and Reproductive Healthcare

SSOTM(O). Size Shape Outline Texture Measurements (Origin)

STI. Sexually Transmitted Infection

STOP. Surgical Termination of Pregnancy

TAUS. Transabdominal Ultrasound

TGC. Time Gain Compensation

TI. Thermal Index

TOP. Termination of Pregnancy

TVUS. Transvaginal Ultrasound

US. Ultrasound

WRMSD. Work-Related Musculo-Skeletal Disorders

Index

abdominal circumference (AC), second trimester pregnancy dating, 123–24
abdominal ectopic pregnancy, 146–47
abdominal X ray, perforation complications with IUC/IUS, 167–68
abnormal uterine bleeding (AUB)
  adenomyosis and, 202–4
  assessment, 209–10
  case studies, 214–17
  causes of, 209
  coagulopathy, 208
  contraception and, 211–13
  endometrial pathology, 208
  fibroids and, 202–6
  guidelines for, 47
  iatrogenic causes, 208–9
  with IUCs, 169–70, 208–9
  malignancy and hyperplasia, 204–7
  management of, 211–14
  in non-pregnant reproductive age women, 201–9
  ovulation dysfunction, 208
  PALM-COEIN classification system, 201–9
  in perimenopausal women, 218–19, 220–22
  polyps and, 201–3
  in postmenopausal women, 6–7
  ultrasound imaging of, 201–17
abortion
  case study of, 131–33
  complications of, 131–33
  IUC in situ and, 169
  miscarriage management and, 129–30
  ultrasound imaging and, 115, 130–31
absorption, acoustic shadowing, 41
acoustic gel, ultrasound generation and echo reception, 30–34
acoustic impedance, reflection and, 33
acoustic shadowing, 39–43
  IUC implantation, 171–72
  subdermal implant imaging, 153–55
acrania, imaging of, 125–29
adenomyosis

abnormal uterine bleeding and, 202–4
  imaging of, 91–95, 183–85
  in perimenopausal women, 220–22
  uterine enlargement and, 87
adipose tissue. See also obesity
  implant imaging and, 157
adnexal imaging
  adnexal torsion, 113
  benign masses, 98–102, 113
  case example, 109
  classification of masses, 101
  cyst contents, 98–101
  ectopic pregnancy diagnosis, 142–47
  gynaecological cancer, 227–30
  heterotopic pregnancy, 148–47
  menopausal status and mass assessment, 108
  transvaginal ultrasound pathology diagnosis, 28, 58–60
adnexal torsion, ultrasound imaging of, 113
ADNEX risk calculator, 48, 107–8, 227–30
ALARA (as low as reasonably achievable) principle, ultrasound exposure limits and, 10–11, 239
amenorrhea, 201
  Asherman's syndrome, 184
  IUC/IUS imaging and, 169–72
  menstruation and, 201
  perimenopause and, 218–19
  polycystic ovarian syndrome and, 195
  prepuberty and, 60–61
  uterine imaging and, 52–54, 59–60, 183–84
American Institute of Ultrasound in Medicine, 7
'amniotic bands,' differential diagnosis, 97–100
amniotic sac, pregnancy ultrasound and detection of, 117–18
androgens, polycystic ovarian syndrome and, 197
anechogenic cysts, 98–101
angiogenesis, ultrasound diagnosis of, 6
anteverted uterus, ultrasound examinations, 50–51

anti-Mullerian hormone (AMH), 184–86, 218–19
antral follicular count (AFC), 184–86, 189–90, 218–19
AP diameter, uterine measurement, 52–54
'Application of Echo-ranging Techniques to the Determination of Structure of Biological Tissues' (Wild and Reid), 1–2
arcuate uterus, 93–98
arm structure, implant imaging and, 155
artefacts
  refraction/edge shadowing, 41
  ultrasound imaging, 39–41
A-scan imaging, development of, 1–3
Asherman's syndrome, 184
assisted reproductive technology (ART), ultrasound and, 182–83
auditable standards for ultrasounding imaging, 246
axial uterus, imaging in perimenopausal women of, 220–22
azoospermia, ultrasound detection of, 183

"bagel" sign, ectopic pregnancy diagnosis, 142–47
baseline settings
  Doppler imaging, 24
  guidelines for, 13–15
bicornuate uterus, 93–98, 183–84
  abortion and, 130–31
biopsy procedures
  endometrial pathology, 225–27
  in polycystic ovarian syndrome, 196–97
biparietal diameter (BPD), second trimester pregnancy dating, 121–24
bladder distention
  history of imaging with, 3
  non-gynaecological pathology imaging, 233
  pregnancy ultrasound procedures, 115–16
  transabdominal assessment, 52–55
blood flow analysis, uterine vascularity, 66–67

blood vessels, implant imaging
and, 157–58
B-mode (brightness modulated)
operation, 22–26
body mass index (BMI)
infertility management and, 192–93
transabdominal imaging and, 52–55
ultrasound absorption and, 21–22
bone, ultrasound images of, 9–11
breakthrough bleeding, causes
of, 208–9
breastfeeding, cavity size and, 78–84
breast imaging, history of, 1–2
Bridson, Julie-Michelle, 8–43, 49–72,
234–39, 241–46
Briggs, Paula, 182–93, 195–200
British Medical Ultrasound
Society, 7, 234
Safety Publications of, 10–11
Brown, Louise, 191
Brown, Tom, 1–3

Ca125 assessment, 48
borderline ovarian tumors, 228–29
ovarian pathology differential
diagnosis, 106–9
Campbell, Stuart, 3
cancer. See also gynaecological cancer
non-gynaecological, imaging of, 233
risk factors, 208–7
carcinoembryonic antigen (CEA), 48
cerebellum assessment, second
trimester pregnancy
dating, 121–24
cervix
ectopic pregnancy in, 145–47
IUC/IUS placement and, 164–67
subfertility and health of, 182
chaperones, for ultrasound imaging
procedures, 239
chorionicity, multiple
pregnancies, 124–25
cineloop function, 21–22
clinical cases
abnormal uterine bleeding, 214–17
adenexal imaging, 109
contrast sonohysterography
imaging, 75–83
Doppler imaging, 27–30
endometrial pathology in, 225–27
infertility, 192–93
IUC/IUS devices, 174–80
non-epithelial ovarian
malignancies, 231–33
ovarian cancer pathology, 227–30
polycystic ovary and polycystic
ovarian syndrome, 198–99
pregnancy termination, 131–33
reporting and recording guidelines
in, 245

clomiphene citrate, ovulation
induction with, 191, 193–94
coagulopathies, abnormal uterine
bleeding, 208
colour flow imaging (CFI). See also
Doppler imaging
Doppler principle, 26
ectopic pregnancy diagnosis,
142–47, 148
infertility and, 182–83
retained products diagnosis, 28–29
communication skills
diagnostic communications, 45–46
emotional responses of patients, 46
patient preparation, 46
results disclosure, 46
treatment or follow up plans, 46–47
ultrasound assessment, 45–48
community clinics
quality control for ultrasound
in, 234
ultrasound assessment in, 6–7
competency evaluation, quality
control in ultrasound imaging
and, 234–35
compound imaging, subdermal
implants, 153–55
congenital uterine anomalies, 93–98
contraceptive implants. See also
intrauterine contraceptive
devices (IUC)
arm structure images, 155
case study, 151–52
complications, imaging in
management of, 161
deep insertion, avoidance of, 161
impalpable implants,
151–52, 159–61
location, 152–53
progestogen-only subdermal
implants, 151–62
ultrasound assessment of, 6–7
ultrasound imaging, 153–55
contrast sonohysterography
abnormal uterine bleeding,
209–10
cavity dimensions, 78–84
clinical cases, 75–76
endometrial imaging, 75–76
fibroid assessment, 76–83
in situ IUC imaging, 78–86
lesion assessment, 76–80
in perimenopausal women,
220–22
technique, 73–75
Controlled Ovarian Hyperstimulation
(COH), 182–83, 191
copper-containing IUCs, 50–51, 102–5,
163–65, 166–67
cornual pregnancy, 143–44

corpus luteum (CL)
anatomy of, 70–71
ectopic pregnancy in, 145
infertility imaging and, 186–88, 189
transvaginal ultrasound diagnosis, 28
crown rump length (CRL)
miscarriage diagnosis and, 127–29
pregnancy dating and, 118–20
second trimester pregnancy
dating, 120–24
crystal drop out, transducer care
and, 12–13
Cul-de-sac imaging, 70–71
Curie, Pierre, 1
curved array transducers, 15–20

data entry, guidelines for, 13–15
decidual cysts, ectopic pregnancy
and, 139–45
Depo provera, cavity size in women
on, 78–84
depth control, 21, 36
dermoid ovarian cyst, 110–12
diagnostic communication
guidelines, 45–46
unexpected pregnancy loss, 47
Diasonography, 1–3
dichorionic diamniotic (DCDA)
twins, 124–25
Dickson, Jane, 201–17
dilatation evacuation, ultrasound
during, 131
direct contact imaging, 1–3
discriminatory zone concept, ectopic
pregnancy, 148
Donald, Ian, 1–3
Doppler, Christian, 3
Doppler imaging
clinical cases using, 27–30
colour flow imaging, 26
development of, 3
ectopic pregnancy diagnosis,
142–47, 148
endometrial pathology, 225–27
infertility and, 182–83
operating modes, 23–27
pregnancy and contraindications
in, 239
pre-sets, common errors, 24
double decidual sign, ectopic
pregnancy, 139–45
double uterus, imaging of, 93–98
"doughnut" sign, ectopic pregnancy
diagnosis, 142–47
Duncan, Colin, 197
Dussik, Karl Theo, 1–2
dysgerminomas, 231–33

early pregnancy
abnormal findings in, 125–29

dating in, 118–20
diagnosis in ART of, 192
guidelines for ultrasound in, 127
transvaginal ultrasound and, 4–7
ultrasound imaging and, 3, 117–18
Easton, Karen, 45–48, 135–49
echogenic ring
ectopic pregnancy and, 139–45
pregnancy ultrasound and, 116–18
echo reception, ultrasound
generation, 30–34
echoscope, history of, 1–2
'eclipse sign,' implant imaging, 153–55
ECLIPSE study, abnormal uterine
bleeding, 211–14
ectopic pregnancy. See also heterotopic
pregnancy
beta human chorionic
gonadotropin, 148–49
clinical presentation, 135–36
diagnosis, 138
discriminatory zone concept, 148
epidemiology, 135
infertility and risk of, 192
IUC in situ and, 169
locations for, 138
progesterone levels in, 148–49
risk factors, 135
signs and symptoms, 136–38
transvaginal ultrasound and, 4–7
treatment of, 149
ultrasound imaging of,
115–16, 138–43
uncommon locations, 145–47
electromagnetic waves, ultrasound
and, 1–2
embryonic detection
crown rump length (CRL), 118–20
pregnancy ultrasound and, 117–18
emotional responses of patients,
management of, 46
endocavity transducers, 15–20
endometriomas, 110–12
follow-up imaging of, 113–14
endometriosis
infertility and, 188
ovarian cysts and, 110–12
endometritis
abnormal uterine bleeding and, 208
infertility and, 184
endometrium and endometrial
thickness
abnormal uterine bleeding, 209–10
abnormal uterine bleeding and, 208
adenomyosis, 91–95
cancer risk factors, 208–7
contrast sonohysterography imaging
of, 75–76
ectopic pregnancy in, 139–45
gynaecological cancer and, 225

imaging in perimenopausal women
of, 220–22
infertility imaging, 183–85,
189–90, 191–92
intracavitary pathology and, 73
malignancy and hyperplasia
and, 204–7
measurement of, 66, 95–97, 196–97
pathological analysis, 225–27
perimenopausal histology
and, 219–20
in polycystic ovarian
syndrome, 196–97
in postmenopausal women, 63
premenopausal women, 61–65
transabdominal imaging, 54
ultrasound assessment of, 6–7
endo-myometrial border, cancer and
disruption of, 225–27
endothelin-1, abnormal uterine
bleeding and production of, 208
endovaginal sonography
tubal patency assessment, 4–7
uterine assessment with, 6–7
epithelial cancer
invasive ovarian epithelial
malignancies, 229–31
transvaginal ultrasound diagnosis
of, 29–30
equipment for ultrasound
'adopted' equipment, quality issues
and, 236
guidelines for using, 13–15
overview, 8–10
system controls, 20–28
system pre-sets, 14–16
ergonomics of ultrasound
imaging, 12–13
quality control and, 236–37
estradiol contraceptives, abnormal
uterine bleeding and, 211–13
estrogen, polycystic ovarian syndrome
and, 197
exposure limits, ultrasound safety
and, 10–11

failed contraception, unexpected
pregnancy loss and, 47
fallopian tubes
benign pathology, 102–5
cancer pathology in, 232–33
ectopic pregnancy in, 135, 138, 143–44
infertility imaging and, 182, 188, 190
transvaginal ultrasound of, 58–60
tube-ovarian abscess, 105–6
fascia, implant imaging and, 157
female reproductive system
abnormal uterine bleeding and, 201–9
infertility and investigation
of, 183–89

femur length, second trimester
pregnancy dating, 123–24
fetal cardiac activity, pregnancy
ultrasound and, 117–18
fetal cephalometry
second trimester pregnancy
dating, 121–24
ultrasound technology for, 3
fetal heartbeat, M-mode operation, 23
fetal pole, ectopic pregnancy
assessment and, 139–45
fibrinolytics, abnormal uterine
bleeding with, 211–14
fibroid imaging
abnormal uterine bleeding, 202–6
contrast sonohysterography, 76–83
Doppler imaging, 28
FIGO classification, 87–89
infertility investigation, 183–85
IUC/IUS complications and, 76–83,
87–89, 168–69
leiomyoma classification
system, 202–6
malpositioning of IUC and, 169–71
myometrial fibroids, 87
in perimenopausal women, 220–22
field of view (FOV)
image formation and, 17–18
sector angle, 36–37
transabdominal imaging, 52–55
transducer classification and, 15–20
FIGO classification system
fibroids, 87–89
invasive ovarian epithelial
malignancies, 229–31
flexion of uterus, ultrasound
examinations, 50–51
Flexi T 300 IUC, 170–71
fluid (pelvic)
ectopic pregnancy diagnosis
and, 139–45
endometrial pathology and, 225–27
infertility imaging and, 188–89
in pelvis, 70
ultrasound images of, 9–11
fluid infusion sonography (FIS), basic
principles, 73
Focused Ultrasound Training
Standards, 234–35
focus settings, 21, 37
follicle stimulating hormone (FSH)
injections, infertility
management, 191
perimenopause and, 218–19
polycystic ovarian syndrome, 197
follicular growth monitoring
clomiphene citrate, 191
infertility imaging and, 189–90
normal ovaries, 67–69
transvaginal ultrasound and, 4–7

253

follow-up procedures
  communication of, 46–47
  ovarian benign masses, 113–14
footprint size, transducer classification
  and, 15–20
four-dimensional ultrasound,
  development of, 3
frame production, image generation
  and, 30–31
frame rates
  basic principles, 30–31
  focus zones and, 37
frozen embryo transfer
  case studies in, 192–93
  in vitro fertilisation, 192
frozen images, 21
  transabdominal imaging, 52–55
FSRH Guidelines, abnormal uterine
  bleeding, 211–13

gain
  overall gain, 21–22, 36
  power and, 36
gel infusion (GIS)
  contrast sonohysterography, 73–75
  endometrial pathology, 225–27
gestational age
  second trimester pregnancy
    dating, 120–24
  ultrasound assessment of, 6–7
gestational trophoblastic
  disease, 126–29
Goldstein, Steven R., 218–24
granulosa cell tumours, 231–33
gray scale imaging
  basic principles, 8–10
  history of, 1–3
ground glass cysts, 98–101
gynaecological cancer
  borderline ovarian tumors, 228–29
  endometrial pathology, 225–27
  fallopian tube pathology, 232–33
  incidence and prevalence, 225
  invasive ovarian epithelial
    malignancies, 229–31
  myometrial pathology and, 227
  non-epithelial ovarian
    malignancies, 231–33
  ovarian pathology, 227–30
  ultrasound imaging of,
    29–30, 225–33
gynaecology, ultrasound development
  and, 4–7
GyneFix® IUC, 78–84, 171–72

haemoperitoneum, ectopic pregnancy
  diagnosis, 139–45
haemorrhagic cysts, 98–101, 109–10
Haider, Zara, 163–73
harmonics, 38–39

head circumference, second trimester
  pregnancy dating, 121–24
Hertz frequency unit, ultrasound
  imaging and, 8–10
heterotopic pregnancy, 148–47
high frequency linear transducer, for
  implant imaging, 153–55
Hillaby, Kathryn, 225–33
hirsuitism, polycystic ovarian
  syndrome and, 197, 198–99
histological assessment
  abnormal uterine bleeding,
    211–14
  perimenopause, 219–20
hormonal intrauterine systems.
  See also progestogen-only
    subdermal implants
  abnormal uterine bleeding, 211–13
  classification, 163–65
  endometrium imaging and, 75–76
  ovarian cysts and, 67–69
  positioning of, 166–67
  uterine fibroids and, 76–83,
    87–89, 168–69
hormone replacement cycles, in vitro
  fertilisation, 192
human chorionic gonadotropin (HCG)
  levels. See also serum beta human
    chorionic gonadotropin (β-hCG)
    assessment
  interpretation of, 116
  as ovulation trigger, 191
Hurley & Leoni TVUS procedure, 183
hydatidiform mole, 126–29
  transvaginal ultrasound and, 4–7
hydrosalpinx, fallopian tube
  pathology, 102–5

image archiving and reporting
  archiving guidelines, 241–42
  examination outcomes, 242–45
  governance and auditable
    standards, 246
  labeling requirements, 241
  overview, 241–46
  quality control and, 236–37
image formation, field of view
  and, 17–18
image management systems
  (IMS), 236–37
image optimisation, 13–15, 34, 239
Imaging Services Accreditation
  Scheme (ISAS), 234
impalpable subdermal implants,
  imaging of, 151–52, 159–61
industrial flaw technology, ultrasound
  and, 1–3
infection control
  quality control in imaging and, 238
  transducer care and, 12–13

infertility
  case studies, 192–93
  controlled ovarian hyperstimulation,
    in vitro fertilisation, 191
  ectopic pregnancy and, 135
  endometriosis and, 188
  endometrium monitoring, 191–92
  female reproductive system, 183–89
  incidence of, 182
  male reproductive system, 183
  ovulation induction monitoring, 191
  ovulation investigation, 189–90
  pelvic effusion and, 188–89
  pelvic organ assessment, 190
  transvaginal ultrasound and, 4–7
  ultrasound for investigation and
    management of, 182–93
inflammation, abnormal uterine
  bleeding and, 208
informed consent, for ultrasound
  imaging procedures, 239
Instsillagel (anesthetic), 171–73
insulin resistance, polycystic ovarian
  syndrome, 197
interactive imaging, ectopic pregnancy
  diagnosis, 142–43
interdecidual sac sign, pregnancy
  ultrasound and, 116–18
International Endometrial Tumour
  Analysis (IETA) group, 66
International Ovarian Tumour
  Assessment (IOTA ADNEX)
  classification, 48, 106–9, 227–30
International Society of Ultrasound in
  Obstetrics and Gynaecology, 7
interstitial pregnancy, 143–44
intracavitary pathology
  endometrial thickness and, 73
  FIGO fibroid classification, 87–89
intradecidual sac sign, in ectopic
  pregnancy, 139–45
intramural fibroids, FIGO
  classification, 87–89
intrauterine contraceptive devices
  (IUC and IUS). See also
  progestogen-only subdermal
  implants
  abnormal uterine bleeding with,
    169–70, 208–9, 211–14
  case studies, 174–80
  cavity size and, 78–84
  complications with, 163,
    167–70, 180
  contrast sonohysterography, in situ
    imaging, 78–86
  difficult fittings, 172–73,
    174–75, 178
  expulsion of, 168–69, 171–72
  frameless IUCs, 171–72
  frame size, 170–71

malpositioning of, 169–71, 177
pain or unscheduled bleeding
with, 169–70
patterns in use of, 163
perforation complications,
167–68, 175
in postmenopausal women, 61
pregnancy with, 115–16, 169, 179
removal of, 174, 176
scanning for positioning of, 164–67
sub-optimal placement, 47–48
types of, 163–65
ultrasound assessment of,
6–7, 163–73
intrauterine insemination (IUI), 191
'The Investigation of Abdominal
Masses with Pulsed Ultrasound'
(Donald, McVicar and
Brown), 1–3
in vitro fertilisation (IVF)
complications, 182–83
controlled ovarian hyperstimulation
for, 191
ectopic pregnancy and, 135, 148–47
frozen embryo transfer, 192
hormone replacement cycles, 192
stimulated cycle for, 191–92

Jadelle® (Norplant-2), 151–52, 154
Jaydess® IUC, 166–67, 169
Jurkovic, D., 6–7

Kovacs, Gab, 182–93, 195–200
Kratochwil, Alfred, 4–7

Langevin, Paul, 1
laparoscopic salpingectomy, ectopic
pregnancy, 149
leiomyofibromata. See fibroid imaging
leiomyomas
imaging of, 87
sub classification system, 202–6
leiomyosarcoma, ultrasound
imaging of, 89
lesion assessment, contrast
sonohysterography, 76–80
Levonorgestrel IUS. See also
progestogen-only subdermal
implants
ovarian cysts and, 67–69
Lewis, Pat, 1–7
linear array scanners, 2–3
transducers, 15–20
long axis, uterine measurement, 52–54
luteinising hormone (LH), polycystic
ovarian syndrome and, 197

male reproductive system, infertility
and investigation of, 183
malignant pelvic disease

abnormal uterine bleeding
and, 204–7
differential diagnosis, 29–30, 106–9
Doppler imaging of, 29–30
manuals, for system optimisation, 34
manufacturers' support, system
optimisation and, 34
mature cystic teratoma, 110–12
maximum transverse diameter, uterine
measurement, 52–54
McVicar, John, 1–3
mean sac diameter (MSD)
abnormal findings in early
pregnancy, 125–29
miscarriage diagnosis and, 127–29
pregnancy ultrasound and, 116–18
Mechanical Index (MI), 10–11
power settings, 34–35
menopause, defined, 218–19
menstrual bleeding, abnormalities
in, 201
methotrexate, ectopic pregnancy
treatment, 149
miscarriage
complications of, 131–33
diagnostic criteria, 127–29
ectopic pregnancy, 145–47
false positive diagnostic rates,
129t7.1
management of, 129–30
patient interaction following, 47
transvaginal ultrasound and, 4–7
ultrasound diagnosis of, 3
M-mode (motion-mode) operation, 23
monochorionic twins, 124–25
Morisson's pouch, ectopic pregnancy
diagnosis, 139–45
Müllerian ducts, imaging of,
93–98, 183–84
multiple pregnancies, ultrasound
diagnosis of, 3, 124–25
multiple-zone focusing, 37
muscle, implant imaging and, 157
myomas, imaging of, 87
myometrium
benign pathology, imaging of, 87
ectopic pregnancy and, 143–44
endometrial pathology and, 225–27
gynaecological cancer and, 227
IUC/IUS perforation in, 167–68
scarring of, 89–94

National Cervical Screening
Programme, 209–10
Neal, Donald, 1–2
needle-lift technique, subdermal
implant removal, 159–61
nerves, implant imaging and, 158–59
neural tube disorders, imaging
of, 125–29

Nexplanon®, 151–52, 154
NICE Guidance on Pain and Bleeding
in Early Pregnancy, 47

obesity
gynaecological cancer risk and, 225
imaging in perimenopausal women
and, 220–22
IUC fitting and, 172–73
polycystic ovarian syndrome and,
195–200
quality control in ultrasound
imaging and increase
in, 235–36
transabdominal imaging and, 52–55
ultrasound absorption and, 21–22
O'Brien, Paul, 151–62
obstetrics, ultrasound development
and, 3
occipital frontal diameter (OFD),
second trimester pregnancy
dating, 121–24
oocyte retrieval, transvaginal
ultrasound and, 4–7
oophorectomy, ectopic pregnancy
and, 149
open technique, subdermal implant
removal, 159
operators of ultrasound equipment
ergonomics and quality control
for, 236–37
guidelines for, 12–13
modes of operation, 22–27
training and competency
assesssment for, 12–13, 234–35
oral contraceptives
abnormal uterine bleeding and, 211–13
polycystic ovarian syndrome
management and, 198–99
ovarian cysts
assessment of, 67–69, 98–101
benign masses, 109–12
dermoid cyst, 110–12
ectopic pregnancy and, 145
endometriosis and, 110–12
follow-up imaging of, 113–14
haemorrhagic, 109–10
infertility imaging and, 186–88
pathology, 227–30
simple cysts, 109
ovarian hyper stimulation syndrome
(OHSS), 182–83, 191
ovaries
adnexal torsion, 113
benign masses, imaging of, 109–12
borderline tumors, imaging
of, 228–29
cancer pathology in, 227–30
differential diagnosis, benign/
malignant pathology, 106–9

ovaries (*cont.*)
ectopic pregnancy in, 145
infertility imaging and, 184–88
invasive epithelial
malignancies, 229–31
measurement of, 70–72
non-epithelial malignancies, 231–33
normal ovaries, 67–69
in polycystic ovarian syndrome, 196
transabdominal ultrasound, 54–55
transvaginal ultrasound of, 58–60
tube-ovarian abscess, 105–6
ultrasound diagnosis of, 6, 48
overall gain, 21–22, 36
ovulation
abnormal uterine bleeding and
disorders of, 208
induction, monitoring of,
191, 193–94
infertility imaging and, 182, 189–90
perimenopause and irregularity
of, 218–19

PALM-COEIN system,
abnormal uterine bleeding
classification, 201–9
parametrial cysts, imaging of, 105–7
patient interaction
clinician's knowledge of patient, 46
diagnostic communications, 45–46
emotional responses of patients, 46
intimate examinations, informed
consent and chaperones, 239
patient perceptions of condition, 46
reporting and recording of results
and, 242–45
treatment or follow-up plans,
communication of, 46–47
ultrasound generation, 31–34
pelvic actinomycosis, 102–5
IUC/IUD complications and, 180
tube-ovarian abscess, 105–6
pelvic anatomy
benign pathology, imaging of, 87–114
fluid assessment, 70
indications for ultrasound
assessment, 49–50
infertility assessment, 190
post-menopausal changes in, 61
in prepuberty, 60–61
reporting and recording of
anomalies in, 242–45
systematic examination, 50–51
transabdominal assessment, 52–55
transvaginal ultrasound imaging,
55–57, 183
ultrasound scanning techniques and
normal findings, 49–72
pelvic infection, IUC complications
and, 170, 180

pelvic masses
tube-ovarian abscess, 105–6
ultrasound diagnosis of, 6
perforation complications with
IUC/IUS, imaging of, 167–68
perimenopausal women
clinical application of ultrasound
in, 220–22
histological assessment of, 219–20
limitations of ultrasound imaging
in, 222–23
ultrasound imaging in, 218–24
peritoneal inclusion cysts, imaging
of, 105–7
phased array scanners, 2–3
piezo-electric elements
history, 1
image formation in ultrasound,
9–11, 30–34
Pillai, Mary, 49–72, 73–79, 87–114,
115–33, 174–80
'pincer' grip for transducers, 12–13
placental imaging
multiple pregnancies, 124–25
ultrasound technology for, 3
plasminogen activator, abnormal
uterine bleeding and
production of, 208
polycystic ovarian syndrome (PCOS)
case studies, 198–99
infertility imaging and, 186,
192–93
management guidelines, 195–98
pathophysiology of, 197
ultrasound assessment, 48, 195–200
polycystic ovary (PCO)
case studies, 198–99
diagnosis and management, 195–200
polyps (endometrial)
abnormal uterine bleeding
and, 201–3
contrast sonohysterography,
73, 75–76
endometrial thickness and, 6–7
extent of lesion, 76–80
fibroid classification and, 87–89
infertility and, 183–85
polycystic ovarian syndrome and,
195
three-dimensional imaging, 39–40
'pop-out' technique, progestogen-
only subdermal implant
removal, 151–52
positive predictive value (PPV),
ectopic pregnancy adnexal
findings, 143–44
post cystic enhancement (PCE), 41–42
postmenopausal bleeding
endometrial pathology and, 225–27
ultrasound assessment of, 6–7

postmenopausal women
endometrial pathology in, 225–27
endometrial thickness in, 66
endometrium in, 63
ovarian anatomy in, 67–69
pelvic anatomy in, 61
Pouch of Douglas, imaging of,
70–71, 189–90
power Doppler, 27–28
'power' grip for transducers, 12–13
power output, ultrasound
imaging, 21–22
power settings
gain and, 36
management of, 34–35
pregnancy, ultrasound in. *See also* early
pregnancy
abnormal findings in early
pregnancy, 125–29
complications management
using, 131–33
dating of pregnancy and, 118–20
Doppler contraindications in, 239
examination protocol, 116–18
human chorionic gonadotropin
(HCG) levels and, 116
IUC in situ and, 169, 179
multiple pregnancy, 124–25
overview of, 115
second trimester dating, 120–24
service operational issues, 115–16
unexpected pregnancy loss, 47
pregnancy of uncertain viability
(PUV), 127–29
pregnancy of unknown location
(PUL), 115–16
ectopic pregnancy and, 138
management of, 149
pregnancy testing, ultrasound
following, 115–16
premenopausal women, endometrium
in, 61–65
prepuberty, pelvic anatomy in, 60–61
pre-sets
Doppler operating modes, 24
power settings, 34–35
ultrasound equipment, 14–16
progesterone levels, ectopic
pregnancy, 148–49
progestogen-only subdermal implants.
See also hormonal intrauterine
systems
arm structure images, 155
case study, 151–52
complications, imaging in
management of, 161
impalpable implants,
151–52, 159–61
location, 152–53
ultrasound imaging, 153–55

prostacyclin, abnormal uterine bleeding and production of, 208
prostaglandin E$_2$, abnormal uterine bleeding and production of, 208
prostaglandin F$_{2\alpha}$, abnormal uterine bleeding and production of, 208
"pseudosac"
    ectopic pregnancy assessment and, 139–45
    pregnancy ultrasound and, 116–18
pulsed-wave (PW)/Spectral Doppler, operating modes, 24–27
pulse-echo effect, ultrasound generation, 30–31
pulse-echo return time (PERT), ultrasound generation, 30–31
pulse repetition frequency (PFR), Doppler imaging, 24

quality control
    'adopted' ultrasound equipment, 236
    examination techniques, 239
    'fitness for purpose' principle, 235–37
    governance and auditable standards, 246
    image archiving and reporting, 236–37
    image quality optimisation, 13–15, 34, 239
    infection control and, 238
    interventions and actions relating to, 246
    intimate examinations, informed consent and chaperones, 239
    requests and justifications for imaging and, 237–38
    safety issues, 239
    scanning environment, 236–37
    selection criteria, ultrasound systems, 235–36
    standard operating procedures/ protocols/guidelines, 237
    training and updating and, 234–35
    for transducers, 236
    in ultrasound imaging, 234–39

RADAR (radio detection and ranging), 1–2
read zoom, 37–38
real-time imaging
    development of, 2–3
    transvaginal ultrasound and, 4–7
received echos, patient interaction, 34
recto-uterine space, 70–71, 189–90
reflection, patient interaction and, 33
refraction/edge shadowing artefact, 41
Reid, John, 1–2
results of ultrasound imaging
    communication of, 46
    reporting and recording procedures, 242–45

retained products
    abortion and, 131–33
    Doppler ultrasound diagnosis, 28–29
retroverted uterus, ultrasound examinations, 50–51
reverberation, 43
'ring of fire' (corpus luteum), 70–71
Risk of Malignancy Index (RMI), 48
    ovarian differential diagnosis, benign/malignant pathology, 106–9
Roche Cobas® analyzer, 148–49
Rokitansky nodule, 110–12
Rokitansky (MRKH) syndrome, 183–84
Rotterdam criteria, 195
Royal College of Obstetrics and Gynaecology, 117–18, 234
Royal College of Radiologists, 234–35, 242–45

safety, in ultrasound imaging, 10–11, 239
saline infusion (SIS), contrast sonohysterography, 73–75
salpingography, tubal patency assessment, 4–7
scan converter, development of, 1–3
scanning techniques
    quality control, 236–37, 239
    transabdominal imaging, 52–55
scar ectopic pregnancy, 146–47
scattering, patient interaction, 33
second trimester pregnancy dating, 120–24
septate uterus, imaging of, 93–98, 183–84
Sertoli-Leydig tumours, 231–33
serum beta human chorionic gonadotropin (β-hCG) assessment
    ectopic pregnancy diagnosis, 135, 138, 139–45, 148–49
    reference ranges, 148–49
sex hormone binding globulin (SHBG), polycystic ovarian syndrome, 197
sex steroid hormones, polycystic ovarian syndrome and, 197
sexually transmitted diseases (STDs), fallopian tube pathology, 102–5
"s gign," fallopian tube patency and, 188
signal processing, patient interaction, 34
Society of Radiographers, 234
SONAR (sound navigation and ranging), 1–2
sperm count, subfertility and, 182
SSOTMO mnemonic, pelvic assessment, 58

Standard Operating Procedures (SOPs), ultrasound imaging quality controls and, 237
"STRAW + 10" consensus, 218–19
subchorionic fluid, pregnancy imaging and, 124–25
subchorionic haematoma, abnormal findings in early pregnancy, 125–29
subfertility. See infertility
submucus fibroids, FIGO classification, 87–89
subserous fibroids, FIGO classification, 87–89
synechiae
    endometrium in premenopausal women, 63
    imaging of, 97–100
system boot-up, guidelines for, 13–15
system controls
    depth control, 36
    field of view/sector angle, 36–37
    focus, 37
    gain/power interplay, 36
    harmonics, 38–39
    image optimisation, 34
    interplay between, 38–39
    overview of, 20–28
    power settings, 34–35
    time gain compensation, 36
    zoom, 37–38

teratomas, 231–33
theca cell tumours, 231–33
Thermal Index (TI), 10–11
    power settings, 34–35
three-dimensional ultrasound
    development of, 3
    malpositioning of IUC and, 169–71
    system controls, 39–40
    uterine assessment and, 6–7
time gain compensation (TGC), 21–24, 36
training programs
    for operators of ultrasound equipment, 12–13
    quality control in ultrasound imaging and, 234–35
    ultrasound technology, 7
transabdominal ultrasound (TAUS)
    endometrial assessment, 54
    history of, 17–18
    IUC fitting and, 169–71, 172–73
    non-gynaecological pathology, 233
    ovarian assessment, 54–55
    pelvic assessment, 52–55
    in pregnancy, 115–16
transducers
    classification of, 15–20
    components of, 15–20

frame production, 30–31
for implant imaging, 153–55
infection control and care of, 12–13
quality control for, 236
ultrasound generation and echo reception, 30–34
transrectal ultrasound, history of, 1–2
transvaginal ultrasound (TVUS)
abnormal uterine bleeding, 209–10
adenomyosis, 202–4
artefacts, 39–41
corpus luteum diagnosis, 28
ectopic pregnancy diagnosis, 135, 139–45
female reproductive system, infertility investigations, 183–89
fibroid diagnosis, 28, 202–6
gynaecological cancer and, 225
gynaecological cancer imaging and, 29–30
history of, 1–2, 4–7
intimate examinations, informed consent and chaperones, 239
IUC/IUS positioning using, 164–67
malignant pelvic disease diagnosis, 29–30
malpositioning of IUC and, 169–71
non-gynaecological pathology, 233
pelvic assessment, 55–57
in perimenopausal women, 220–22
polycystic ovarian syndrome, 195–96, 198–99
in pregnancy, 115–16
reflection and, 33
retained products diagnosis, 28–29
three-dimensional imaging, 39–40
transducer components, 19–20
uterine clot diagnosis, 29

treatment plans, communication of, 46 47
trilaminar appearance, endometrium in premenopausal women, 61–65
tubo-ovarian abscess (TOA), 105–6
two-dimensional (2D) imaging
basic principles, 8–10
B-mode operation, 22–26
history of, 1–3
M-mode operation, 23
stages of image formation, 30–31

UK National Institute for Health and Care Excellence, 117–18
Ulipristal Acetate, 183–85, 211–14
ultrasound imaging
basic principles of, 8–10
equipment for, 8–10
ergonomics, 12–13
evolution in medicine of, 1–3
formation of images, 9–11
gynaecological cancer imaging, 29–30, 225–33
history in gynaecology of, 4–7
impalpable implants, 151–52, 159–61
intrauterine contraception, 163–73
operational modes, 22–27
perimenopausal women, 218–24
polycystic ovarian syndrome, 195–200
progestogen-only subdermal implants, 151–62
quality control in, 234–39
requests and justifications for, 237–38
safety issues, 10–11
stages of image formation, 30–31

U-technique, subdermal implant removal, 151–52, 159
uterine masses
clot diagnosis, Doppler imaging of, 29
ultrasound diagnosis of, 6
uterus
congenital anomalies, 93–98, 172–73, 183–84
evaluation guidelines, 58–61
measurement of, 52–54, 59–60, 70–72, 164–67
myometrium imaging, 87
in perimenopausal women, imaging of, 220–22
in polycystic ovarian syndrome, 196–97
subfertility and health of, 182
transabdominal imaging, 52–54
ultrasound images of, 9–11
vascularity, 66–67, 95–97

Vaniqa®, 198

Wild, John, 1–2
work-related musculo-skeletal disorders, ultrasound imaging ergonomics and, 236–37
World Health Organisation (WHO), endometrial malignancy and hyperplasia classification, 204–7, 218–19
write zoom, 37–38

yolk sac assessment, pregnancy ultrasound and, 116–18

zoom, 21
zoom controls, 37–38